# Advances in ERCP

*Editor*

ADAM SLIVKA

# GASTROINTESTINAL ENDOSCOPY CLINICS OF NORTH AMERICA

www.giendo.theclinics.com

*Consulting Editor*
CHARLES J. LIGHTDALE

October 2015 • Volume 25 • Number 4

**ELSEVIER**

1600 John F. Kennedy Boulevard • Suite 1800 • Philadelphia, Pennsylvania, 19103-2899

http://www.theclinics.com

**GASTROINTESTINAL ENDOSCOPY CLINICS OF NORTH AMERICA Volume 25, Number 4**
**October 2015 ISSN 1052-5157, ISBN-13: 978-0-323-40084-8**

Editor: Kerry Holland
Developmental Editor: Donald Mumford

Gastrointestinal Endoscopy Clinics of North America (ISSN 1052-5157) is published quarterly by Elsevier Inc., 360 Park Avenue South, New York, NY 10010-1710. Months of issue are January, April, July, and October. Business and Editorial Offices: 1600 John F. Kennedy Blvd., Suite 1800, Philadelphia, PA, 19103-2899. Periodicals postage paid at New York, NY and additional mailing offices. Subscription prices are $335.00 per year for US individuals, $486.00 per year for US institutions, $175.00 per year for US students and residents, $370.00 per year for Canadian individuals, $576.00 per year for Canadian institutions, $465.00 per year for international individuals, $576.00 per year for international institutions, and $245.00 per year for Canadian and foreign students/residents. To receive student/resident rate, orders must be accompanied by name of affiliated institution, date of term, and the signature of program/residency coordinator on institution letterhead. Orders will be billed at individual rate until proof of status is received. Foreign air speed delivery is included in all Clinics subscription prices. All prices are subject to change without notice. **POSTMASTER:** Send address change to Gastrointestinal Endoscopy Clinics of North America, Elsevier Health Sciences Division, Subscription Customer Service, 3251 Riverport Lane, Maryland Heights, MO 63043. **Customer Service: 1-800-654-2452 (US). From outside the United States, call 1-314-447-8871. Fax: 1-314-447-8029. E-mail: JournalsCustomerService-usa@elsevier.com (for print support) or JournalsOnlineSupport-usa@elsevier.com (for online support).**

Reprints. For copies of 100 or more, of articles in this publication, please contact the Commercial Reprints Department, Elsevier Inc., 360 Park Avenue South, New York, NY 10010-1710. Tel. 212-633-3874; Fax: 212-633-3820; E-mail: reprints@elsevier.com.

Gastrointestinal Endoscopy Clinics of North America is covered in Excerpta Medica, MEDLINE/PubMed (Index Medicus), and MEDLINE/MEDLARS.

# Contributors

## CONSULTING EDITOR

### CHARLES J. LIGHTDALE, MD
Professor of Medicine, Division of Digestive and Liver Diseases, Columbia University Medical Center, New York, New York

## EDITOR

### ADAM SLIVKA, MD, PhD
Professor of Medicine, Associate Chief of the Division, Gastroenterology, Hepatology, and Nutrition; Director of the GI Service Line, University of Pittsburgh Medical Center, Pittsburgh, Pennsylvania

## AUTHORS

### MAJID A. ALMADI, MBBS, FRCPC, MSc (Clinical Epidemiology)
Division of Gastroenterology, King Khalid University Hospital, King Saud University Medical City, King Saud University, Riyadh, Saudi Arabia; Division of Gastroenterology, The McGill University Health Center, Montreal General Hospital, McGill University, Montréal, Quebec, Canada

### ALAN N. BARKUN, MD, CM, FRCPC, MSc (Clinical Epidemiology)
Divisions of Gastroenterology and Clinical Epidemiology, The McGill University Health Center, Montreal General Hospital, McGill University, Montréal, Quebec, Canada

### JEFFREY S. BARKUN, MD, CM, FRCS, MSc
Division of General Surgery, The McGill University Health Centre, McGill University, Montréal, Quebec, Canada

### KENNETH F. BINMOELLER, MD
Director, Interventional Endoscopy Services, California Pacific Medical Center, San Francisco, California

### ROHIT DAS, MD
Fellow, Division of Gastroenterology, Hepatology and Nutrition, University of Pittsburgh Medical Center, Pittsburgh, Pennsylvania

### JACQUES DEVIÈRE, MD, PhD
Head, Medical Surgical, Department of Gastroenterology, Hepatopancreatology and Digestive Oncology, Erasme University Hospital; Professor of Medicine, Université Libre de Bruxelles, Brussels, Belgium

### JEFFREY J. EASLER, MD
Division of Gastroenterology and Hepatology, Indiana University School of Medicine, Indianapolis, Indiana

**B. JOSEPH ELMUNZER, MD**
Associate Professor of Medicine, Division of Gastroenterology and Hepatology, Medical University of South Carolina, Charleston, South Carolina

**VICTORIA GÓMEZ, MD**
Assistant Professor of Medicine, Division of Gastroenterology, Mayo Clinic, Jacksonville, Florida

**GREGORY HABER, MD**
Director, Division of Gastroenterology; Director, The Center for Advanced Therapeutic Endoscopy, Lenox Hill Hospital, New York, New York

**MICHEL KAHALEH, MD**
Professor of Medicine, Chief of Endoscopy, Division of Gastroenterology and Hepatology, Weill Cornell Medical College, New York, New York

**RICHARD A. KOZAREK, MD**
Division of Gastroenterology, Executive Director, Digestive Disease Institute, Virginia Mason Medical Center, Clinical Professor of Medicine, University of Washington, Seattle, Washington

**ANISH MAMMEN, MD**
Advanced Fellow, Lenox Hill Hospital, New York, New York

**GEORGIOS I. PAPACHRISTOU, MD**
Associate Professor, Division of Gastroenterology, Hepatology and Nutrition, University of Pittsburgh Medical Center, Pittsburgh, Pennsylvania

**BRET T. PETERSEN, MD**
Professor of Medicine, Division of Gastroenterology, Mayo Clinic, Rochester, Minnesota

**DUVVUR NAGESHWAR REDDY, MD, DM**
Director, Chairman, Asian Institute of Gastroenterology, Hyderabad, India

**AMRITA SETHI, MD**
Assistant Professor of Medicine, Division of Digestive and Liver Diseases, Columbia University Medical Center, New York, New York

**RAJ J. SHAH, MD, FASGE, AGAF**
Professor of Medicine, University of Colorado School of Medicine, Director, Pancreaticobiliary Endoscopy, University of Colorado Anschutz Medical Campus, Aurora, Colorado

**STUART SHERMAN, MD**
Division of Gastroenterology and Hepatology, Indiana University School of Medicine, Indianapolis, Indiana

**AARON J. SMALL, MD, MSCE**
Division of Gastroenterology, Digestive Disease Institute, Virginia Mason Medical Center, Seattle, Washington

**IOANA SMITH, MD**
Internal Medicine Resident, Division of Gastroenterology and Hepatology, University of Alabama at Birmingham, Birmingham, Alabama

**RUPJYOTI TALUKDAR, MD**
Clinical Pancreatologist and Clinician Scientist, Asian Healthcare Foundation, Asian Institute of Gastroenterology, Hyderabad, India

**FRANK WEILERT, MD**
Waikato Hospital, Waikato District Health Board, Hamilton, New Zealand

**MING-MING XU, MD**
Gastroenterology Fellow, Division of Digestive and Liver Diseases, Columbia University Medical Center, New York, New York

**DHIRAJ YADAV, MD, MPH**
Associate Professor, Division of Gastroenterology, Hepatology and Nutrition, University of Pittsburgh Medical Center, Pittsburgh, Pennsylvania

# Contents

Many devices and techniques have been developed to assist in cases of difficult biliary cannulation. Guidewire-assisted cannulation has become the first-line technique for biliary cannulation. Precut sphincterotomy can be safe and effective if used soon after encountering difficulty. Pancreatic duct stents are an important adjunct to reduce the risk of post–endoscopic retrograde cholangiopancreatography pancreatitis in difficult access. Ultimately, cannulation success of greater than 95% and complication rates of less than 5% is the standard that endoscopists doing ERCP should achieve.

 Video of native papilla as seen with Billroth II reconstruction during endoscopy with use of a clear cap accompanies this article

ERCP in surgically altered anatomy requires the endoscopist to fully understand the procedural goals and the reconstructed anatomy before proceeding. Altered anatomy presents a variety of challenges unique to enteroscopy, and others related to accessing the biliary or pancreatic duct from unusual orientations. Both side-viewing and forward-viewing endoscopes, as well as single and double balloon techniques, are available for ERCP in these settings. Endoscope selection largely depends on the anatomy and length of reconstructed intestinal limbs. Endoscopist experience with performing ERCP in surgically altered anatomy is the most important factor for determining outcomes and success rates.

Biliary disease is a common cause of acute pancreatitis. Risk stratification for persistent pancreatobiliary obstruction is important for selecting a treatment approach. Most common bile duct stones are extracted with standard endoscopic techniques. However, prior foregut surgery, stones with extreme morphologic attributes, and at difficult positions within the biliary system are technically challenging and predict a need for advanced biliary endoscopic techniques. Surgical common bile duct exploration at the time of cholecystectomy is appropriate in centers with experience. We outline the options and approach for the clinician to successfully identify and manage patients with symptomatic choledocholithiasis with or without biliary pancreatitis.

Postendoscopic retrograde cholangiopancreatography pancreatitis is a common and potentially devastating complication of endoscopic retrograde cholangiopancreatography. Advances in risk-stratification, patient selection, procedure technique, and prophylactic interventions have substantially improved the ability to prevent this complication. This article presents the evidence-based approaches to preventing postendoscopic retrograde cholangiopancreatography pancreatitis and discusses timely research questions in this important area.

Recurrent acute pancreatitis (RAP) is a challenging condition that can lead to chronic pancreatitis and long-term morbidity. Etiology-based treatment can potentially have an impact on the natural history of RAP and its progression to chronic pancreatitis. In cases of divisum-associated RAP and idiopathic RAP, several studies have been performed to evaluate the efficacy of endoscopic therapy in alleviation of symptoms and frequency of AP events. This review discusses the literature available on these topic as well as touching on the role of endoscopic therapy in smoldering acute pancreatitis.

This article reviews the diagnosis and management of sphincter of Oddi dysfunction (SOD), including the various factors to consider before embarking on endoscopic therapy for SOD. Selection starts with patient education to include possible patient misconceptions related to symptoms caused by the pancreaticobiliary sphincter as well as reinforcing the risks associated with the diagnosis and therapy. The likelihood of relief of recurrent abdominal pain attributed to SOD is related to the classification of SOD type and a crucial consideration before considering endoscopic therapy in light of recent evidence.

Extracorporeal shock wave lithotripsy is recommended as the first-line therapy for large (>5-mm) obstructive pancreatic ductal stones. Dominant pancreatic duct strictures should be initially managed with a wide-bore single plastic stent with 3 monthly exchanges for a year, even in asymptomatic patients. Recent studies have evaluated multiple plastic and self-expanding covered metal stents for refractory pancreatic ductal stricture. Pancreatic pseudocysts should be treated endoscopically with or without endoscopic ultrasound guidance.

Cholangioscopy was first performed in the 1970s. We now use the term cholangiopancreatoscopy (CP) to reflect the wider application of these miniature reusable dual-operator "mother-daughter" endoscope systems and now fully disposable and digital single-operator optical catheters for evaluating the biliary or pancreatic duct. Cholangioscopy is an established modality for the management of large biliary stones and for the diagnosis and exclusion of biliary tumors. Pancreatoscopy is increasingly being performed to treat difficult pancreatic duct stones and may be used to distinguish malignant from benign ductal pathology. This review covers available CP technologies, indications, technique, efficacy, and complications.

Within the past two decades, major progress has been made in biliary endoscopy both with stenting and with ablative therapy. A primary goal in patients with malignant biliary lesions who are not candidates for surgery is to provide localized and efficient necrosis of the lesions. This article summarizes the current literature on biliary tumor ablation with photodynamic therapy and radiofrequency ablation. Prognosis, treatment technique, potential complications, treatment efficacy, and controversies are discussed.

 Video of single-step endoscopic ultrasound–guided gallbladder stenting with a cautery-equipped stent delivery system for the lumen-apposing stent accompanies this article

Endoscopic retrograde cholangiopancreatography (ERCP) is the primary approach to drain an obstructed pancreatic or biliary duct. Failed biliary drainage is traditionally referred for percutaneous transhepatic biliary drainage or surgical bypass, which carry significantly higher morbidity and mortality rates compared with ERCP and transpapillary drainage. Endoscopic ultrasound provides a real-time imaging platform to access and deliver therapy to organs and tissues outside of the bowel lumen. The bile and pancreatic ducts can be directly accessed from the stomach and duodenum, offering an alternative to ERCP when this fails or is not feasible.

# GASTROINTESTINAL ENDOSCOPY CLINICS OF NORTH AMERICA

**THE CLINICS ARE AVAILABLE ONLINE!**
Access your subscription at:
www.theclinics.com

# Foreword

# Advances in Therapeutic Endoscopic Retrograde Cholangiopancreatography: Benefits Far Outweigh the Small Risks

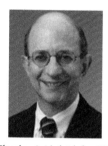

Charles J. Lightdale, MD
*Consulting Editor*

When endoscopic retrograde cholangiopancreatography (ERCP) was initially performed in the late 1960s and early 1970s, it was intended to be a purely diagnostic tool.[1] Even then, this hybrid procedure combining endoscopy with fluoroscopy was felt to be among the most difficult endoscopic procedures, and it was not without its complications. In a survey conducted in 1974 by the American Society for Gastrointestinal Endoscopy, the complication rate was 2.2%, considerably higher than for other endoscopic methods. Soon, endoscopists learned how to reduce complications, for example, by giving antibiotics to patients with biliary sepsis and by decreasing dye injection pressure when imaging the pancreatic ducts.

In the mid-1970s, therapeutic ERCP burst upon the endoscopic scene, most notably endoscopic sphincterotomy, with associated devices for removing ductal stones and placing stents for palliation of malignancy. As imaging with ultrasound, computed tomography, and MRI, MRCP improved; diagnostic ERCP has decreased except for the most difficult diagnostic problems, while therapeutic ERCP has continued to grow. It is estimated that currently more than 500,000 ERCP procedures are performed annually in the United States.

The great benefits of therapeutic ERCP have been clearly shown in many biliary and pancreatic diseases, where they have greater success than radiologic interventions, and success equal to many open and laparoscopic surgical procedures with considerably less morbidity. The most recent challenge to ERCP, however, has been the demonstrated transmission of multidrug-resistant organisms via the duodenoscopes

Gastrointest Endoscopy Clin N Am 25 (2015) xiii–xiv
http://dx.doi.org/10.1016/j.giec.2015.07.002
1052-5157/15/$ – see front matter © 2015 Published by Elsevier Inc.

used for ERCP despite stringent cleaning and disinfection. The culprit appears to be the complex elevator system used to guide instruments during ERCP. All the GI societies in the United States have cooperated with instrument manufacturers, hospitals, and the US Food and Drug Administration (FDA) to recommend carrying out even more aggressive cleaning, disinfection, and sterilization of duodenoscopes coupled with continuous testing and monitoring for bacterial contamination. One thing is clear: these incidents are very infrequent. In the words of the FDA leadership: "Fortunately, the vast majority of ERCPs are conducted without incident and often to the patient's great benefit. For most patients, the benefits of this potentially life-saving procedure far outweigh the risks of possible infection."[2] Patients likely to benefit from ERCP should have these issues thoroughly discussed during the informed consent process.

It is most opportune that we have an issue of the *Gastrointestinal Endoscopy Clinics of North America* dedicated to "Advances in Endoscopic Retrograde Cholangiopancreatography." The Guest Editor is Adam Slivka, MD, PhD, widely known as a thought-leader in the field, and one who insists on data to guide endoscopic practice. He has chosen topics that brightly illustrate the wide advances made by ERCP in recent years and has corralled a dream-team of skilled specialists as authors. The huge benefits of modern ERCP are evident in every article. This issue should have wide appeal to gastroenterologists at all levels, as well as surgeons, radiologists, and all those interested in liver and pancreatic diseases.

Charles J. Lightdale, MD
Division of Digestive and Liver Diseases
Columbia University Medical Center
161 Fort Washington Avenue
New York, NY 10032, USA

E-mail address:
cjl18@cumc.columbia.edu

## REFERENCES

1. Edmonson JM. History of the instruments for gastrointestinal endoscopy. Gastrointest Endosc 1991;37(Suppl):S27–56.
2. Maisel W. Bacterial infections associated with duodenoscopes: FDA's actions to better understand the problem and what can be done to mitigate it. FDA Voice 2015. [Epub ahead of print].

# Preface

# Advances in Endoscopic Retrograde Cholangiopancreatography

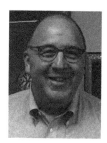

Adam Slivka, MD, PhD
*Editor*

Endoscopic retrograde cholangiopancreatography (ERCP) has evolved over the last four decades into a therapeutic procedure for a variety of pancreaticobiliary conditions. Recently, there have been a number of technologic and pharmacologic advances that have impacted the timing, indications, success, and safety of ERCP. Furthermore, as we evolve to value-based medicine, we have to prove not only that we can perform a procedure but also when we should perform it and balance risk, benefits, and cost against alternative treatment strategies. Fortunately for ERCP, many alternatives are higher risk, less successful radiologic and surgical interventions and ERCP remains well-poised to provide continued value for our patients. The authors who agreed to contribute to this issue of *Gastrointestinal Endoscopy Clinics of North America* represent an international who's who in ERCP, and I am personally grateful to each one of them for agreeing to participate. All aspects of pancreaticobiliary endoscopy are covered in conceptual and technical detail. The articles are truly outstanding, and this issue will be an invaluable resource for endoscopists at all levels of training and experience, including fellows, practitioners, and even Master Endoscopists.

Gastrointest Endoscopy Clin N Am 25 (2015) xv–xvi
http://dx.doi.org/10.1016/j.giec.2015.07.001
1052-5157/15/$ – see front matter © 2015 Published by Elsevier Inc.

giendo.theclinics.com

I hope you enjoy reading and referencing this issue as much as I enjoyed putting it together, and I, again, extend my warmest thanks to the contributing authors.

Adam Slivka, MD, PhD
University of Pittsburgh Medical Center
M-Level C-Wing
Presbyterian University Hospital
200 Lothrop Street
Pittsburgh, PA 15213, USA

E-mail address:
Slivkaa@upmc.edu

# Difficult Biliary Access
## Advanced Cannulation and Sphincterotomy Technique

Anish Mammen, MD[a], Gregory Haber, MD[b],*

## KEYWORDS

- ERCP • Biliary cannulation • Advanced cannulation technique
- Guidewire-assisted cannulation • Precut sphincterotomy
- Needle knife sphincterotomy • Transpancreatic septotomy

## KEY POINTS

- Many devices and techniques have been developed to assist in cases of difficult biliary cannulation.
- Guidewire-assisted cannulation has become the first-line technique for biliary cannulation.
- Precut sphincterotomy can be safe and effective if used soon after encountering difficulty.
- Pancreatic duct (PD) stents are an important adjunct to reduce the risk of post–endoscopic retrograde cholangiopancreatography (ERCP) pancreatitis (PEP) in difficult access.
- Ultimately, cannulation success of greater than 95% and complication rates of less than 5% is the standard that endoscopists doing ERCP should achieve.

## INTRODUCTION

ERCP was originally developed almost half a century ago as a diagnostic tool for pancreaticobiliary disorders.[1] It has been proved to be an effective procedure over the years,[2] not without associated complications. With the development of noninvasive and minimally invasive diagnostic alternatives such as magnetic resonance cholangiopancreatography and endoscopic ultrasonography (EUS), ERCP has evolved from being primarily a diagnostic modality to almost entirely a therapeutic procedure. Selective deep cannulation of the common bile duct (CBD) or PD with guidewire access is required for successful therapeutic interventions. At times, this can be difficult for even the most experienced endoscopists. Many advanced techniques have been developed to overcome the difficulties encountered when attempting biliary cannulation.

[a] Lenox Hill Hospital, 100 East 77th St., New York, NY 10075, USA; [b] Division of Gastroenterology, The Center for Advanced Therapeutic Endoscopy, Lenox Hill Hospital, 100 East 77th St., New York, NY 10075, USA
* Corresponding author.
E-mail address: ghaber@nshs.edu

Gastrointest Endoscopy Clin N Am 25 (2015) 619–630
http://dx.doi.org/10.1016/j.giec.2015.06.007
1052-5157/15/$ – see front matter © 2015 Elsevier Inc. All rights reserved.

## GUIDEWIRE-ASSISTED CANNULATION

Guidewire-assisted cannulation has quickly become the standard technique to improve biliary cannulation with the intent of reducing complications.[3] The technique involves cannulating the papilla with gentle probing of a guidewire preloaded in a papillotome. The guidewire is then advanced up the duct without injecting contrast; this can be done either by initially advancing the guidewire out of the papillotome a few millimeters before commencing cannulation or by engaging the tip of the papillotome in the papillary orifice before advancing the guidewire. The former is preferred when there is a small punctum or a stenotic papillary orifice, but the latter is a much more reliable approach, as seating the tip of the papillotome in the mucosal orifice provides a stable platform to begin wire manipulation. Manipulation of the guidewire can be handled by an assistant or the endoscopist. The choice is highly personal depending in large part on the experience of the assistant and the prior experience of working together on a large number of cases. Most endoscopists prefer to control the wire by gently probing in a staccato fashion to advance through the sphincter orifice and up the CBD. A straight-tipped wire is best to start with, and the author prefers the 0.025-in-caliber wire, which has a malleable tip with sufficient stiffness along the body of the wire for pushability. Buckling of the wire within a few centimeters of advancement may be due to passage into the cystic duct takeoff in the CBD or a branch duct in the PD. When in doubt, the position of the guidewire can be confirmed with fluoroscopy by injecting a small amount of contrast before advancing the papillotome deeply into the duct.

Several early studies found that guidewire-assisted cannulation technique increased the percentage of successful cannulations while decreasing the risk of PEP.[4–7] Postulated mechanisms for improved outcomes included less papillary trauma and edema, as well as avoidance of contrast, which may increase hydrostatic pressure within the duct, induce an inflammatory response to the chemical constituents, or introduce bacteria into the PD. A recent meta-analysis of 12 randomized controls trials (RCTs) showed that guidewire-assisted cannulation significantly reduced PEP compared with traditional contrast-assisted cannulation technique (relative risk [RR], 0.51; 95% confidence interval [CI], 0.32–0.82). In addition, guidewire-assisted cannulation technique was associated with greater primary cannulation success (RR, 1.07; 95% CI, 1.00–1.15), fewer precut sphincterotomies (RR, 0.75; 95% CI, 0.60–0.95), and no increase in other ERCP-related complications.[8]

Unfortunately, guidewire-assisted cannulation has not been a panacea, as newer studies have not substantiated this analysis of earlier trials. A prospective randomized multicenter study involving 400 consecutive patients compared wire-guided cannulation with traditional contrast-guided cannulation. Although wire-guided cannulation was found to significantly shorten cannulation and fluoroscopy times, it did not decrease the incidence of PEP.[9] Another prospective comparative-intervention single-center study of 1249 patients found no significant difference in the rate or severity of PEP between the guidewire and contrast-assisted groups. In fact, there was actually a trend toward increased risk of pancreatitis in the guidewire-assisted group, but the risk of severe pancreatitis occurred more often in the contrast injection group. No significant difference in the characteristics of the 2 groups, including prophylactic pancreatic stenting, was found to explain this trend.[10] A prospective multicenter randomized controlled crossover trial of 322 patients also failed to show any difference in biliary cannulation success or PEP ($P = .40$ and $.95$).[11]

Given that guidewire cannulation has its own risks of false passage, intramural dissection, pancreatic ductal injury, and perforation,[12] one must advance the guidewire carefully, recognizing the potential traumatic impact possible. Currently available guidewires have a soft, hydrophilic leading segment to facilitate passage through a tortuous common channel and minimize trauma. In the author's experience, using a 0.025-in-caliber guidewire with a soft, tapered hydrophilic tip and a stiff shaft may improve cannulation success and decrease complications, although no large studies have directly addressed this.[13,14] Regardless of the guidewire used, placement of a pancreatic stent for PEP prophylaxis should be considered after multiple guidewire insertions into the PD in high-risk patients.[8,15–17]

## PANCREATIC DUCT TECHNIQUES

In situations when the CBD is unable to be cannulated with standard techniques, cannulation of the PD can often be achieved more easily. When the guidewire is inadvertently advanced into the PD, it can be left in the duct to assist through a variety of mechanisms. The wire may help to stabilize the scope position, anchor and straighten the PD and common channel, open up a stenotic papilla, separate the biliary and pancreatic orifices, identify the pancreatic axis, direct a precut incision, and partially occlude the pancreatic orifice to deflect the guidewire into the CBD. Initial studies of double-wire technique were promising. A randomized trial of 53 patients in whom biliary cannulation failed after 10 minutes showed that double-wire technique achieved successful cannulation in 93% of patients as opposed to 58% in the standard biliary technique group.[18] A similar efficacy of 94% successful biliary cannulation was achieved by double guidewire technique in another randomized trial of 70 patients. No differences in complications were observed in either study.

Prolonged manipulation of the wire in the PD is a well-recognized risk factor for PEP. It was thought that early use of the double-guidewire technique may decrease the number of PD cannulations and thus the incidence of PEP as well. However, a single-center cohort study of 50 patients and a multicenter prospective RCT that included 274 patients failed to show a decrease in the rate of PEP. Possible explanations include the degree of guidewire manipulation with the wire in the PD as well as possible penetration or perforation of side branches during cannulation. With the wire already in the PD, it is easy to protect against complications by placing a narrow-caliber pancreatic stent (3F–5F). The efficacy of a prophylactic pancreatic stent in this situation has been demonstrated in randomized control trials.[15,19]

A variation on the double-guidewire cannulation technique involves placing the pancreatic stent immediately after cannulating the PD. This technique allows for better identification of the pancreatic axis and total occlusion of the PD, which then allows for deflection of the guidewire into the CBD. A randomized control trial of difficult biliary cannulation in 87 patients demonstrated a higher rate of successful biliary cannulation in the pancreatic stent-assisted cannulation group than in the double-wire technique group (91% vs 67%). However, more precut sphincterotomies were performed with the pancreatic stent-assisted technique (26% vs 10%), likely accounting for the higher cannulation success.[20] A retrospective study of 76 patients showed similar efficacy (93% success, 21% requiring precut).[21] The placement of a pancreatic stent immediately, although helpful for precut, can often compress the biliary orifice and make standard approaches more difficult. The author only places a pancreatic stent early to protect the PD for intended precut sphincterotomy.[22]

## PRECUT SPHINCTEROTOMY

Precut sphincterotomy was first described by Siegel[23] in 1980 as a technique to create a controlled incision to facilitate biliary cannulation when standard attempts have failed. The term has now come to encompass a broad range of technical variations on the original precut technique as well. The decision to use precut sphincterotomy can depend on multiple factors, including the indication, skill and experience of the endoscopist, and anatomy. The technique is most helpful in unusual or distorted anatomy of the papilla, such as cases of malignancy, impacted stone, or humpback anatomic configuration.[24,25] Precut sphincterotomy is also useful in patients with altered anatomy status post Billroth II or Roux-en-Y anastomosis. Because the papilla is approached from below in these patients, standard sphincterotomes do not align along the biliary axis, which is now in the 5-o'clock position.[26] Use of a plastic cap, when balloon enteroscopy-assisted ERCP is required due to a long afferent limb, can be helpful in positioning and stabilizing the biliary orifice for cannulation.[27]

The most commonly applied precut technique is precut papillotomy (PP), which involves starting the incision from the upper rim or lip of the papillary orifice and extending the cut cephalad in the biliary axis. This technique can be accomplished with various devices but is most frequently performed freehand with a needle knife and commonly referred to as needle-knife sphincterotomy (NKS).

Precut fistulotomy (PF) is another precut technique that involves creating an incision usually at the apex of the bulge created by the intraduodenal bile duct and cutting downward into a dilated duct or to the surface of an impacted stone. PF is theoretically safer as it spares the pancreatic orifice from thermal injury and may decrease the incidence of PEP, but it is predicated on having a dilated intraduodenal segment of bile duct. Lithotripsy was required more often when PF was performed for stone disease versus PP, presumably related to a smaller sphincterotomy, which is not extended to the papillary orifice.[28–30]

Once the CBD has been cannulated, a standard sphincterotome is generally used to extend the sphincterotomy as needed. A small precut incision can also be expanded with a dilation balloon to facilitate the removal of large CBD stones. The balloon diameter is chosen to match the size of the stone but not larger than the native duct. Recent studies and meta-analyses have shown balloon dilation after initial sphincterotomy to be as effective as sphincterotomy alone and to decrease the need for mechanical lithotripsy.[31–35] The balloon dilation technique is discussed further in the article by Dr Sherman elsewhere in this issue.

For many years, precut sphincterotomy was considered high risk and only to be done by experts as a last resort after multiple attempts at standard cannulation had failed.[36–38] The complication rates were high, up to one-third of patients, with increases seen in bleeding, perforation, and pancreatitis. However, the incidence of severe pancreatitis and overall complications was reduced when precut sphincterotomy was performed with prophylactic pancreatic stent placement.[22,39–41]

The negative outcomes in early studies may have been related to the absence of prophylactic measures and limited experience with the technique. More recent studies have demonstrated that precut sphincterotomy is a safe, time-saving, and effective technique.[42–44] A meta-analysis of 6 prospective trials that included 959 patients actually showed that precut (PP and PF) significantly reduced the risk of PEP as well as a trend toward increased biliary cannulation success.[45]

It has been suggested that switching to precut earlier in the procedure may help avoid PEP because the prolonged and repeated attempts at cannulation that typically precede this advanced technique may be responsible for many of the reported complications.[43,46] A retrospective analysis of 2004 patients undergoing ERCP for choledocholithiasis at a single center showed no significant difference in rates of PEP when less than 10 attempts at cannulation were made compared with precut.[44] A meta-analysis of 6 RCTs that included 966 patients undergoing early precut sphincterotomy using various techniques

(PP, PF, Erlangen PP) versus persistent attempts at cannulation using standard techniques has been reported. Overall biliary cannulation rates and total adverse event rates were similar. However, when pancreatitis alone was considered, a significantly lower PEP rate was seen in the early precut group (2.5% vs 5.3%; odds ratio [OR], 0.47; 95% CI, 0.24–0.91).[47] An updated meta-analysis of 7 RCTs with 1039 patients showed a trend toward higher rates of cannulations in the early precut group than in the traditional cannulation group (90% vs 86.3%; OR, 1.98; 95% CI, 0.70–5.65) and a trend toward lower rates of PEP (3.9% vs 6.1%; OR, 0.58; 95% CI, 0.32–1.05), with similar overall complication rates (6.2% vs 6.9%; OR, 0.85; 95% CI, 0.51–1.41).[48]

Even if biliary cannulation fails after initial precut sphincterotomy, repeating the ERCP after 2 days (allowing the inflammation and edema from manipulation of the papilla to resolve) may be an option if the patient's condition permits. Reports of 2 series of patients found that repeat ERCP within 2 to 7 days after failed initial precut sphincterotomy was ultimately successful 82% to 100% of the time, thus justifying a repeat ERCP before considering more invasive approaches such as EUS-guided or percutaneous biliary access.[49,50]

The initial fears regarding precut sphincterotomy have largely been dispelled by a more thorough understanding of the indications, the utility of a pancreatic stent, greater respect for the risks, and better understanding of the anatomic features. Persistance versus precut as a choice is not clear cut but much more a decision based on cannulation skills and familiarity with needle knife principles, with the final decision best made based on anatomic considerations as to what is favorable for precut or not.

## TRANSPANCREATIC SEPTOTOMY

Transpancreatic septotomy (TPS) is a precut technique of cutting through the septum that separates the terminal end of the CBD and PD. Goff[51] first described the technique in 1995 using a standard traction sphincterotome inserted superficially into the PD. The sphincterotome is then oriented in the 11-o'clock position, and an incision is made to expose the biliary orifice or the bile duct itself. Once the ductal septum is cut, biliary cannulation can be reattempted. Advantages of the technique include not having to exchange catheters for a needle-knife device and the ability to better control the depth of incision with a traction-type sphincterotome than with a free-hand needle knife. Retrospective and prospective series have demonstrated the relative efficacy and safety of TPS, although increased rates of PEP have been seen due to direct thermal injury to the pancreatic orifice.[52–57] Placing a PD stent after TPS has been shown to reduce the incidence of PEP.[58]

A prospective multicenter study of 216 patients comparing TPS and NKS found no significant difference in the initial and eventual success rates or the incidence of PEP and overall complications.[59] A recent single-center prospective RCT of 149 patients showed TPS to have a higher biliary cannulation rate (96% vs 84%, $P = .018$), faster cannulation time (193 vs 485 seconds, $P<.001$), and similar incidence of complications as NKS.[60] Another single-center prospective RCT of 71 patients compared TPS with the double-guidewire technique. Biliary cannulation rates and the time to cannulate were similar, but the overall incidence of PEP was significantly lower in the TPS group (11% vs 38%, $P<.01$).[61]

TPS is a viable option, although not commonly used in North America. The success of this approach critically depends on the appropriate cutting current to minimize any coagulation effect and to avoid a deeper cut to prevent pancreatic parenchymal insult. A prophylactic pancreatic stent should be considered after TPS, especially in high-risk patients.[15,58]

## ADDITIONAL VARIATIONS ON PRECUT

A variation on the PP technique involves using a specialized noseless Erlangen-type traction sphincterotome, which takes its name from the birthplace of endoscopic sphincterotomy, Erlangen, Germany.[62] Using a traction sphincterotome is thought to limit complications by allowing better control of the depth of incision compared with a freehand needle-knife device, although limited data exist to support this hypothesis.[63,64]

Intramucosal incision is another variation of the PP technique, first described by Burdick in 2002, that takes advantage of the inadvertent formation of a false tract. Sometimes during bowing of the sphincterotome/cannula and the use of guidewire-facilitated cannulation, inadvertent formation of a false passage occurs in the 11-o'clock direction. The tip of the wire or the sphincterotome punctures the superior aspect of the mucosal canal of the papillary orifice and then tracks submucosally and emerges out of the roof of the papilla. This event is generally considered undesirable; however, Burdick used this false tract formation as an opportunity to achieve selective biliary cannulation by applying an intramucosal incision technique whereby the mucosa is laid open and the pseudotract is incised with the sphincterotome, thus improving exposure of the biliary duct orifice.[65] This technique has some conceptual similarities to TPS, in which a mucosal cut is responsible in large part for improving access to the sphincter lumen. The safety and efficacy of intramucosal incision have been demonstrated in retrospective series.[65–67]

## COMPARING TECHNIQUES

With so many advanced cannulating techniques developed by expert endoscopists over the years, it can be difficult to decide what the next best course of action is when faced with difficult biliary cannulation. Without large comparative RCTs to guide us, disagreement exists even among expert endoscopists. Many switch over to the technique with which they were trained or are most comfortable.

A retrospective analysis of 274 cases was done involving the 3 main precut techniques (NKS, PF, and TPS) when biliary cannulation was not achieved using standard methods. NKS was performed in 129 cases (47.1%), PF in 78 patients (28.5%), and TPS in 67 cases (24.5%). No significant difference was observed in the initial and eventual success rate of biliary cannulation between the 3 groups. PEP developed in 27 cases (20.9%) with NKS and in 15 cases (22.4%) with TPS, compared with 2 cases (2.6%) with PF, which was statistically significant.[30] The difference is likely a reflection of selection bias, in which a grossly dilated intramural duct or impacted stone affords great protection against pancreatitis. Unfortunately, this particular indication for precut occurs the least frequently, although when present provides a safe anatomic approach for PF.

Algorithms have been proposed based on expert opinion to guide escalation of techniques when cannulation initially fails.[44,68] A sequential algorithm for the management of difficult biliary cannulation involving early PF, or early pancreatic guidewire/stent-assisted biliary cannulation in the case of unintentional cannulation of the PD, was studied in a prospective clinical study involving 140 patients. Following the algorithm ultimately achieved 97% successful biliary cannulation with complications comparable with historic data (10% PEP).[69]

## INTRADIVERTICULAR PAPILLA

Unusual or distorted ampullary anatomy can be a major impediment to successful biliary cannulation. The ampulla may be located anywhere around the inferior rim or inside a duodenal diverticulum. Juxtapapillary diverticulum may seem intimidating but does not significantly increase the difficulty of selective biliary cannulation.[70,71] However, intradiverticular papilla can be challenging, with successful cannulation rates lower than for patients without diverticula. Many techniques have been developed to facilitate cannulation by exposing the papillary orifice and aligning the ducts correctly for cannulation. These techniques include balloon dilation of a narrow diverticular rim,[72] injecting saline to lift the papilla out of the diverticulum,[73] cap-assisted forward viewing scope,[74] and endoscopic clipping of the diverticular or peripapillary folds to expose the biliary orifice.[75,76]

The papilla can also be everted by placing a device in the common channel or preferably by placing a guidewire or stent in the PD. Dual accessory approaches are feasible as well, in which a pediatric grasping forceps may be used to pull the papilla within reach of the cannulating sphincterotome or cannula.[77,78] This approach is often cumbersome and demands pediatric (5F) size forceps to allow room for a 7F cannula or sphincterotome. A steerable or swing-tip catheter allows for orienting the catheter along the axis of the CBD, which may be altered within the diverticulum. Precut sphincterotomy has been performed safely and effectively in periampullary diverticulum, but precut techniques should be approached cautiously because of the thinner wall and risk of perforation.[79] A side-saddle diverticulum, in which the papillary runs down the center of the diverticulum, is particularly amenable to a safe precut attempt.

## DEVICES

The most fundamental change in ERCP instrumentation in recent years has been the introduction of short-wire systems.[80,81] One RCT showed significant reduction in device exchange time and stent insertion time, while showing a trend to shorter total procedure time, fluoroscopy time, and cannulation time.[82] The main benefit of the short-wire systems is the ability of the endoscopist to control the guidewire, thus theoretically decreasing the risk of PEP. However, studies to date have not shown this to be the case. Long-wire systems have also been adapted to give the endoscopist similar control over the guidewire. Moreover, all devices work with long-wire systems, whereas less commonly used accessories may not have short-wire compatibility. Although short-wire platforms have quickly spread in popularity to be used by a slight majority of endoscopists in the United States (54%), most high-volume endoscopists (>200 ERCPs per year) still prefer long-wire systems (58%).[3]

The advent of endoscopic submucosal dissection (ESD) technique necessitated the creation of a whole new set of endoscopic tools to precisely dissect the submucosa off of the muscularis. Expert endoscopists are now exploring the utility of these specialized devices in other applications. A specialized electrocautery device, the dual knife, was used in place of a needle knife to perform PP in 18 patients with difficult access. Selective CBD cannulation was achieved in 100% of the cases, and only 1 (5.6%) developed pancreatitis.[83]

The Iso-tome, a modified needle-knife papillotome with an insulated round tip, resembles another specialized ESD device, the insulation tip knife. The tip of the knife/papillotome is insulated to block electrical discharge from the incision needle and prevent unintended electrical damage to the pancreas. The semicircular tip also acts like a hook that is helpful in cases of spontaneous choledochoduodenal fistulas or after an artificial one has already been created with a needle knife.[84,85] More studies are needed before the safety and efficacy of these new tools can be assessed.

## SUMMARY

Data comparing the various techniques and associated outcomes should be evaluated within the context of the inclusion criteria of the various studies. It is certain that there is a much greater understanding of the anatomy of the papilla as well as the risks associated with patient and device variables. The most helpful interpretation of the results from the prospective trials has been the recognition of the appropriateness of different approaches in different anatomic configurations. The decision to use one technique versus another mainly depends on patient anatomy, endoscopist experience, and whether wire cannulation of the pancreas is easily achieved.

The old adage "Don't look a gift horse in the mouth" applies to ERCP as well. If the guidewire goes into the PD more than 2 to 3 times, then use pancreatic stent-assisted cannulation or precut technique. If a false tract is created, then open up the submucosal tunnel to expose the ductal orifices. If there is a bulging choledochal cyst eminently suitable for a PF, then that is the best approach. Once again, it is not a single RCT, or even a meta-analysis, that should determine what is to be done in an individual case, but using the knowledge garnered from these trials, the endoscopist should custom design an approach suitable to the situation.

Ultimately, cannulation success of greater than 95% and complication rates of less than 5% should be a standard that endoscopists doing ERCP should achieve.

## REFERENCES

1. McCune WS, Shorb PE, Moscovitz H. Endoscopic cannulation of the ampulla of Vater: a preliminary report. Ann Surg 1968;167(5):752–6.
2. Freeman ML, Nelson DB, Sherman S, et al. Same-day discharge after endoscopic biliary sphincterotomy: observations from a prospective multicenter complication study. The Multicenter Endoscopic Sphincterotomy (MESH) Study Group. Gastrointest Endosc 1999;49(5):580–6.
3. Coté GA, Keswani RN, Jackson T, et al. Individual and practice differences among physicians who perform ERCP at varying frequency: a national survey. Gastrointest Endosc 2011;74(1):65–73.e12.
4. Lella F, Bagnolo F, Colombo E, et al. A simple way of avoiding post-ERCP pancreatitis. Gastrointest Endosc 2004;59:830–4.
5. Artifon EL, Sakai P, Cunha JE, et al. Guidewire cannulation reduces risk of post-ERCP pancreatitis and facilitates bile duct cannulation. Am J Gastroenterol 2007; 102:2147–53.
6. Lee TH, Park do H, Park JY, et al. Can wire-guided cannulation prevent post-ERCP pancreatitis? A prospective randomized trial. Gastrointest Endosc 2009; 69(3 Pt 1):444–9.
7. Cheung J, Tsoi KK, Quan WL, et al. Guidewire versus conventional contrast cannulation of the common bile duct for the prevention of post-ERCP pancreatitis: a systematic review and meta-analysis. Gastrointest Endosc 2009;70:1211–9.
8. Tse F, Yuan Y, Moayyedi P, et al. Guide wire-assisted cannulation for the prevention of post-ERCP pancreatitis: a systematic review and meta-analysis. Endoscopy 2013;45(8):605–18.
9. Kawakami H, Maguchi H, Mukai T, et al. A multicenter, prospective, randomized study of selective bile duct cannulation performed by multiple endoscopists: the BIDMEN study. Gastrointest Endosc 2012;75(2):362–72.
10. Mariani A, Giussani A, Di Leo M, et al. Guidewire biliary cannulation does not reduce post-ERCP pancreatitis compared with the contrast injection technique in low-risk and high-risk patients. Gastrointest Endosc 2012;75(2):339–46.
11. Kobayashi G, Fujita N, Imaizumi K, et al. Wire-guided biliary cannulation technique does not reduce the risk of post-ERCP pancreatitis: multicenter randomized controlled trial. Dig Endosc 2013;25(3):295–302.

12. Freeman ML, Guda NM. ERCP cannulation: a review of reported techniques. Gastrointest Endosc 2005;61:112–25.
13. Diehl DL. Benefits of 0.025" guidewires for ERCP. Surg Endosc 2014;28(7):2243.
14. Halttunen J, Kylänpää L. A prospective randomized study of thin versus regular-sized guidewire in wire-guided cannulation. Surg Endosc 2013;27(5):1662–7.
15. Freeman ML. Pancreatic stents for prevention of post-endoscopic retrograde cholangiopancreatography pancreatitis. Clin Gastroenterol Hepatol 2007;5(11): 1354–65.
16. Choudhary A, Bechtold ML, Arif M, et al. Pancreatic stents for prophylaxis against post-ERCP pancreatitis: a meta-analysis and systematic review. Gastrointest Endosc 2011;73:275–82.
17. Mazaki T, Mado K, Masuda H, et al. Prophylactic pancreatic stent placement and post-ERCP pancreatitis: an updated meta-analysis. J Gastroenterol 2014;49(2): 343–55.
18. Maeda S, Hayashi H, Hosokawa O, et al. Prospective randomized pilot trial of selective biliary cannulation using pancreatic guide-wire placement. Endoscopy 2003;35(9):721–4.
19. Ito K, Fujita N, Noda Y, et al. Can pancreatic duct stenting prevent post-ERCP pancreatitis in patients who undergo pancreatic duct guidewire placement for achieving selective biliary cannulation? J Gastroenterol 2010;45(11):1183–91.
20. Coté GA, Mullady DK, Jonnalagadda SS, et al. Use of a pancreatic duct stent or guidewire facilitates bile duct access with low rates of precut sphincterotomy: a randomized clinical trial. Dig Dis Sci 2012;57(12):3271–8.
21. Coté GA, Ansstas M, Pawa R, et al. Difficult biliary cannulation: use of physician-controlled wire-guided cannulation over a pancreatic duct stent to reduce the rate of precut sphincterotomy (with video). Gastrointest Endosc 2010;71(2): 275–9.
22. Kubota K, Sato T, Kato S, et al. Needle-knife precut papillotomy with a small incision over a pancreatic stent improves the success rate and reduces the complication rate in difficult biliary cannulations. J Hepatobiliary Pancreat Sci 2013; 20(3):382–8.
23. Siegel JH. Precut papillotomy: a method to improve success of ERCP and papillotomy. Endoscopy 1980;12(3):130–3.
24. Larkin CJ, Huibregtse K. Precut sphincterotomy: indications, pitfalls, and complications. Curr Gastroenterol Rep 2001;3(2):147–53.
25. Linder S, Söderlund C. Factors influencing the use of precut technique at endoscopic sphincterotomy. Hepatogastroenterology 2007;54:2192–7.
26. Haber GB. Double balloon endoscopy for pancreatic and biliary access in altered anatomy (with videos). Gastrointest Endosc 2007;66(3 Suppl):S47–50.
27. Trindade AJ, Mella JM, Slattery E, et al. Use of a cap in single-balloon enteroscopy-assisted endoscopic retrograde cholangiography. Endoscopy 2015; 47(5):453–6.
28. Mavrogiannis C, Liatsos C, Romanos A, et al. Needle-knife fistulotomy versus needle-knife precut papillotomy for the treatment of common bile duct stones. Gastrointest Endosc 1999;50:334–9.
29. Abu-Hamda EM, Baron TH, Simmons DT, et al. A retrospective comparison of outcomes using three different precut needle knife techniques for biliary cannulation. J Clin Gastroenterol 2005;39:717–21.
30. Katsinelos P, Gkagkalis S, Chatzimavroudis G, et al. The three types of precut sphincterotomy have no different overall CBD cannulation rates; SPF reduces post-ERCP pancreatitis risk. Dig Dis Sci 2012;57(12):3286–92.

31. Jun BG, Lee TH, Jeong S, et al. One-step transfistula large versus conventional balloon dilation following precut fistulotomy in difficult biliary cannulation for the removal of biliary stones: a multicenter retrospective study. J Gastroenterol Hepatol 2014;29(7):1551–6.

32. Teoh AY, Cheung FK, Hu B, et al. Randomized trial of endoscopic sphincterotomy with balloon dilation versus endoscopic sphincterotomy alone for removal of bile duct stones. Gastroenterology 2013;144(2):341–5.

33. Yang XM, Hu B. Endoscopic sphincterotomy plus large-balloon dilation vs endoscopic sphincterotomy for choledocholithiasis: a meta-analysis. World J Gastroenterol 2013;19(48):9453–60.

34. Madhoun MF, Wani S, Hong S, et al. Endoscopic papillary large balloon dilation reduces the need for mechanical lithotripsy in patients with large bile duct stones: a systematic review and meta-analysis. Diagn Ther Endosc 2014;2014:309618.

35. Xu L, Kyaw MH, Tse YK, et al. Endoscopic sphincterotomy with large balloon dilation versus endoscopic sphincterotomy for bile duct stones: a systematic review and meta-analysis. Biomed Res Int 2015;2015:673103.

36. Cotton PB. Precut papillotomy-a risky technique for experts only. Gastrointest Endosc 1989;35:578–9.

37. Harewood GC, Baron TH. An assessment of the learning curve for precut biliary sphincterotomy. Am J Gastroenterol 2002;97:1708–12.

38. Kasmin FE, Cohen D, Batra S, et al. Needle knife sphincterotomy in a tertiary referral center: efficacy and complications. Gastrointest Endosc 1996;44:48–53.

39. Freeman ML, Guda NM. Prevention of post-ERCP pancreatitis: a comprehensive review. Gastrointest Endosc 2004;59(7):845–64.

40. Loperfido S, Angelini G, Benedetti G, et al. Major early complications from diagnostic and therapeutic ERCP: a prospective multicenter study. Gastrointest Endosc 1998;48:1–10.

41. Masci E, Mariani A, Curioni S, et al. Risk factors for pancreatitis following endoscopic retrograde cholangiopancreatography: a meta-analysis. Endoscopy 2003;35:830–4.

42. Tang SJ, Haber GB, Kortan P, et al. Precut papillotomy versus persistence in difficult biliary cannulation: a prospective randomized trial. Endoscopy 2005;37(1):58–65.

43. Manes G, Di Giorgio P, Repici A, et al. An analysis of the factors associated with the development of complications in patients undergoing precut sphincterotomy: a prospective, controlled, randomized, multicenter study. Am J Gastroenterol 2009;104(10):2412–7.

44. Testoni PA, Giussani A, Vailati C, et al. Precut sphincterotomy, repeated cannulation and post-ERCP pancreatitis in patients with bile duct stone disease. Dig Liver Dis 2011;43(10):792–6.

45. Gong B, Hao L, Bie L, et al. Does precut technique improve selective bile duct cannulation or increase post-ERCP pancreatitis rate? A meta-analysis of randomized controlled trials. Surg Endosc 2010;24(11):2670–80.

46. Freeman ML, DiSario JA, Nelson DB, et al. Risk factors for post-ERCP pancreatitis: a prospective, multicenter study. Gastrointest Endosc 2001;54:425–34.

47. Cennamo V, Fuccio L, Zagari RM, et al. Can early precut implementation reduce endoscopic retrograde cholangiopancreatography-related complication risk? Meta-analysis of randomized controlled trials. Endoscopy 2010;42:381–8.

48. Navaneethan U, Konjeti R, Venkatesh PG, et al. Early precut sphincterotomy and the risk of endoscopic retrograde cholangiopancreatography related complications: an updated meta-analysis. World J Gastrointest Endosc 2014;6(5):200–8.

49. Pavlides M, Barnabas A, Fernandopulle N, et al. Repeat endoscopic retrograde cholangiopancreaticography after failed initial precut sphincterotomy for biliary cannulation. World J Gastroenterol 2014;20(36):13153–8.
50. Fiocca F, Fanello G, Cereatti F, et al. Early 'shallow' needle-knife papillotomy and guidewire cannulation: an effective and safe approach to difficult papilla. Therap Adv Gastroenterol 2015;8(3):114–20.
51. Goff JS. Common bile duct pre-cut sphincterotomy: transpancreatic sphincter approach. Gastrointest Endosc 1995;41:502–5.
52. Goff JS. Long-term experience with the transpancreatic sphincter pre-cut approach to biliary sphincterotomy. Gastrointest Endosc 1999;50:642–5.
53. Akashi R, Kiyozumi T, Jinnouchi K, et al. Pancreatic sphincter precutting to gain selective access to the common bile duct: a series of 172 patients. Endoscopy 2004;36:405–10.
54. Chan CH, Brennan FN, Zimmerman MJ, et al. Wire assisted transpancreatic septotomy, needle knife precut or both for difficult biliary access. J Gastroenterol Hepatol 2012;27(8):1293–7.
55. Huang L, Yu QS, Zhang Q, et al. Comparison between double-guidewire technique and transpancreatic sphincterotomy technique for difficult biliary cannulation. Dig Endosc 2015;27(3):381–7.
56. Miao L, Li QP, Zhu MH, et al. Endoscopic transpancreatic septotomy as a precutting technique for difficult bile duct cannulation. World J Gastroenterol 2015; 21(13):3978–82.
57. Kahaleh M, Tokar J, Mullick T, et al. Prospective evaluation of pancreatic sphincterotomy as a precut technique for biliary cannulation. Clin Gastroenterol Hepatol 2004;2:971–7.
58. Sakai Y, Tsuyuguchi T, Sugiyama H, et al. Transpancreatic precut papillotomy in patients with difficulty in selective biliary cannulation. Hepatogastroenterology 2011;58:1853–8.
59. Wang P, Zhang W, Liu F, et al. Success and complication rates of two precut techniques, transpancreatic sphincterotomy and needle knife sphincterotomy for bile duct cannulation. J Gastrointest Surg 2010;14:697–704.
60. Zang J, Zhang C, Gao J. Guidewire-assisted transpancreatic sphincterotomy for difficult biliary cannulation: a prospective randomized controlled trial. Surg Laparosc Endosc Percutan Tech 2014;24(5):429–33.
61. Yoo YW, Cha SW, Lee WC, et al. Double guidewire technique vs transpancreatic precut sphincterotomy in difficult biliary cannulation. World J Gastroenterol 2013; 19(1):108–14.
62. Rabenstein T, Schneider HT, Hahn EG, et al. 25 years of endoscopic sphincterotomy in Erlangen: assessment of the experience in 3498 patients. Endoscopy 1998;30:A194–201.
63. Binmoeller KF, Seifert H, Gerke H, et al. Papillary roof incision using the Erlangen-type pre-cut papillotome to achieve selective bile duct cannulation. Gastrointest Endosc 1996;44:689–95.
64. Palm J, Saarela A, Makela J. Safety of Erlangen precut papillotomy: an analysis of 1044 consecutive ERCP examinations in a single institution. J Clin Gastroenterol 2007;41:528–33.
65. Burdick JS, London A, Thompson DR. Intramural incision technique. Gastrointest Endosc 2002;55:425–7.
66. Misra SP, Dwivedi M. Intramural incision technique: a useful and safe procedure for obtaining ductal access during ERCP. Gastrointest Endosc 2008;67: 629–33.

67. Goenka MK, Rai VK. Burdick's technique for biliary access revisited. Clin Endosc 2015;48(1):20–3.
68. Bakman YG, Freeman ML. Difficult biliary access at ERCP. Gastrointest Endosc Clin N Am 2013;23(2):219–36.
69. Lee TH, Hwang SO, Choi HJ, et al. Sequential algorithm analysis to facilitate selective biliary access for difficult biliary cannulation in ERCP: a prospective clinical study. BMC Gastroenterol 2014;14:30.
70. Tham TC, Kelly M. Association of periampullary duodenal diverticula with bile duct stones and with technical success of endoscopic retrograde cholangiopancreatography. Endoscopy 2004;36:1050–3.
71. Chang-Chien CS. Do juxtapapillary diverticula of the duodenum interfere with cannulation at endoscopic retrograde cholangiopancreatography? A prospective study. Gastrointest Endosc 1987;33:298–300.
72. Tóth E, Lindström E, Fork FT. An alternative approach to the inaccessible intradiverticular papilla. Endoscopy 1999;31:554–6.
73. Sherman S, Hawes RH, Lehman GA. A new approach to performing endoscopic sphincterotomy in the setting of a juxtapapillary duodenal diverticulum. Gastrointest Endosc 1991;37:353–5.
74. Myung DS, Park CH, Koh HR, et al. Cap-assisted ERCP in patients with difficult cannulation due to periampullary diverticulum. Endoscopy 2014;46:352–5.
75. Huang CH, Tsou YK, Lin CH, et al. Endoscopic retrograde cholangiopancreatography (ERCP) for intradiverticular papilla: endoclip-assisted biliary cannulation. Endoscopy 2010;42(Suppl 2):E223–4.
76. Cappell MS, Mogrovejo E, Manickam P, et al. Endoclips to facilitate cannulation and sphincterotomy during ERCP in a patient with an ampulla within a large duodenal diverticulum: case report and literature review. Dig Dis Sci 2015; 60(1):168–73.
77. Tantau M, Person B, Burtin P, et al. Duodenal diverticula and ERCP: a new trick. Endoscopy 1996;28:326.
78. Fujita N, Noda Y, Kobayashi G, et al. ERCP for intradiverticular papilla: two devices-in-one-channel method. Gastrointest Endosc 1998;48:517–20.
79. Park CS, Park CH, Koh HR, et al. Needle-knife fistulotomy in patients with periampullary diverticula and difficult bile duct cannulation. J Gastroenterol Hepatol 2012;27(9):1480–3.
80. ASGE Technology Committee, Shah RJ, Somogyi L, et al. Short-wire ERCP systems. Gastrointest Endosc 2007;66(4):650–7.
81. Reddy SC, Draganov PV. ERCP wire systems: the long and the short of it. World J Gastroenterol 2009;15(1):55–60.
82. Draganov PV, Kowalczyk L, Fazel A, et al. Prospective randomized blinded comparison of a short-wire endoscopic retrograde cholangiopancreatography system with traditional long-wire devices. Dig Dis Sci 2010;55(2):510–5.
83. Liu F, Liu J, Li Z. New role of the dual knife for precut papillotomy in difficult bile duct cannulation. Dig Endosc 2013;25(3):329–32.
84. Park SH, Kim HJ, Park DH, et al. Pre-cut papillotomy with a new papillotome. Gastrointest Endosc 2005;62(4):588–91.
85. Cho YS, Park SH, Jun BG, et al. New technique of endoscopic sphincterotomy with Iso-tome® to incise the distal papillary roof in patients with choledocholiths and choledochoduodenal fistula. Gut Liver 2015;9(2):231–8.

# Endoscopic Retrograde Cholangiopancreatography in Surgically Altered Anatomy

Victoria Gómez, MD[a], Bret T. Petersen, MD[b],*

## KEYWORDS

- Endoscopic retrograde cholangiopancreatography
- Surgically altered bowel anatomy • Enteroscopy • Gastrojejunostomy
- Roux-en-Y reconstruction • Biliopancreatic limb

## KEY POINTS

- Performance of endoscopic retrograde cholangiopancreatography (ERCP) in the patient with surgically altered bowel anatomy requires clear understanding of the common surgical rearrangements and thorough knowledge of the patient's specific surgical history. Endoscope selection is largely based on understanding the patient's postoperative anatomy, including the presence and lengths of afferent, efferent, or Roux limbs, and the type of biliary drainage present (ie, intact papilla vs bilioenteric/pancreaticoenteric anastomosis).

- Alterations that leave the biliary and pancreatic drainage intact at the major papilla (Roux-en-Y gastric bypass, Billroth II procedure, and others) necessitate either traversal of a long limb of gut using an end-viewing instrument, with a difficult approach to the papilla from below, or invasive entry to the excluded stomach to gain traditional access to the papilla from above using a side-viewing duodenoscope.

- Alterations that use a surgical biliary or pancreatic anastomosis to jejunum (Whipple procedure; Roux limb hepaticojejunostomy, and so on) generally necessitate long limb access with an end-viewing instrument.

- Device selection is largely dependent on the bilioenteric or pancreaticoenteric communication and on the caliber and length of the endoscope selected.

*Continued*

**Video of native papilla as seen with Billroth II reconstruction during endoscopy with use of a clear cap accompanies this article at http://www.giendo. theclinics.com/**

---

Disclosures/Conflicts of Interest/Funding: Dr V. Gómez has nothing to disclose. Dr B.T. Petersen: consultant Boston Scientific.
[a] Division of Gastroenterology, Mayo Clinic, Jacksonville, FL, USA; [b] Division of Gastroenterology, Mayo Clinic, 200 First Street Southwest, Rochester, MN 55905, USA
* Corresponding author.
*E-mail address:* Petersen.bret@mayo.edu

Gastrointest Endoscopy Clin N Am 25 (2015) 631–656
http://dx.doi.org/10.1016/j.giec.2015.06.001
1052-5157/15/$ – see front matter © 2015 Elsevier Inc. All rights reserved.

giendo.theclinics.com

*Continued*

- The length and mobility (vs fixation) of bowel needing to be traversed and the endoscopist's experience are 2 dominant factors related to the overall success of ERCP via altered bowel anatomy.
- The success rates, risks, benefits, and planned sequence of alternatives to performance of ERCP in altered anatomy should be thoroughly reviewed with the patient and family. Further studies comparing the different methods for access to the biliary and pancreatic systems are necessary in order to guide clinicians in choosing the most effective, safe, and least costly approach.

## INTRODUCTION

Since the first reports of endoscopic retrograde cholangiopancreatography (ERCP) in the late 1960s, the procedure has matured into an important yet standard modality for management of pancreatic and biliary disease.[1] Similarly, gastric and biliopancreatic surgery has progressed beyond longstanding procedures for malignant conditions, to commonplace intestinal alterations for liver transplantation and bariatric management. Patients undergoing these various rearrangements are equally or more susceptible to postoperative issues related to biliary stones, dyskinesia, and periampullary neoplasm. Moreover, bilio-enteric and pancreato-enteric anastomoses are subject to stenosis, with associated stone disease or infection. ERCP success rates exceeding 95% are commonplace in patients with normal gastrointestinal (GI) anatomy, whereas patients with surgically altered anatomy pose a greater challenge.[2] In this article, the most common surgical alterations in upper intestinal anatomy (**Table 1**), and selection of appropriate routes, endoscopes, and accessories for performance of ERCP in these settings, are discussed.

**Table 1**
**Common surgical operations and corresponding biliopancreatic anatomy pertinent to performance of ERCP**

| Operation | Biliary and Pancreatic Drainage |
|---|---|
| Billroth<br>  Billroth I gastroduodenostomy<br>  Billroth II gastrojejunostomy | Intact papilla |
| Subtotal or total gastrectomy<br>  with Roux-en-Y anastomosis | Intact papilla |
| RYGB | Intact papilla |
| Gastroenteric anastomosis<br>  (side-to-side gastrojejunostomy) | Intact papilla |
| Whipple operation (pancreatoduodenectomy)<br>  Classic (with antrectomy)<br>  Pylorus preserving | Separate new bilioenteric and<br>  pancreatoenteric anastomoses |
| Roux-en-Y hepaticojejunostomy | New bilioenteric anastomosis |
| Cholecystojejunostomy | Pancreatic flow at major/minor papilla intact |
| Choledochoduodenostomy | Side-to-side or end to side bilioenteric<br>  anastomosis |
| Choledochojejunostomy | Biliary continuity at major papilla<br>  may be intact as well |

## TERMINOLOGY

Before performing an ERCP in the patient with surgically altered anatomy, the endoscopist should have a clear understanding of the surgical history of the patient, including the nature and, ideally, the lengths of enteric limbs and the type of pancreatobiliary reconstruction, if any. The terms afferent, efferent, Roux-en-Y, and pancreatobiliary limbs are often used interchangeably and incorrectly. *Afferent* and *efferent* describe limb rearrangements in which a gastrojejunostomy, duodenojejunostomy, or other loop-type bypass operation is performed (**Fig. 1A**).[3] The *afferent limb* refers to the portion of intestine that drains upstream contents (bile, pancreatic juice and other proximal intestinal secretions) *toward* the gastrojejunostomy; the *efferent limb* refers to the portion of jejunum that carries these contents downstream and *away* from the gastrojejunostomy.

The Roux-en-Y operation was named after the Swiss surgeon César Roux, who in 1892 developed a Y-shaped intestinal reconstruction to decompress an obstructed stomach.[4] With this configuration, the jejunum is divided, and the distal limb is brought up to drain an organ or focal pathologic abnormality, such as an obstructed stomach or pancreas, a proximal gastric pouch, the liver, or a pseudocyst. This limb is referred to as the *Roux limb* (see **Fig. 1B**).[3] In most Roux-en-Y applications, the native duodenum and proximal 20 to 40 cm of jejunum are left intact and the jejunal end is anastomosed to the side of the Roux limb 40 to 150 cm downstream from the jejunal disruption, thus forming the opposite limb of the Y from the Roux limb. Whichever limb carries food downstream can be referred to as the *alimentary limb* (same as the Roux limb in Roux-en-Y gastric bypass [RYGB] anatomy, but the native duodenojejunal limb

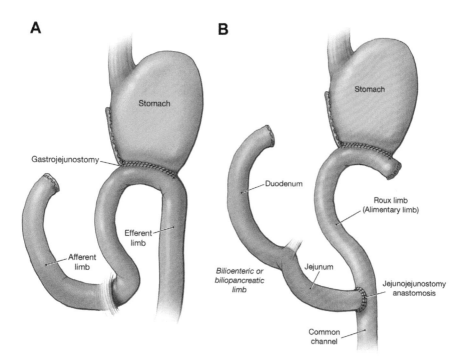

**Fig. 1.** (*A*) Gastrojejunostomy reconstruction. (*B*) Roux-en-Y reconstruction. (Used with permission of Mayo Foundation for Medical Education and Research, Rochester, MN. All rights reserved.)

following Roux-en-Y hepaticojejunostomy).[3] Whichever limb carries the biliary and pancreatic drainage can be called the biliary, pancreatic, or biliopancreatic limb. This limb may be the native upper gut, as in RYGB anatomy or the Roux limb following hepaticojejunostomy or pancreaticojejunostomy. The section of jejunoileum distal to the junction of the 2 Y limbs is termed the common channel. Meticulous use of terminology is important for clinical endoscopy reports, which provide vital information to referring physicians and surgeons.

It is also helpful to distinguish surgical alterations that involve anastomoses of the biliary or pancreatic junction to the intestine (see **Table 1**) from those in which flow through the native papilla is left intact, because this may influence anticipation of success and selection of preferred routes and endoscopic accessories.

## PREPARATION FOR ENDOSCOPIC RETROGRADE CHOLANGIOPANCREATOGRAPHY: A CHECKLIST FOR THE ENDOSCOPIST

Beyond the usual review of indications and appropriateness of ERCP for a given patient, additional considerations (**Box 1**) include review of prior operative reports, paying attention to the type of reconstruction, length of surgically created limbs of intestine, and types of anastomoses.[5–10] If certain aspects of the anatomy are unclear, it may be helpful to review the operative report with a surgical colleague or the

---

**Box 1**
**Checklist for the endoscopist preparing for endoscopic retrograde cholangiopancreatography in a patient with surgically altered anatomy**

1. Review operative reports
   - Understand the postoperative anatomy and lengths of reconstructed limbs
   - Clarify whether biliopancreaticenteric anastomoses were created
   - Review postoperative anatomy with surgical colleagues if necessary
2. Review all available radiologic, laboratory, and clinical information
   - Identify and verify the indications and goals of procedure
3. Select appropriate sedation and patient position
   - Consider anesthesia-assisted sedation or general anesthesia, given usually prolonged duration of procedure
   - Supine, prone, or left lateral
4. Select the most appropriate endoscope and accessories
   - Forward viewing endoscope versus side-viewing duodenoscope
   - Standard length versus longer endoscope
   - Single- versus double-balloon overtube versus other accessories to facilitate intubation
   - Therapeutic (duodenoscope/adult colonoscope) versus standard accessory channel
   - Straight versus angled catheters and wires, standard versus enteral length
   - ± Clear cap at scope tip
5. Informed consent with patient and family
   - Goals, risks, benefits of procedure
   - Honest acknowledgment of endoscopic success rates, alternatives for management of problem (ie, observation, other access to papilla, IR surgery)

performing surgeon. All available radiologic studies, such as cross-sectional imaging and upper GI contrast studies, should be reviewed when considering the preprocedure likelihood of a disease process being present and the estimated success rate of reaching, cannulating, and treating the suspected biliary or pancreatic pathologic condition. Most ERCPs performed on patients with surgically altered anatomy are for postoperative biliary issues, such as bilioenteric anastomotic strictures, recurrent cholangitis, and common bile duct stones.[11] Fewer pancreatic interventions have been reported, and interventional procedures are usually in patients who have undergone a pancreatoduodenectomy or Whipple procedure.[12] ERCPs in surgically altered anatomy are often prolonged procedures, so assistance from an anesthesiologist should be considered for the safety and comfort of the patient.[13] Fluoroscopy is often used during these procedures to facilitate deep intubation of long limbs and endoscope tip orientation toward the biliary system. Hence, placement of the patient in a supine or left oblique position can assist with navigation, when appropriate consideration is given to airway protection. Endoscope and accessory selection will be addressed in the discussion of individual anatomic challenges. An overview of endoscope and device compatibilities is available in **Table 2**. Working with one's local representatives for ERCP device manufacturers is another great resource. Finally, the patient and appropriate family members should be thoroughly counseled on not only the goals, risks, and benefits of the procedure but also the overall likelihood of endoscopic success and the various alternatives for management, including observation, referral to another center or endoscopist, other means for access to the papilla, interventional radiology (IR), or surgery.

Several key components of ERCP in long limb anatomy directly affect the feasibility and success of the procedure, including the ability to (1) intubate the enteric anastomoses (eg, esophagojejunal, gastrojejunal, or duodenojejunal, or Roux-en-Y enteroenteric); (2) navigate the length of the respective enteral limbs (afferent, Roux, and native duodenojejunal limbs) to reach the papilla or biliary anastomoses; (3) cannulate the respective duct of interest; and (4) accomplish appropriate therapy for the findings identified.[10,11,14] Review of a mental checklist or similar process is central to ensuring a safe and successful procedure.

## ENDOSCOPIC RETROGRADE CHOLANGIOPANCREATOGRAPHY IN ALTERED BOWEL ANATOMY WITHOUT ALTERATION OF BILIOPANCREATIC ANATOMY
### Gastric Reconstructive Procedures

Partial to complete gastric resection or bypass is often performed for the management of benign and malignant conditions, including the operative treatment of obesity. The 3 most common anatomic rearrangements following gastric resection or bypass are the Billroth I, Billroth II, and Roux-en-Y reconstructions.

### Billroth I reconstruction
Theodor Billroth was a leading European surgeon of the nineteenth century who performed one of the first antrectomies in 1881 in which the patient survived.[15,16] Billroth I and II procedures are performed for reconstruction after partial gastrectomy. With the advent of acid-suppressing therapy and recognition of *Helicobacter pylori*, they are both far less common than in previous generations. The Billroth I entails a distal gastrectomy/antrectomy, with an anastomosis of the gastric remnant to the duodenum (**Fig. 2**).[17] This anatomy is the most physiologic type of reconstruction after a distal gastric resection because it restores normal gastroduodenal continuity.[18] Because of the loss of the superior duodenal angle, the duodenum is straightened, and the major and minor duodenal papillae are closer to the stomach. Performance of ERCP in patients with Billroth I anatomy is minimally different from ERCP in those with intact

**Table 2**
**Compatibility of endoscopes and endoscopic retrograde cholangiopancreatography accessories**

| Endoscope | Working Length (cm) | Caliber of Biopsy Channel (mm) | Compatible Stents and Accessories | Considerations |
|---|---|---|---|---|
| Therapeutic duodenoscope | 124 | 4.2 | • All stents including 11.5 Fr<br>• All ERCP accessories | • Elevator facilitates access and interventions<br>• Best used for Billroth I/II and some post-Whipple anatomy<br>• Caution with traversing small bowel as stiffness yields risk for jejunal perforation |
| Adult colonoscope | 168 | 3.7 | • Up to 10-Fr plastic stents (ensure to keep side flaps down when passing through biopsy channel)<br>• Most ERCP accessories: check length before use | • Lack of elevator<br>• Best used for Billroth II, post-Whipple, or short Roux limb anatomy<br>• Stiffness may preclude depth of intubation in jejunum |
| Pediatric colonoscope | 168 | 3.2 | • Up to 7-Fr stents<br>• Most ERCP accessories: check length before use | • Lack of elevator<br>• Realistically limited to 7-Fr plastic and selected metal stents |
| Single-balloon enteroscope<br>Double-balloon enteroscope | 200<br><br>200/220 | 2.8<br><br>2.8 | • Up to 7-Fr plastic stents: use care with side flaps<br>• Requires use of long guidewires | • Lack of elevator<br>• Best used for RYGB and other long length Roux-en-Y anatomy<br>• Ensure adequate length of all standard nonenteroscopy devices as many ERCP accessories are insufficiently long<br>• NOTE: Shorter enteroscope model with a working length of 152 cm is commercially available (EN-450T5; Fujinon, Inc) and permits passage of standard ERCP accessories, but is not routinely available in most endoscopy units |

gastroduodenal anatomy. A duodenoscope is still used. Loss of the pylorus and the superior duodenal angle may reduce stability of the endoscope when in the straight or short position, with repeated slippage back toward the stomach. This slippage can usually be overcome by application of slight inward tension on the endoscope, stabilization of intubation depth at the patient's teeth, or use of a medium to long endoscope position with slight looping in the stomach.[19] Once cannulation has been achieved, all standard therapeutic maneuvers performed in the conventional ERCP without altered anatomy can be performed in the patient with Billroth I reconstruction.

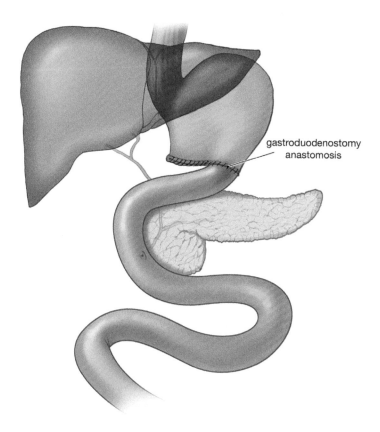

gastroduodenostomy
anastomosis

**Fig. 2.** Billroth I reconstruction. (Used with permission of Mayo Foundation for Medical Education and Research, Rochester, MN. All rights reserved.)

### Billroth II reconstruction

The Billroth II reconstruction after a gastric resection is one of the most commonly performed procedures for cancer of the stomach and is also performed for operative treatment of duodenal ulcer disease when a gastric resection is necessary.[20] The distal stomach is resected and the remnant stomach is anastomosed to the proximal jejunum in an end-to-side fashion, with closure of the proximal duodenal stump (**Fig. 3**). The single gastrojejunal anastomosis at the distal end of the gastric remnant yields entry to side-by-side afferent and efferent lumens with a saddle of jejunal mucosa between them. The orientation of the anastomosis and the position of the jejunal loop in relation to the transverse colon (retrocolic—through the transverse mesocolon vs antecolic—anterior to the transverse colon) are dependent on the patient's anatomy and pathologic condition and the preference of the surgeon. The Polya method (see **Fig. 3**A) uses a wide (>6 cm) anastomosis to the entire gastric opening, whereas the Hofmeister method yields a smaller diameter anastomosis between the greater curvature of the gastric opening and the jejunum (see **Fig. 3**B).[20] Sometimes the end of the gastric remnant is closed and a gastrojejunal side-to-side anastomosis is created in the gastric remnant proximal to the closed end of the gastric remnant.

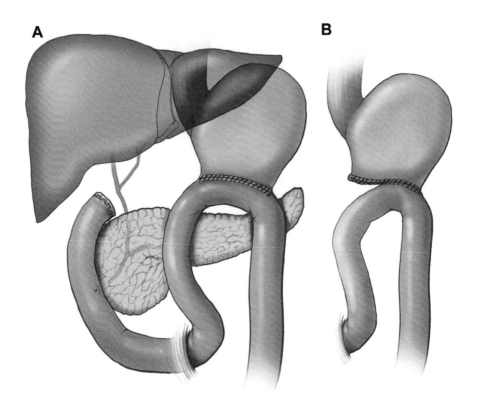

**Fig. 3.** (*A*) Billroth II reconstruction: Polya method. (*B*) Billroth II reconstruction: Hofmeister method. (Used with permission of Mayo Foundation for Medical Education and Research, Rochester, MN. All rights reserved.)

Because of bile reflux into the gastric remnant after a Billroth II reconstruction, a side-to-side jejunojejunostomy between the afferent and efferent limbs is sometimes created to divert the bile away from the remaining stomach. This procedure is known as the Braun procedure (**Fig. 4**).[21] Endoscopically, this anastomosis will be found in either the afferent or the efferent limb approximately 15 to 20 cm from the gastrojejunostomy. Billroth II anatomy approximates that of the loop gastrojejunostomy performed for distal gastric or proximal duodenal obstruction without resection, so most remarks about afferent limb entry and cannulation in Billroth II anatomy also pertain there.

In Billroth II anatomy, the afferent limb of the duodenum and proximal jejunum often enter the stomach at an acute angle, while the efferent limb of jejunum drains in somewhat more linear fashion from the gastric lumen. Hence, the afferent jejunal limb is more often the leftward oriented lumen on the greater curve or posterior wall, from the patient's perspective.[22]

Both the forward (gastroscope or colonoscope) and the side-viewing endoscopes (duodenoscope) with a standard or large-diameter accessory channel can be used to achieve and successfully cannulate the biliary tree in the setting of a Billroth II reconstruction. Overtubes or smaller channel enteroscopes are rarely needed. Papillary cannulation is facilitated by use of the duodenoscope, which is the preferred instrument in experienced hands, but in many circumstances the length or fixation of the

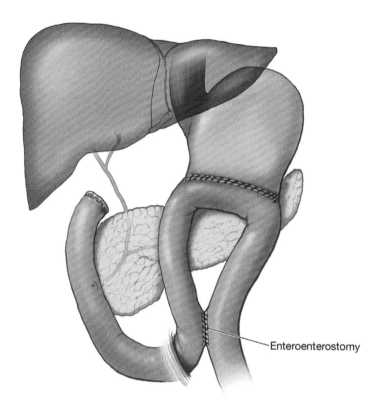

Enteroenterostomy

**Fig. 4.** Billroth II reconstruction with Braun enteroenterostomy. (Used with permission of Mayo Foundation for Medical Education and Research, Rochester, MN. All rights reserved.)

afferent limb requires use of more flexible or longer end-viewing instruments. Larger series studies of ERCP in Billroth II anatomy have demonstrated success rates using duodenoscopes for reaching the papilla and for selective biliary cannulation of 70% to 97% and 60% to 91%, respectively.[23–25] Entry from stomach to the afferent limb carries a risk of anastomotic or jejunal perforation, particularly with torque entry of the duodenoscope. Advantages of forward-viewing endoscopes, most of which are less rigid than duodenoscopes, include greater ease of entry to the afferent loop and safety of deep intubation to the level of the papilla. Cannulation rates as high as 81% to 87% have been reported using forward-viewing endoscopes in this patient population.[24,26] Forward and side-viewing endoscopes were compared in a prospective, randomized trial of ERCP in 45 patients with Billroth II anatomy. Cannulation rates were higher (87% vs 68%) with the use of gastroscopes.[26] However, these results must be interpreted with caution, as all cannulation failures in the duodenoscope group (N = 7) were due to the inability to reach the papilla as a result of intestinal perforations, difficulty in entering the afferent limb, or abdominal pain during insertion. Therefore, factors related to endoscopic skills and comfort level of the endoscopist as well as anatomic factors related to the surgical reconstruction will guide the endoscopist in selecting the appropriate endoscope.[27,28]

The afferent and efferent limbs can often be differentiated by visualization of bile and observation of motility on initial entry. The afferent limb should contain more bile, with motility propulsing toward the lens. The proximal end of the afferent limb is characterized by a blind stump of flat mucosa, with or without an obvious closure line, scars, staples, or sutures.[10] Fluoroscopy can help clarify the direction of the endoscope if the correct lumen or extent of intubation is in question. Demonstration of the endoscope in, or heading toward, the right upper quadrant and the liver suggests entry into the afferent limb. Evidence of a biliary aerogram is uncommon with an intact papilla but may prove useful. Advancement of a slippery wire and a biliary occlusion balloon ahead of the endoscope can confirm the correct limb while also characterizing and facilitating advancement through acutely angulated loops of jejunum. Occasionally repositioning the patient in the supine position allows hand compression over the abdomen to reduce loops formed by the endoscope.

Once in the duodenum, the duodenoscope provides a superior view of the papilla from below, compared with the eccentric view seen with forward-viewing endoscopes. Availability of an elevator also facilitates device manipulation, although overuse contributes to inadvertent pancreatic cannulation. The major papilla is commonly found near the 12 o'clock position of the visual field when a duodenoscope is used in a patient in the left lateral decubitus position, and eccentrically at the 3 to 6 o'clock position when a forward-viewing endoscope is used. Visualization and approach to the papilla from below with any end-viewing instrument are facilitated by use of a clear plastic cap affixed to the endoscope (**Fig. 5**, Video 1).[29,30] Compression of the duodenal angle between the second and third portion and of periampullary folds enables a slightly more distant and useful view of the papilla than can be achieved with a bare endoscope tip.

When viewed from below using a duodenoscope, the paths of the bile duct and the pancreatic duct can be confusing, because they are upside down from standard views seen with normal antegrade positioning of the side-viewing instrument. The apex of the ampulla and the upward directed bile duct lie at 5 to 6 o'clock in the visual field, rather than the usual 12 o'clock. The pancreatic duct penetrates from the midpoint of the papilla at a slight angle.[24,31] Hence, standard cannulas with an upward curve toward 12 o'clock in the visual field will orient predominantly into the pancreas. This dilemma can best be overcome by retracting the lens to the angle between second and third portion and viewing the papilla from a distance while passing a straightened catheter and a nonangled guidewire directly upward in a vertical axis aligned with the bile duct, avoiding or limiting use of the elevator, which redirects devices into the pancreas.

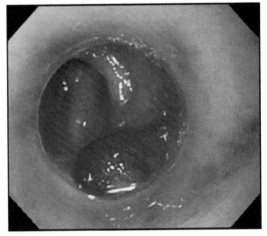

**Fig. 5.** Native papilla as seen with Billroth II reconstruction during endoscopy with use of a clear cap.

Once into the bile duct, cholangiography is straightforward, but therapy, beginning with performance of sphincterotomy, requires accommodation to the upside down view. A variety of inverted, upside down, and "shark-fin" sphincterotomes have been described, but sphincterotomy is generally most safely and easily accomplished by insertion of a 5- or 7-Fr temporary biliary stent for use as a guide to needle-knife incision.[10,19,24,31-36] Success rates as high as 95% have been reported with the over-the-stent needle-knife technique in one series, and with a low complication rate (5%).[36] Free-hand needle-knife sphincterotomy is occasionally required if cannulation cannot be achieved; however, this approach carries increased risk of periampullary perforation. Balloon sphincteroplasty, or dilation of the intact or partially incised sphincter, can reduce the risk of full sphincter incision, but dilation of an intact papilla heightens the risk of pancreatitis in some patients.[37-39] Balloon dilation catheters do not require changing the angle used to approach the papilla, and furthermore, usually come in a sufficient length for use with even longer endoscopes, such as single- and double-balloon enteroscopes, making them widely available in most endoscopy suites. In addition, balloon dilation may be more appealing rather than sphincterotomy in patients with increased risk of bleeding. In a single-center study in which 34 patients with bile duct stone and a previous Billroth II gastrectomy were randomized to ERCP with a side-viewing duodenoscope and either endoscopic sphincterotomy (EST) or endoscopic balloon dilation (EBD), there were no statistically significant differences in the rates of bile duct stone removal (14/18 patients in EST group vs 14/16 in EBD group, $P = 1.00$), use of mechanical lithotripsy (4 EST procedures vs 3 EBD procedures, $P = 1.00$), or early complications (7 EST procedures vs 3 EBD procedures, $P = .27$).[38] Three patients in the EST group experienced bleeding requiring blood transfusions, and one patient in the EBD group developed mild pancreatitis. Thus, although both EST and EBD are options, both carry a small, yet present, risk of complications that are unique to each technique. Additional studies have shown satisfactory cannulation rates with balloon dilation alone, with either duodenoscope or forward-viewing endoscopes, with success rates ranging from 83% to 92%.[39,40] Dilation of the papilla combined with guidewire-assisted needle-knife papillotomy is another option that has also been described as successful.[41]

### Subtotal gastrectomy or gastric bypass with Roux-en-Y anastomosis

All Roux-en-Y anastomoses to the esophagus or proximal gastric remnants, whether performed with extended gastric resection or gastric bypass, pose similar challenges for performance of ERCP. Total or subtotal gastrectomy with Roux-en-Y anastomosis is usually performed as a primary oncologic procedure, or in some circumstances, as salvage of a complicated gastric bypass. Roux limb anastomosis to more generous proximal gastric segments is occasionally done in revision of a previous Billroth resection to reduce troublesome bile reflux gastritis or esophagitis.[42] The length of a non-bariatric alimentary Roux limb is typically at least 40 cm in length from the esophagojejunal or gastrojejunal anastomosis to the jejunojejunal anastomosis at the base of the Y (**Fig. 6**). Hence, no bile should be present in the remnant stomach or esophagus, regardless of patency of the biliary tree.

RYGB is the most frequently performed operation for morbid obesity in the United States and Canada, accounting for 60% of all obesity operations.[43-45] This operation, which combines gastric restriction with minimal malabsorption, creates a very small-volume gastric pouch (less than 30 mL or 1 oz.), a small 10- to 12-mm side-to-side anastomosis between the pouch and the jejunum, and a variable length Roux limb.[43,44] The distal stomach is left in situ but does not communicate with the proximal stomach. Distally, it remains in continuity with the duodenum. The jejunum is divided

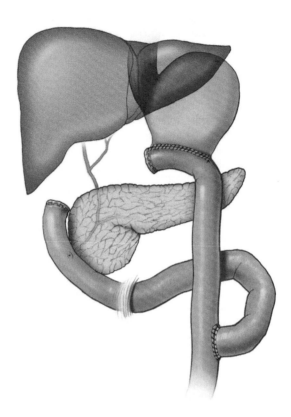

**Fig. 6.** Subtotal gastrectomy with Roux-en-Y reconstruction. (Used with permission of Mayo Foundation for Medical Education and Research, Rochester, MN. All rights reserved.)

typically 30 to 60 cm distal to the ligament of Treitz and the native biliopancreatic limb and Roux limb are anastomosed 75 to 150 cm beyond the gastrojejunostomy **(Fig. 7)**.[46] Long (>100 cm) or very long-limb (>150 cm) Roux-en-Y reconstructions are often performed in revisional bariatric operations in patients with inadequate weight loss or as a primary procedure for very obese patients (body mass index ≥50).

The need for ERCP after RYGB is not uncommon because cholelithiasis induced by rapid weight loss after bariatric surgery can occur in up to 30% of patients.[47,48] These patients are at risk of cholecystitis, choledocholithiasis, ascending cholangitis, and pancreatitis.[49] Cholecystectomy during bariatric surgery is not routinely performed and is an ongoing debate in the surgical community.[49,50] Similarly, papillary stenosis is thought to be more common after gastric bypass and requires performance of biliary sphincterotomy during ERCP.

ERCP through shorter nonbariatric Roux limbs can often be accomplished with pediatric or adult colonoscopes, or even a duodenoscope in rare cases, fashioned some years ago. Use of single- or double-balloon enteroscopes often facilitates ease and efficiency of complete intubation, however. Standard long-limb ERCP following RYGB for bariatric purposes usually requires use of an enteroscope with dedicated balloon or spiral overtubes. Aside from ease of complete intubation, endoscope selection influences the selection of devices and stents available for passage through the long 2.8-mm or 3.8-mm channels. Some but not all standard ERCP devices can reach

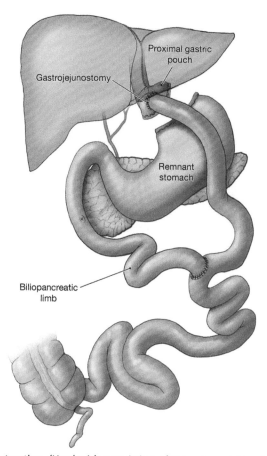

**Fig. 7.** RYGB reconstruction. (Used with permission of Mayo Foundation for Medical Education and Research. All rights reserved.)

through pediatric and adult colonoscopes. Specialty length devices are required for the use through dedicated enteroscopes. Dedicated enteroscopes and pediatric colonoscopes have 2.8-mm channels that can only accommodate 7-Fr plastic stents, whereas adult colonoscopes have 3.8-mm channels, enabling passage of up to 10-Fr stents (see **Table 2**). Some metal biliary stents can be placed through a pediatric colonoscope, whereas others require the larger channel of the adult instrument. No metal stents are available for passage through enteroscopes.

In most cases, both the gastrojejunostomy and the jejunojejunal Roux limb anastomoses are fashioned in side-to-side fashion (**Fig. 8**). If so, care must be taken to avoid attempting to intubate beyond the length of the short blind limb on the far side of an anastomosis. At the jejunojejunostomy, the alimentary lumen continues downstream as a common channel, without traversing the anastomosis, while advancement upstream through the native pancreatobiliary limb requires traversing the anastomosis. Clear visualization of the anastomosis and exploration of 1 or 2 lumens on its far side enables upstream passage toward the duodenum. This angle is often quite acute and may be difficult to negotiate. The same techniques described in Billroth II anatomy, using balloons, guidewires, fluoroscopy, and visualization of bile, can assist in characterization of the correct limb and traversal of acutely angulated turns. If entry to the

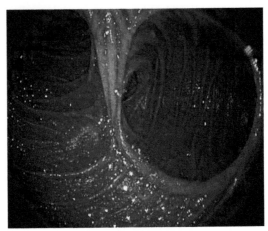

**Fig. 8.** Side-to-side jejunojejunal anastomosis. Note the presence of 3 lumens, corresponding to the common channel on the left, the biliopancreatic limb on the far right, and a blind jejunal limb in the center.

incorrect limb is suspected, extending a guidewire or occlusion balloon into the limb while the endoscope is withdrawn can assist with identifying the proper limb at the jejunojejunal anastomosis. Alternatively, biopsy of the wrong limb just beyond the anastomosis allows prompt confirmation if it is repeatedly entered. Frequently, a 180-degree turn is required to intubate the biliopancreatic limb. If the biliopancreatic limb is very acutely angulated, passage of a balloon catheter and long guidewire deeply into the limb can be used to lessen the angle and provide countertraction.[51] Common enteroscopy techniques are usually required to fully intubate RYGB anatomy to the level of the papilla, using alternating endoscope advancement and fixation, overtube advancement, balloon fixation, and reduction of the length and looping of the intubated bowel.

As in Billroth II anatomy, traversal of the acutely angled ligament of Treitz and the third part of the duodenum yields entry to the descending duodenum. Usually the endoscope passes up to the duodenal bulb and the underside of the pylorus, requiring careful inspection during withdrawal until the papilla is visualized. Rotation of the endoscope to orient the papilla at the bottom of the screen facilitates passage of accessories in an en face upward direction. Again, as described in Billroth II anatomy, identification and entry to the papilla are facilitated by use of a clear plastic cap on the endoscope; this should be standard for all long limb ERCPs with intact papillae. Angulation and unstable endoscope positions impair access to the papilla, so careful positioning of overtubes and stabilization by balloon inflation, if available, are helpful. Sphincterotomy can be carried out in a similar fashion to Billroth II anatomy, with placement of a biliary stent over a guidewire, followed by needle-knife sphincterotomy over the stent, or as previously described, partial sphincterotomy followed by balloon dilation of the papilla can be performed.

Conventional side-viewing duodenoscopes and forward-viewing colonoscopes are usually not adequate for performing ERCP in patients with long Roux-en-Y anatomy (ie, post-RYGB surgery), and therefore, enteroscopes are used. A large, multicenter study from 8 US tertiary-care referral centers evaluated outcomes of ERCP in patients with long-limb surgical bypass anatomy using single-balloon enteroscopy (SBE), double-balloon enteroscopy (DBE), and rotational overtube enteroscopy.[52] Enteroscopy and ERCP success were defined as accessing the papilla or bilio-/pancreatoenteric anastomosis and completion of the intended ERCP intervention, respectively. Entero-scopy success was achieved in 71% of patients (92/129) and ERCP success in 88% of patients (81/92). By intention-to-treat analysis, ERCP was successful in 63% of pa-tients (81/129). ERCP success rates did not differ among the enteroscopy techniques ($P = .878$). Almost half of the patient cohort had post-RYGB anatomy (N = 63), for which enteroscopy and ERCP success were achieved in 76% (48/63) and 62% (39/63) of patients, respectively, without statistically significant differences with regards to enteroscopy technique. Enteroscopy and ERCP success rates were also similar be-tween post-RYGB patients versus non-RYGB patients. In a systematic review by Skinner and colleagues,[53] enteroscopy and ERCP success in patients with prior RYGB using overtube-assisted enteroscopy was 80% (230/289) and 70% (187/266), respectively. These success rates were lower when compared with patients with Bill-roth II anatomy, pancreatoduodenectomy, and Roux-en-Y hepaticojejunostomy. The decision to use single versus double balloon, for the most part, depends on availability of enteroscopes at a particular endoscopy center and local expertise.

For cannulation, a long (450 cm) guidewire with a hydrophilic tip to allow exchange of accessories once cannulation is achieved is recommended. Many ERCP accessories are not long enough to pass through the 2-m enteroscopes, and although these acces-sories can be custom ordered, many endoscopy units are not able to stock these addi-tional tools. Alternatively, a shorter double balloon enteroscope is commercially available (EC-450BI5; Fujinon Inc, Saitama, Japan), with a working length of 152 cm and biopsy channel diameter of 2.8 mm. This enteroscope enables use of all standard ERCP accessories; however, it is not routinely available in most endoscopy units.

Sometimes, even in the hands of the most experienced endoscopists, enteroscopy-assisted ERCP in the setting of post-RYGB is still unsuccessful. Several alternative techniques have been described for performance of ERCP in long-limb patients, most dedicated to gaining antegrade access to the papilla, as during ERCP in normal anatomy. When an excluded but intact stomach remains in continuity with the duo-denum, access to the distal stomach equates to normal access to the papilla. This ac-cess can be accomplished via a gastrostomy to the excluded stomach using any of several methods, including percutaneous endoscopic gastrostomy (PEG) via Russell technique after retrograde enteroscope advancement into the remnant stomach; lapa-roscopic surgical gastrostomy tube or gastrotomy, through which a duodenoscope can be introduced for same session ERCP; IR-guided percutaneous gastrostomy placement; or endoscopic ultrasound (US) -guided inflation or contrast instillation through the proximal gastric pouch to the excluded stomach for assistance with PEG via IR techniques.[54–58] Although these approaches are attractive and usually successful, many require maturation of the gastrostomy tract, delaying ERCP up to 4 weeks. In contrast, percutaneous-assisted transprosthetic endoscopic therapy (PATENT) allows for single-session ERCP via enteroscopy access to the remnant stomach, followed by direct PEG using Russell technique with T-tag gastric immobili-zation, dilation of the PEG tract, placement and balloon expansion of a fully-covered esophageal metal stent across the tract, and antegrade ERCP through the gastrotomy stent and the gastroduodenum.[59] Following ERCP, a 24-Fr gastrostomy tube is placed through the stent, and the stent is removed after being sectioned longitudinally. A small case series of 5 RYGB patients with suspected sphincter of Oddi dysfunction under-went ERCP using PATENT, during which biliary sphincterotomy was performed in all patients, with subsequent normalization of liver enzymes in 4 patients.[60] One mild adverse event occurred, in which a sphincterotomy-induced perforation was sus-pected and treated by placement of a fully covered biliary self-expanding metal stent, which was subsequently removed.

Important factors, such as hospital resources, endoscopist skills, and patient anatomy, play an integral role in deciding the optimal method for reaching the papilla and performing therapy in patients with RYGB anatomy. In a single-center retrospective study comparing 24 single-session laparoscopy-assisted ERCPs to 32 DBE/SBE-ERCPs in patients with RYGB anatomy, the surgical approach was superior in reaching the papilla (100% vs 72%, $P$ = .005), cannulation (100% vs 59%, $P$<.001), and performance of therapy (100% vs 59%, $P$<.001).[61] There were no differences in postprocedure hospital stay or complication rates. On both univariate and multivariate analysis, however, an overall limb length of 150 cm or longer, defined as Roux limb + biliopancreatic limb (from ligament of Treitz to jejunojejunal anastomosis), was associated with a lower therapeutic success with balloon-assisted enteroscopy (BAE)-ERCP ($P$ = .024). Furthermore, a cost analysis model demonstrated increased costs when using BAE-ERCP as the initial approach in these patients. The authors concluded that patients with Roux + biliopancreatic limbs of 150 cm or longer be considered first for laparoscopic-assisted ERCP. Further studies comparing the alternative methods for ERCP in post-RYGB patients are needed.

## ENDOSCOPIC RETROGRADE CHOLANGIOPANCREATOGRAPHY IN ALTERED BOWEL ANATOMY WITH ALTERATION OF BILIOPANCREATIC ANATOMY
### Whipple Operation (Pancreatoduodenectomy)

A Whipple resection or pancreatoduodenectomy is the most common operation performed for many diseases of the head of pancreas and for periampullary malignancy. The standard Whipple resection consists of a gastric antrectomy, cholecystectomy, removal of the distal common bile duct, head of pancreas, duodenum, proximal jejunum, and regional lymph nodes, with reconstructive gastrojejunostomies, hepaticojejunostomies, and pancreaticojejunostomies (**Fig. 9**A). Currently, most surgeons perform the pylorus-preserving pancreatoduodenectomy, in which antrectomy is avoided in favor of duodenal transection 1 to 3 cm distal to the pylorus (see **Fig. 9**B). This modification preserves function of the stomach and pylorus and maintains postoperative gastric emptying closer to normal.[62,63] The pancreatic and biliary anastomoses are created 45 to 60 cm proximal to the gastric or duodenal anastomosis,

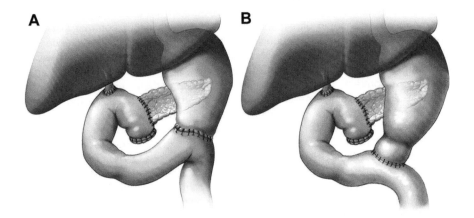

**Fig. 9.** (*A*) Standard pancreatoduodenectomy (Whipple operation). (*B*) Pylorus-preserving pancreatoduodenectomy. (Used with permission of Mayo Foundation for Medical Education and Research, Rochester, MN. All rights reserved.)

depending on the position of the jejunal loop relative to the mesocolon and surgeon preference. The pancreaticojejunostomy is found at the blind end of the afferent limb and the choledochojejunostomy is found about 5 to 10 cm downstream from there. Rarely, the biliojejunal and pancreaticojejunal anastomoses are made into separate Roux limbs. Formal review of the anatomy of the reconstructions should prevent confusion during the endoscopy.

Historically, success rates for cannulation of the pancreatic duct in patients with post-Whipple anatomy are extremely low, because of both difficulty in reaching the most proximal end of the afferent limb and challenging identification and access to the tiny, often subtle, pancreatic duct opening of less than 3 mm.[64,65] Use of secretin stimulation of pancreatic secretion and methylene blue dye spraying on the perianastomotic mucosa can aid in identifying flow from the small pancreatic os. Fortunately, most patients requiring ERCP have indications related to biliary obstruction due to bilioenteric stricture or choledocholithiasis. Noninvasive evaluation using magnetic resonance cholangiopancreatography before ERCP is helpful for determining which patients may benefit from pancreatic or biliary endotherapy and which may benefit from alternative methods for gaining access to either ductal system.

Both side-viewing and forward-viewing endoscopes can be used to reach the pancreatic and biliary anastomoses, with the expertise level of the endoscopist, length of afferent limb, and extent of angulations due to adhesions being the rate limiting factors when choosing an appropriate instrument. In one study, 51 patients with prior pancreatoduodenectomy (22 classic Whipple, 29 pylorus-preserving Whipple) underwent a total of 88 ERCPs with initial use of a standard duodenoscope (44 attempts at ERC, 37 attempts at ERCP, and 7 attempts at ERCP).[65] Technical success rates were significantly lower for pancreatic access than for biliary access (8% vs 84%, $P<.001$), and overall success of ERCP for assessment of the pancreatic, biliary, or both anastomoses was only 51% (45 of the 88 procedures). Failures were related to strictures of the pancreatic anastomosis, excessive looping of the endoscope, benign strictures or adhesions, excessive length, or metastatic obstruction of the afferent limb. In 13 of 21 failed intubations of the afferent limb, switching to an adult or pediatric variable-stiffness colonoscope enabled a successful ERCP. Data for BAE-ERCP in post-Whipple patients have shown promising outcomes. In a single-center study of 28 post-Whipple patients, overall success of reaching the hepaticojejunostomy was 96.4% (27/28) with either standard or short SBE (93.8% and 91.7%, respectively).[66] Thus, equipment availability and experience of the endoscopist are key factors when deciding which endoscope to use for ERCP.

As with Billroth II anatomy, entry to the modified stomach, or the duodenal bulb in pylorus sparing anatomy, yields a view of a single anastomosis with 2 enteral lumens representing the upstream afferent biliopancreatic limb and the downstream efferent limb to the distal GI tract. Recognition and navigation of the afferent limb have previously been discussed. Once in the proximal afferent limb, the end-to-side hepaticojejunostomy can be located, often at the outer wall of the apex of a luminal turn downward toward the pancreatic opening. Fluoroscopic review of endoscope tip movement can facilitate orientation toward the underside of the liver and, if the anastomosis is patent, an air cholangiogram can often be identified (**Fig. 10**). However, strictured anastomoses can easily be missed if the endoscopist does not spend adequate time inspecting the mucosa for subtle findings, such as disruption of normal small bowel mucosal folds, punctate scars, or the presence of bile or pus. When the duct cannot be located, injection of contrast into the jejunal lumen can also aid in identifying the anastomosis. Access to the bile or pancreatic ducts can be obtained with straight-tipped catheters and accessories (**Fig. 11**).

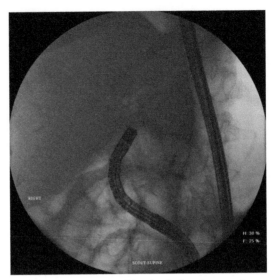

**Fig. 10.** Stenosed hepaticojejunostomy with air cholangiogram in a patient with post-Whipple anatomy. Visualization of air in the biliary tree aided in identifying the hepaticojejunostomy anastomosis during endoscopy.

Management of chronic complications after Whipple resection is difficult and may use endoscopic or surgical interventions. Operative treatments are limited to repeat resection with reanastomosis of the ducts to the jejunal limb, or total pancreatectomy.[67] Endoscopic treatment of biliary strictures and stones can be carried out using most ERCP accessories. EUS-guided methods have also been described in situations where ERCP with forward-viewing endoscopes failed to reach or access the biliary or the pancreatic orifice.[68] EUS-guided transgastric access to the pancreatic duct has been used for concurrent treatment of duct obstruction using antegrade (ie,

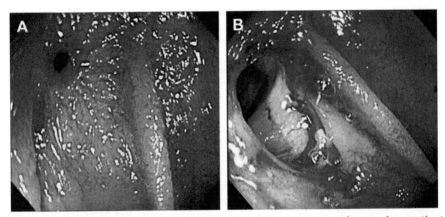

**Fig. 11.** (A) Hepaticojejunostomy anastomotic stenosis as seen on endoscopy in a patient with post-Whipple anatomy. (B) Hepaticojejunostomy anastomosis after balloon dilatation. A postdilatation tear of the anastomotic rim was present on one side; however, fluoroscopic images showed no evidence for either contrast or air leakage at this level.

transgastric), retrograde, or rendezvous techniques, with standard oblique-viewing and forward-viewing echoendoscopes.[67,69–72] The process entails EUS visualization, transgastric needle puncture, and contrast injection into the pancreatic duct, followed by advancement of a guidewire, dilation of the tract, and antegrade or retrograde stent placement into the duct and across strictures. These alternative techniques have proven more successful than long-limb retrograde access for therapy for pancreatic strictures or stones.

### Roux-en-Y Hepaticojejunostomy Reconstruction

When bile flow through the native extrahepatic bile duct is disrupted by pathologic condition, injury, or surgery, and continuity cannot be reconstructed via a duct-to-duct anastomosis, biliary-enteric communication can be re-established by anastomosis of a jejunal Roux limb to the proximal biliary tree. The length of remaining extrahepatic duct dictates whether this yields a choledochojejunostomy or a true hepaticojejunostomy to the ductal bifurcation at the base of the liver. Most Roux-en-Y hepaticojejunostomy operations transect and ligate the distal extrahepatic bile duct (**Fig. 12**). Occasionally, for benign distal obstruction, the extrahepatic duct is left intact and a side-to-side choledochojejunal anastomosis is constructed.

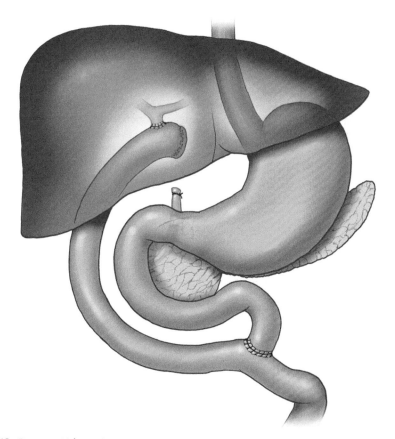

**Fig. 12.** Roux-en-Y hepaticojejunostomy reconstruction. (Used with permission of Mayo Foundation for Medical Education and Research, Rochester, MN. All rights reserved.)

Common indications for Roux limb drainage of the biliary tree include benign distal biliary strictures, such as obstructing chronic pancreatitis, cholangiocarcinoma, liver transplantation, and iatrogenic bile duct injury. Biliary access in this anatomy uses enteroscopy techniques analogous to other Roux limb procedures and cannulation techniques analogous to other bilioenteric anastomoses, such as post-Whipple anatomy. In contrast, the pancreatic os at the major papilla is preserved in this anatomy, so pancreatic access is gained in the usual fashion with a standard duodenoscope and ERCP methods.

Because of significant looping that occurs within the intact stomach, colonoscopes and enteroscopes are preferred when biliary access is desired. A large, retrospective study from the Mayo Clinic reported on 199 ERCPs performed in 90 liver transplant patients with Roux-en-Y biliary anastomoses.[73] Variable stiffness adult or pediatric colonoscopes and SBE were used to perform ERC. Although there was no statistical difference in reaching the Roux limb among the 3 endoscope groups (91.4% vs 89.5% vs 83.6% for SBE, adult colonoscope, and pediatric colonoscope, respectively; overall $P = .42$), success rates were all significantly higher with SBE than with a pediatric colonoscope for biliary cannulation (75.9% vs 58.5%, $P = .05$), therapeutic outcome (71.4% vs 53.8%, $P = .01$), and procedural outcome (75.9% vs 56.4%, $P = .03$). Although similar differences were found when SBE was compared with adult colonoscopes, the findings did not reach statistical significance (all $P$ values >.22). Of 25 failed ERCs with adult colonoscopes, exchange to SBEs resulted in procedural success in 4 of 4 attempts, and of 22 failures with use of a pediatric colonoscope, exchange for an SBE resulted in success in 3 of 4 cases.

Once the Roux limb is successfully accessed, the bilioenteric anastomosis can be found 3 to 5 cm downstream from the end of the limb (no upstream pancreatic anastomosis). Depending on the location of bile duct resection, one or more openings may be seen anastomosed to the jejunum. As described in previous sections, if endoscopic visualization of the bilioenteric anastomosis is not successful, appreciation of an air cholangiogram on fluoroscopy can facilitate localizing the anastomosis and may help with clinical decision making.

## ADVERSE EVENTS RELATED TO ENDOSCOPIC RETROGRADE CHOLANGIOPANCREATOGRAPHY IN SURGICALLY ALTERED ANATOMY

ERCP in surgically altered anatomy may be associated with both usual and additional risks compared with standard ERCP. Post-ERCP pancreatitis is not likely in patients with reconstructed biliary anatomy when ERCP is performed for biliary therapy. For ERCP that requires use of small bowel enteroscopes, the rate of complications range from 0% to 19%.[74] Perforation of the intestine is the most common serious complication and can occur at any point along the intubated intestinal tract. Most common sites of perforation are at the bilioenteric anastomosis and enteroenteric anastomoses, but intestinal tears and perforation can occur secondary to traction injury at angulations in the traversed limb of intestine. Patients requiring nonemergent ERCP soon after surgical rearrangements of the upper intestine should wait at least 2 weeks to allow the anastomoses to heal properly and avoid disrupting sutures and reconstructions.[75] In settings where an intact papilla is cannulated and sphincterotomy is required, an unstable position of the enteroscope can result in poorly controlled manipulation of the sphincterotome, with increased risk of perforation or bleeding.[74] Transient fever and pain from post-ERCP cholangitis and pancreatitis are relatively common, but usually resolve with conservative care and a course of antibiotics.[76] Barotrauma is a unique complication in the setting of a closed loop system, in which the enteroscope and balloon overtube obstruct the proximal end of the blind bilioenteric limb during air insufflation. Without the ability to spontaneously decompress around the endoscope, air leakage through areas of weakness along the tract can occur.[74] Therefore, $CO_2$ insufflation should be used and the endoscopist should limit the amount of air insufflated during the endoscopy. Discussion of the major potential complications should be reviewed in depth with the patient before the procedure, and any suspicion for these potential complications should warrant further investigations, including cross-sectional imaging, hospitalization, and even surgical consultation if necessary.

**Table 3**
**Summary of recommended endoscopes and cannulation methods based on type of surgical reconstruction**

| Operation | Recommended Endoscope | Cannulation Methods |
|---|---|---|
| Billroth I | Therapeutic duodenoscope | Standard ERCP techniques |
| Billroth II | Therapeutic duodenoscope<br>Colonoscope<br>• Consider using clear cap at end of endoscope to facilitate better visualization of papilla | • Over-the-stent needle-knife technique<br>• S-shaped sphincterotome<br>• Sphincteroplasty<br>• Free-hand needle-knife (more difficult and higher risk of complications) |
| Subtotal gastrectomy with Roux-en-Y/RYGB | Enteroscope<br>• SBE<br>• DBE<br>Colonoscope<br>Alternative methods for accessing papilla (particularly if long Roux and biliopancreatic limbs)<br>• Laparoscopic-assisted creation of a gastrostomy or gastrotomy (the latter allowing for single-session ERCP)<br>• Enteroscopy-assisted PEG<br>• Radiologic-guided percutaneous gastrostomy<br>• EUS-guided gastrostomy through gastric pouch<br>• PATENT<br>  ○ Allows for single session ERCP | Similar to Billroth II ERCP<br>Ensure sufficient length of accessories when using enteroscope |
| Whipple procedure (both classic and pylorus-preserving method) | Colonoscope<br>Enteroscope<br>Therapeutic duodenoscope (for shorter limbs)<br>Forward-viewing gastroscope<br>Alternative methods for accessing the PD<br>• EUS-guided methods<br>• Percutaneous | PD difficult to find<br>Straight catheters can be used to cannulate the bilio-enteric or pancreato-enteric anastomosis |
| Roux-en-Y hepaticojejunostomy | Enteroscope<br>Colonoscope (for shorter Roux limbs) | Straight catheters can be used to cannulate the bilioenteric anastomosis |

*Abbreviation:* PD, pancreatic duct.

## SUMMARY

In summary, success of ERCP in the presence of altered bowel anatomy, defined as the ability to *reach* the papilla or biliary/pancreatic anastomosis, to *access* the duct of interest, and to *provide endoscopic therapy*, requires complete knowledge of the reconstructed anatomy, availability of specialty instruments and devices, and expertise with techniques of deep small intestinal endoscopic intubation. When determining which endoscopic device or approach to use, an understanding of the anatomy of afferent, efferent, and Roux (when applicable) limb lengths and the type of biliary drainage (ie, intact papilla vs bilioenteric/pancreaticoenteric anastomosis) are 2 major factors to consider. A summary of recommended endoscopes and cannulation methods based on type of surgical reconstruction is provided in **Table 3**. Although clinical studies have demonstrated varying success rates for reaching the bilioenteric anastomosis and provision of therapy, the experience of the endoscopic team may be the most important factor related to the overall success of ERCP in altered bowel anatomy. The risks, benefits, and alternatives to device-assisted ERCP should be thoroughly reviewed with the patient and endoscopy team, because serious adverse events, including intestinal perforation, are a reality. Alternative methods to perform ERCP, such as EUS-guided transgastric entry to the biliary tree or the pancreatic duct, or transcutaneous entry to the excluded stomach and the duodenum using enteral stents, EUS or laparoscopic-assisted methods, have been described, but further studies comparing these different methods to standard ERCP are necessary in order to guide clinicians in choosing the most effective, safe, and least costly approach.

## ACKNOWLEDGMENTS

The authors sincerely acknowledge the contributions of Michael G. Sarr, MD, Professor of Surgery at the Mayo Clinic in Rochester, Minnesota, for his assistance with reviewing the medical illustrations and descriptions of the surgical procedures discussed in this article.

## SUPPLEMENTARY DATA

Supplementary data related to this article can be found online at http://dx.doi.org/10.1016/j.giec.2015.06.001.

## REFERENCES

1. Lee McHenry GL. Four decades. In: Baron TH, editor. ERCP. 2nd edition. Philadelphia (PA): Elsevier Saunders; 2013. p. 2–9.
2. Suissa A, Yassin K, Lavy A, et al. Outcome and early complications of ERCP: a prospective single center study. Hepatogastroenterology 2005;52:352–5.
3. Herron DM, Roohipour R. Bariatric surgical anatomy and mechanisms of action. Gastrointest Endosc Clin N Am 2011;21:213–28.
4. Deitel M. César Roux and his contribution. Obes Surg 2007;17:1277–8.
5. Adler DG, Baron TH, Davila RE, et al. ASGE guideline: the role of ERCP in diseases of the biliary tract and the pancreas. Gastrointest Endosc 2005;62:1–8.
6. Maple JT, Ben-Menachem T, Anderson MA, et al. The role of endoscopy in the evaluation of suspected choledocholithiasis. Gastrointest Endosc 2010;71:1–9.
7. Maple JT, Ikenberry SO, Anderson MA, et al. The role of endoscopy in the management of choledocholithiasis. Gastrointest Endosc 2011;74:731–44.

8. Anderson MA, Appalaneni V, Ben-Menachem T, et al. The role of endoscopy in the evaluation and treatment of patients with biliary neoplasia. Gastrointest Endosc 2013;77:167–74.
9. Anderson MA, Fisher L, Jain R, et al. Complications of ERCP. Gastrointest Endosc 2012;75:467–73.
10. Feitoza AB, Baron TH. Endoscopy and ERCP in the setting of previous upper GI tract surgery. Part I: reconstruction without alteration of pancreaticobiliary anatomy. Gastrointest Endosc 2001;54:743–9.
11. Moreels TG. Altered anatomy: enteroscopy and ERCP procedure. Best Pract Res Clin Gastroenterol 2012;26:347–57.
12. Feitoza AB, Baron TH. Endoscopy and ERCP in the setting of previous upper GI tract surgery. Part II: postsurgical anatomy with alteration of the pancreaticobiliary tree. Gastrointest Endosc 2002;55:75–9.
13. Lichtenstein DR, Jagannath S, Baron TH, et al. Sedation and anesthesia in GI endoscopy. Gastrointest Endosc 2008;68:815–26.
14. Moreels TG. ERCP in the patient with surgically altered anatomy. Curr Gastroenterol Rep 2013;15:343.
15. Favara DM. Theodor Billroth: a surgeon for the 21st century. Am Surg 2014;80: 1192–5.
16. Pach R, Orzel-Nowak A, Scully T. Ludwik Rydygier–contributor to modern surgery. Gastric Cancer 2008;11:187–91.
17. Tavakkolizadeh A, Ashley SW. Operations for peptic ulcer. In, Shackelford's surgery of the alimentary tract. Philadelphia (PA): Elsevier Saunders; 2013.
18. Evers M. Gastric resection: Billroth I. In, Atlas of general surgery techniques. Philadelphia: Saunder Elseviers; 2010.
19. Lichtenstein D. Post-surgical anatomy and ERCP. Tech Gastrointest Endosc 2007;9:114–24.
20. Evers M. Gastric resection: Billroth II. In, Atlas of general surgery techniques. Philadelphia: Saunders Elsevier; 2010.
21. Olbe L, Becker HD. Partial gastrectomy with Billroth II resection and alternative methods. In, Surgery of the stomach. Berlin: Springer-Verlage; 1987.
22. Aabakken L, Holthe B, Sandstad O, et al. Endoscopic pancreaticobiliary procedures in patients with a Billroth II resection: a 10-year follow-up study. Ital J Gastroenterol Hepatol 1998;30:301–5.
23. Cicek B, Parlak E, Disibeyaz S, et al. Endoscopic retrograde cholangiopancreatography in patients with Billroth II gastroenterostomy. J Gastroenterol Hepatol 2007;22:1210–3.
24. Lin LF, Siauw CP, Ho KS, et al. ERCP in post-Billroth II gastrectomy patients: emphasis on technique. Am J Gastroenterol 1999;94:144–8.
25. Faylona JM, Qadir A, Chan AC, et al. Small-bowel perforations related to endoscopic retrograde cholangiopancreatography (ERCP) in patients with Billroth II gastrectomy. Endoscopy 1999;31:546–9.
26. Kim MH, Lee SK, Lee MH, et al. Endoscopic retrograde cholangiopancreatography and needle-knife sphincterotomy in patients with Billroth II gastrectomy: a comparative study of the forward-viewing endoscope and the side-viewing duodenoscope. Endoscopy 1997;29:82–5.
27. Costamagna G. ERCP and endoscopic sphincterotomy in Billroth II patients: a demanding technique for experts only? Ital J Gastroenterol Hepatol 1998;30:306–9.
28. Demarquay JF, Dumas R, Buckley MJ, et al. Endoscopic retrograde cholangiopancreatography in patients with Billroth II gastrectomy. Ital J Gastroenterol Hepatol 1998;30:297–300.

29. Lee YT. Cap-assisted endoscopic retrograde cholangiopancreatography in a patient with a Billroth II gastrectomy. Endoscopy 2004;36:666.

30. Park CH, Lee WS, Joo YE, et al. Cap-assisted ERCP in patients with a Billroth II gastrectomy. Gastrointest Endosc 2007;66:612–5.

31. Lo S. ERCP in surgically altered anatomy. In, ERCP. 2nd edition. Philadelphia (PA): Elsevier Saunders; 2013.

32. Hintze RE, Veltzke W, Adler A, et al. Endoscopic sphincterotomy using an S-shaped sphincterotome in patients with a Billroth II or Roux-en-Y gastrojejunostomy. Endoscopy 1997;29:74–8.

33. Elton E, Hanson BL, Qaseem T, et al. Diagnostic and therapeutic ERCP using an enteroscope and a pediatric colonoscope in long-limb surgical bypass patients. Gastrointest Endosc 1998;47:62–7.

34. Ricci E, Bertoni G, Conigliaro R, et al. Endoscopic sphincterotomy in Billroth II patients: an improved method using a diathermic needle as sphincterotome and a nasobiliary drain as guide. Gastrointest Endosc 1989;35:47–50.

35. Sumegi J. Endoscopic retrograde cholangio-pancreatography after conventional Billroth II resection. Orv Hetil 2004;145:2425–30 [in Hungarian].

36. van Buuren HR, Boender J, Nix GA, et al. Needle-knife sphincterotomy guided by a biliary endoprosthesis in Billroth II gastrectomy patients. Endoscopy 1995;27: 229–32.

37. Dickey W, Jacob S, Porter KG. Balloon dilation of the papilla via a forward-viewing endoscope: an aid to therapeutic endoscopic retrograde cholangiopancreatography in patients with Billroth-II gastrectomy. Endoscopy 1996;28:531–2.

38. Bergman JJ, van Berkel AM, Bruno MJ, et al. A randomized trial of endoscopic balloon dilation and endoscopic sphincterotomy for removal of bile duct stones in patients with a prior Billroth II gastrectomy. Gastrointest Endosc 2001;53:19–26.

39. Jang HW, Lee KJ, Jung MJ, et al. Endoscopic papillary large balloon dilatation alone is safe and effective for the treatment of difficult choledocholithiasis in cases of Billroth II gastrectomy: a single center experience. Dig Dis Sci 2013; 58:1737–43.

40. Lee TH, Hwang JC, Choi HJ, et al. One-step transpapillary balloon dilation under cap-fitted endoscopy without a preceding sphincterotomy for the removal of bile duct stones in Billroth II gastrectomy. Gut Liver 2012;6:113–7.

41. Kim TN, Lee SH. Endoscopic papillary large balloon dilation combined with guidewire-assisted precut papillotomy for the treatment of choledocholithiasis in patients with Billroth II gastrectomy. Gut Liver 2011;5:200–3.

42. Eagon JC, Miedema BW, Kelly KA. Postgastrectomy syndromes. Surg Clin North Am 1992;72:445–65.

43. Stellato TA, Crouse C, Hallowell PT. Bariatric surgery: creating new challenges for the endoscopist. Gastrointest Endosc 2003;57:86–94.

44. Khashab MA, Okolo PI 3rd. Accessing the pancreatobiliary limb and ERCP in the bariatric patient. Gastrointest Endosc Clin N Am 2011;21:305–13.

45. Santry HP, Gillen DL, Lauderdale DS. Trends in bariatric surgical procedures. JAMA 2005;294:1909–17.

46. Trahan M. Roux-en-Y gastric bypass (open and laparoscopic). In, Atlas of general surgery techniques. Philadelphia: Saunders Elsevier; 2010.

47. Lee CW, Kelly JJ, Wassef WY. Complications of bariatric surgery. Curr Opin Gastroenterol 2007;23:636–43.

48. Nagem R, Lazaro-da-Silva A. Cholecystolithiasis after gastric bypass: a clinical, biochemical, and ultrasonographic 3-year follow-up study. Obes Surg 2012;22: 1594–9.

49. Monkhouse SJ, Morgan JD, Norton SA. Complications of bariatric surgery: presentation and emergency management–a review. Ann R Coll Surg Engl 2009; 91:280–6.

50. Benarroch-Gampel J, Lairson DR, Boyd CA, et al. Cost-effectiveness analysis of cholecystectomy during Roux-en-Y gastric bypass for morbid obesity. Surgery 2012;152:363–75.

51. Wang AY, Sauer BG, Behm BW, et al. Single-balloon enteroscopy effectively enables diagnostic and therapeutic retrograde cholangiography in patients with surgically altered anatomy. Gastrointest Endosc 2010;71:641–9.

52. Shah RJ, Smolkin M, Yen R, et al. A multicenter, U.S. experience of single-balloon, double-balloon, and rotational overtube-assisted enteroscopy ERCP in patients with surgically altered pancreaticobiliary anatomy (with video). Gastrointest Endosc 2013;77:593–600.

53. Skinner M, Popa D, Neumann H, et al. ERCP with the overtube-assisted enteroscopy technique: a systematic review. Endoscopy 2014;46:560–72.

54. Lopes TL, Wilcox CM. Endoscopic retrograde cholangiopancreatography in patients with Roux-en-Y anatomy. Gastroenterol Clin North Am 2010;39:99–107.

55. Baron TH, Vickers SM. Surgical gastrostomy placement as access for diagnostic and therapeutic ERCP. Gastrointest Endosc 1998;48:640–1.

56. Goitein D, Gagne DJ, Papasavas PK, et al. Percutaneous computed tomography-guided gastric remnant access after laparoscopic Roux-en-Y gastric bypass. Surg Obes Relat Dis 2006;2:651–5.

57. Tekola B, Wang AY, Ramanath M, et al. Percutaneous gastrostomy tube placement to perform transgastrostomy endoscopic retrograde cholangiopancreaticography in patients with Roux-en-Y anatomy. Dig Dis Sci 2011;56:3364–9.

58. Attam R, Leslie D, Freeman M, et al. EUS-assisted, fluoroscopically guided gastrostomy tube placement in patients with Roux-en-Y gastric bypass: a novel technique for access to the gastric remnant. Gastrointest Endosc 2011;74:677–82.

59. Baron TH, Song LM. Percutaneous assisted transprosthetic endoscopic therapy (PATENT): expanding gut access to infinity and beyond! (with video). Gastrointest Endosc 2012;76:641–4.

60. Law R, Wong Kee Song LM, Petersen BT, et al. Single-session ERCP in patients with previous Roux-en-Y gastric bypass using percutaneous-assisted transprosthetic endoscopic therapy: a case series. Endoscopy 2013;45:671–5.

61. Schreiner MA, Chang L, Gluck M, et al. Laparoscopy-assisted versus balloon enteroscopy-assisted ERCP in bariatric post-Roux-en-Y gastric bypass patients. Gastrointest Endosc 2012;75:748–56.

62. Traverso LW, Longmire WP Jr. Preservation of the pylorus in pancreaticoduodenectomy. Surg Gynecol Obstet 1978;146:959–62.

63. Farnell MB, Nagorney DM, Sarr MG. The Mayo clinic approach to the surgical treatment of adenocarcinoma of the pancreas. Surg Clin North Am 2001;81: 611–23.

64. Farrell J, Carr-Locke D, Garrido T, et al. Endoscopic retrograde cholangiopancreatography after pancreaticoduodenectomy for benign and malignant disease: indications and technical outcomes. Endoscopy 2006;38:1246–9.

65. Chahal P, Baron TH, Topazian MD, et al. Endoscopic retrograde cholangiopancreatography in post-Whipple patients. Endoscopy 2006;38:1241–5.

66. Itokawa F, Itoi T, Ishii K, et al. Single- and double-balloon enteroscopy-assisted endoscopic retrograde cholangiopancreatography in patients with Roux-en-Y plus hepaticojejunostomy anastomosis and Whipple resection. Dig Endosc 2014;26(Suppl 2):136–43.

67. Kinney TP, Li R, Gupta K, et al. Therapeutic pancreatic endoscopy after Whipple resection requires rendezvous access. Endoscopy 2009;41:898–901.
68. Iwashita T, Yasuda I, Mukai T, et al. Successful management of biliary stones in the hepatic duct after a Whipple procedure by using an EUS-guided antegrade approach and temporary metal stent placement. Gastrointest Endosc 2014;80:337.
69. Nakaji S, Hirata N, Shiratori T, et al. Endoscopic ultrasound-guided pancreaticojejunostomy with a forward-viewing echoendoscope as a treatment for stenotic pancreaticojejunal anastomosis. Endoscopy 2015;47(Suppl 1):E41–2.
70. Bataille L, Deprez P. A new application for therapeutic EUS: main pancreatic duct drainage with a "pancreatic rendezvous technique". Gastrointest Endosc 2002; 55:740–3.
71. Itoi T, Kikuyama M, Ishii K, et al. EUS-guided rendezvous with single-balloon enteroscopy for treatment of stenotic pancreaticojejunal anastomosis in post-Whipple patients (with video). Gastrointest Endosc 2011;73:398–401.
72. Matsubayashi H, Kishida Y, Shinjo K, et al. Endoscopic ultrasound-guided retrograde pancreatic stent placement for the treatment of stenotic jejunopancreatic anastomosis after a Whipple procedure. Endoscopy 2013;45(Suppl 2 UCTN): E435–6.
73. Azeem N, Tabibian JH, Baron TH, et al. Use of a single-balloon enteroscope compared with variable-stiffness colonoscopes for endoscopic retrograde cholangiography in liver transplant patients with Roux-en-Y biliary anastomosis. Gastrointest Endosc 2013;77:568–77.
74. Moreels TG. Endoscopic retrograde cholangiopancreatography in patients with altered anatomy: how to deal with the challenges? World J Gastrointest Endosc 2014;6:345–51.
75. Moreels TG, Hubens GJ, Ysebaert DK, et al. Diagnostic and therapeutic double-balloon enteroscopy after small bowel Roux-en-Y reconstructive surgery. Digestion 2009;80:141–7.
76. Raithel M, Dormann H, Naegel A, et al. Double-balloon-enteroscopy-based endoscopic retrograde cholangiopancreatography in post-surgical patients. World J Gastroenterol 2011;17:2302–14.

# Endoscopic Retrograde Cholangiopancreatography for the Management of Common Bile Duct Stones and Gallstone Pancreatitis

CrossMark

Jeffrey J. Easler, MD*, Stuart Sherman, MD

## KEYWORDS

- Choledocholithiasis • Cholangitis • Biliary pancreatitis • Lithotripsy
- Electrohydraulic lithotripsy • Balloon dilation

## KEY POINTS

- Patients with biliary pancreatitis should be risk stratified for persistent biliary obstruction requiring endoscopic retrograde cholangiopancreatography (ERCP) based on admission biochemical testing and ultrasonography.
- Risk factors for a technically complex stone extraction should be identified before and during ERCP to select the most effective techniques and tools for bile duct clearance.
- Endoscopic balloon papillary dilation is an effective adjunct technique for extraction of complex common bile duct stones.
- Electrohydraulic and laser intraductal lithotripsy with the assistance of cholangioscopy is now emerging as a standard of care intervention for large, complex stone burden.

## SYMPTOMATIC CHOLEDOCHOLITHIASIS AND BILIARY PANCREATITIS: WHEN TO IMAGE, INTERVENE, OR OBSERVE

Apart from alcohol abuse, biliary disease is the most common etiology of acute pancreatitis. Antecedent symptoms of biliary colic, cholelithiasis on imaging, and biochemical liver test abnormalities are important findings on presentation that increase suspicion for acute biliary pancreatitis (ABP). An alanine aminotransferase level 3 times the upper limit of normal is the most specific biochemical abnormality for

Disclosures: None relevant to this article.
Division of Gastroenterology and Hepatology, Indiana University School of Medicine, Indianapolis, IN, USA
* Corresponding author. Indiana University School of Medicine, 550 North University Boulevard, Suite 1634, Indianapolis, IN 46202.
E-mail address: jjeasler@iu.edu

ABP.[1] Beyond conservative measures such as IV fluid resuscitation and enteral nutrition support, establishing or excluding the presence of persistent pancreatobiliary obstruction and cholangitis is central to medical decision making in the early hours of presentation for patients with ABP.[2,3] A recent Cochrane review demonstrated a significant decrease in mortality, local and systemic complications of ABP with early endoscopic retrograde cholangiopancreatography (ERCP; <72 hours from admission) in subgroups of patients with persistent biliary obstruction or cholangitis. However, the benefit of this intervention was not significant for all patients with ABP.[4–6] In this context, a clinician must use and interpret the diagnostic resources at hand to identify patients with biliary pancreatitis who are likely to have symptomatic choledocholithiasis and consequently would benefit from early ERCP.

Biochemical liver testing and transabdominal ultrasonography are often the earliest tools available to stratify patients. Biochemical parameters before laparoscopic cholecystectomy are reliable predictors for concomitant choledocholithiasis at the time of presentation with ABP. Normal liver function tests have a negative predictive value of over 95% for stone disease at ERCP. Total bilirubin (>4 mg/dL) has the highest individual specificity for stone disease.[4] Bilirubin >2 mg/dL, patient age greater than 55 years, and common bile duct dilation on ultrasound (>6 mm, gall bladder in situ) have a 75% probability of predicting choledocholithiasis at the time of ERCP.[7] Options after assessing these early objective findings include ERCP, further imaging modalities with a high degree of accuracy (>90%) for choledocholithiasis or clinical observation (**Fig. 1**). High-risk individuals for persistent biliary obstruction have either "very strong"

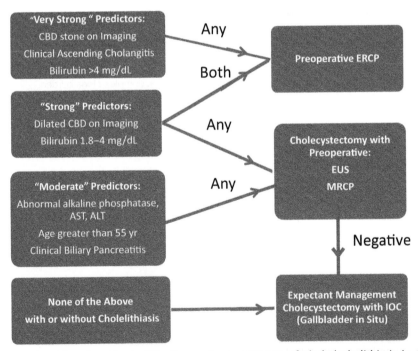

Fig. 1. Algorithm for risk stratification and management of choledocholithiasis in the setting of biliary pancreatitis. ALT, alanine aminotransferase; AST, aspartate aminotransferase; CBD, common bile duct; ERCP, endoscopic retrograde cholangiopancreatography; EUS, endoscopic ultrasonography; IOC, intraoperative cholangiography; MRCP, MR cholangiopancreatography.

(common bile duct stone on transabdominal ultrasound, clinical ascending cholangitis, or bilirubin >4 mg/dL) or multiple "strong" (common bile duct >6 mm with gallbladder in situ on ultrasound, bilirubin level 1.8–4 mg/dL) predictors that suggest ERCP without further imaging is indicated.

Patients with a single "strong" predictor or a combination of "moderate" predictors (any abnormal biochemical liver test other than bilirubin, age 55 or older, and clinical gallstone pancreatitis) benefit from preoperative (if the gallbladder is in situ) imaging (endoscopic ultrasonography or MR cholangiopancreatography) with high levels of sensitivity and specificity. Patients without any predictors may not require any further workup and medical management of acute pancreatitis with observation is most appropriate[2] (see **Fig. 1**).

Finally, a viable option for the management of common bile duct stones include either open or laparoscopic common bile duct exploration at the time of cholecystectomy by an experienced surgeon. A recent Cochrane database review demonstrated no difference in mortality or morbidity and superior clearance of common bile duct stones with open common bile duct exploration compared with preoperative ERCP (8 trials, 733 patients). Similar outcomes between groups were also reported in randomized studies that allocated patients to either laparoscopic common bile duct exploration or preoperative ERCP (5 trials, 580 patients) and studies looking at laparoscopic common bile duct exploration versus postoperative or intraoperative ERCP (3 trials; 166 of 234 patients respectively).[8]

## STANDARD ENDOSCOPIC TECHNIQUES FOR STONE EXTRACTION AND "DIFFICULT" BILE DUCT STONES

Greater than 85% to 90% of common bile duct stones are effectively removed by what are now considered standard endoscopic techniques: biliary sphincterotomy (EST) followed by extraction with a retrieval balloon or basket.[9,10] Risk factors for a technically difficult stone extraction at the time of ERCP have been identified within the context of 1 prospective study. These include age greater than 65, previous gastrojejunostomy, common bile duct stone diameter greater than 15 mm, need for mechanical lithotripsy, distal common bile length below the stone of less than 36 mm, and common bile duct angulation of less than 135°. On multivariable analysis age, distal common bile duct diameter and angulation of the distal common bile duct were significant.[11] Multiple stones (>10), barrel-shaped stones, proximal common bile duct stones, stone extraction in the setting of Mirrizi's syndrome and the presence of distal biliary stricture/primary sclerosing cholangitis are also agreed upon by experts to elevate the technical difficultly of stone extraction[12,13] (**Fig. 2, Table 1**). Patients with "complex" choledocholithiasis may require adjunct techniques for stone extraction, which are discussed elsewhere in this article.

## BILIARY ENDOPROSTHESIS

An approach of temporizing biliary stent placement is required in the setting of multiple or large, complex stones to provide interval biliary drainage, prevent cholangitis, and arrange for further adjunct techniques at subsequent ERCP sessions if complex stone disease was not anticipated or additional endoscopic accessories are not readily available. This technique universally equates to a need for multiple ERCP sessions for clearance of stone burden from the common bile duct. Additionally, this technique has also been evaluated as either a destination intervention or adjunct maneuver to alter the size of stones to facilitate subsequent extraction.

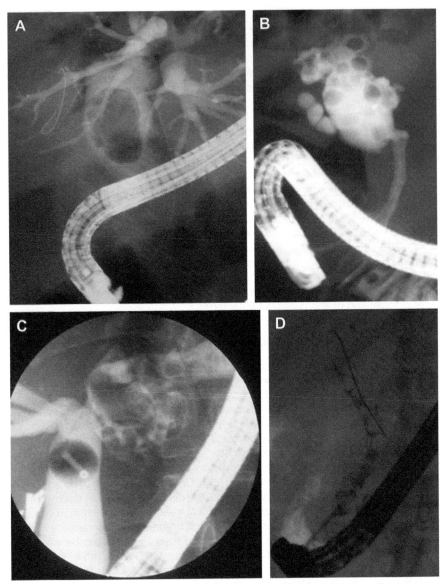

**Fig. 2.** Complex choledocholithiasis. (*A*) A 20-mm stone. (*B*) Stones above a distal stricture. (*C*) Intrahepatic stone burden. (*D*) Multiple common bile duct stones.

As a primary approach, using double pigtail and/or flanged stents for management of large and/or multiple common bile duct stones, retrospective and prospective studies report significant decrease in stone size and number, and increased technical success at subsequent ERCP with overall stone clearance rates approaching 60% to 90% for complex stone burden.[14–17]

A recent randomized, prospective, multicenter study evaluated recommended versus on demand time intervals for exchanges of indwelling biliary stents to manage high-risk patients with choledocholithiasis. Seventy-eight elderly (mean age, 76 years)

**Table 1**
**Risk factors for technically complex endoscopic retrograde cholangiopancreatography stone extraction procedure**

| Category | Risk Factor |
|---|---|
| Clinical | Age >65[a] |
| | Gastroenterostomy anatomy (Pancreaticoduodenectomy, Roux-en-Y gastric bypass, Roux choledochoenterostomy)[a] |
| Stone attributes | Stone size >14 mm |
| | Barrel-shaped, elongated stone |
| | Periampullary position with or without impaction (<36 mm)[a] |
| | Intrahepatic stone(s) |
| | Multiple stones |
| Bile duct morphology | Angulation of the distal common bile duct (<135°)[a] |
| | Redundant, capacious common bile duct |
| | Distal stricture/primary sclerosing cholangitis |
| | Concomitant Mirrizi syndrome |

[a] Evidence-based risk factors, univariate/multivariate analysis (Kim HJ, et al[11]).

patients with large and/or multiple stones (18 mm; mean stone burden of 21 per patient) deemed not to be operative candidates were managed with stent placement without intraductal lithotripsy. They were equally randomized to exchanges performed at set 3-month intervals or "on demand" based on symptoms and monitoring of liver test drawn at 3 month intervals. The incidence of cholangitis during stent therapy was 22% overall, with a greater frequency found in the "on demand" exchange group (36% vs 8%; $P = .03$). Mortality was also higher in the "on demand" group; however, the difference was not significant (8% vs 3%; $P = .62$). Stone clearance was ultimately successful in 58% of patients, without differences between the groups.[15]

A substantial risk of cholangitis is inherent with this overall approach, with studies reporting incidence rates as high as 13% to 38% and endoprosthesis related mortality rates as high as 16%.[14,15,18,19] Lower rates of cholangitis may be associated with set intervals between stent exchanges, shorter duration of stent dwell time to subsequent attempts for clearance, and use of multiple stents.[13,15,16,20]

An initial enthusiasm for the use of ursodeoxycholic acid as an adjunct to biliary endoprosthesis approach has been diminished after a recent randomized, multicenter, prospective study failed to demonstrate incremental benefit to reduction in stone size.[20] Finally, stents with degradable membranes, eluting EDTA and sodium cholate are being evaluated and have demonstrated some promise at the level of ex vivo and animal studies.[21,22]

Biliary endoprosthesis should be considered a temporizing intervention in the vast majority of patients. Owing to substantial rates of associated morbidity and mortality, biliary endoprosthesis as a destination intervention should be considered only in patients unfit for elective surgical, endoscopic, or percutaneous treatments and a short life expectancy.

## ENDOSCOPIC BALLOON PAPILLARY DILATION
### Endoscopic Balloon Papillary Dilation Without Endoscopic Sphincterotomy

First described by Staritz and colleagues[23] as an alternative to biliary sphincterotomy, subsequent randomized studies have reported that papillary balloon dilation has comparable rates of technical success for bile duct clearance as biliary sphincterotomy.[24–26] In recent years, there has been increased enthusiasm for this technique as an alternative to EST in younger patients because endoscopic papillary balloon dilation (EPBD) may preserve the continuity of the biliary sphincter. There is concern for retrograde bacterial colonization of the common bile duct after EST that can result in alteration in bile lithogenicity, biliary "cytotoxicity" and chronic inflammation, and late papillary stenosis that requires further, late interventions. These complications are suspected to occur after either partial or complete transection of the biliary sphincter. Rates of late morbidity can approach 24% after EST, with the delayed expense and inconvenience of need for repeat ERCP procedures to manage these complications. There are now data that suggest that the sphincter of Oddi retains some function after EPBD.[27,28] A recent metaanalysis examined differences of long-term complications between EBPD and EST for common bile duct stones, and reporting the risk of cholecystitis (odds ratio [OR], 0.41; $P$ = .02; n = 6 studies) and stone recurrence after 1 year (OR, 0.48; $P$ = .02; n = 3 studies) to be lower in EPBD groups versus EST across multiple studies.[29]

A metaanalysis of 8 randomized, comparative studies comprising 1106 patients evaluated EPBD versus EST reported a lower rate of initial common bile duct stone removal (pooled relative risk of 0.61; 95% CI, 0.45–0.81) and a greater need for mechanical lithotripsy for EPBD (20.9 vs 14.8%; $P$ = .01), however, calculated a similar ultimate overall rate of technical success because of crossover to sphincterotomy (94% vs 96%; $P$ = .2). Composite early complications were the same between groups (10%), with specific differences being a lower rate of bleeding (0% vs 2%; $P$ = .001) yet high rate of pancreatitis (7.4% vs 4.3%; $P$ = .05) observed in the EPBD group.[30] One death was observed in the EPBD owing to retroperitoneal perforation.

Of particular concern with this technique is a risk for significant morbidity and mortality from severe acute pancreatitis. Balloon dilation of the intact biliary orifice is an established risk factor for post-ERCP pancreatitis (OR, 4.5; $P$ = .0027).[31] The most concerning data are derived from a randomized, controlled trial examining 1 minute duration EPBD versus EST for common bile duct stones. This study reported an overall higher rate of morbidity (18% vs 3%) and severe morbidity (7% vs 0%), reporting 2 deaths owing to severe acute pancreatitis with EPBD. Difficult cannulation was reported in 1 of the 2 that died (>15 attempts at cannulation); however, both patients had small stones (≥6 mm), speaking against technically difficult extraction once access was achieved. The need for invasive procedures, duration of hospitalization stay, and impact on quality of life was also greater in the EPBD group in this study.[27] A second randomized, controlled trial, which was terminated early, also reported a higher rate of morbidity attributable to severe acute pancreatitis in EPBD group (2 vs 0) with a lower rate of technical success (77% vs 100%; $P$ = .010).[24] The increased risk of morbidity owing to acute pancreatitis and metaanalysis level data that suggests that the likelihood of total stone clearance may be lower with EPBD (OR, 0.64–0.90) have tempered enthusiasm for this technique as viable replacement to EST.[29,32]

However, the story of EPBD is further complicated by more recent metaanalysis papers evaluating this topic. A significantly higher incidence of acute pancreatitis after EPBD is reported in studies examining the technique in Western populations, but not in Eastern populations ($P$<.0001 vs $P$ = .08).[29] Beyond variability in outcome metrics and study designs, this difference may be explained by technique (size and duration) of balloon dilation of the biliary orifice, preference in stone extraction techniques, risk factors for post-ERCP pancreatitis, and early differences in the systematic utilization of post-ERCP pancreatitis prophylaxis. Gabexate, a protease inhibitor, is often used for prophylaxis is ERCP centers in Eastern countries. Moreover, a recent study reported a greater degree of technical success (93% vs 80%) and a lesser risk of pancreatitis (5% vs 15%) with 5-minute versus 1-minute EPBD. These differences were significant on multivariable regression analysis (OR, 0.19, and OR, 0.28, respectively).[33] Some authors also suggest that, in carefully selected patients, the use of large EPBD may have advantages.[34–36]

The state of the art for use of this technique is as a viable alternative for stone extraction to EST in patients with Billroth II anatomy owing to the technical difficulty of sphincterotomy and/or coagulopathy (cirrhosis, anticoagulants) to decrease the risk of bleeding associated with sphincterotomy.[36–39] However, despite significant concern for life altering pancreatitis, further consideration may be given to the broader use of EPBD without EST, because it offers a very different profile in terms of complications and enables the biliary sphincter to remain intact after extraction. Prior concerns regarding acute pancreatitis should also now be adjusted for the multiple options that exist for post-ERCP pancreatitis prophylaxis (pancreatic duct stent, rectal indomethacin). One study reported no episodes of post-ERCP pancreatitis after EPBD when a prophylactic pancreas duct stent was inserted, compared with a post-ERCP pancreatitis rate of 6% in the controls (EPBD, no stent); however, this difference was not significant, likely owing to study power.[40] Finally, reproducing the technique of long duration and/or large diameter balloon diameter dilations may alter the risk profile of this procedure.

### Endoscopic Balloon Papillary Dilation after Endoscopic Sphincterotomy

EPBD is now a widely accepted adjunct intervention immediately after EST for extraction of common bile duct stones (**Fig. 3**). Although randomized control trials demonstrated mixed results in terms of the added value of this technique in obviating the need for mechanical lithotripsy, a recent well-designed randomized trial suggests a substantial benefit for large, complex stones.[41–43] One hundred fifty-six patients with choledocholithiasis and a dilated common bile duct (common bile duct ≥13 mm; stone size >15 mm; 80%) were randomized to either a complete EST versus "small" (one-third to one-half the size of the papilla) and EPBD. Balloon dilation was performed to fluoroscopic abolishment of biliary orifice waste and limited to the size of the duct (≥13 mm). The need for mechanical lithotripsy was less for the EPBD–EST group (29% vs 46%; $P$ = .028), which translated to a lower cost based need for additional endoscopic accessories ($5025 vs $6005; $P$ = −.034).[44]

A recent metaanalysis of 6 randomized studies (835 patients) evaluating large balloon dilation (≥12 mm) with EPBD after EST versus EST alone for the management of stones 10 mm or larger demonstrated similar efficacy with stone clearance at first session (OR, 1.02; $P$ = .92), reduction in need for mechanical lithotripsy (OR, 0.26; $P$ = .02), lower risk of complications (perforation OR 0.48; $P$ = .05), without differences in rates of post-ERCP pancreatitis (0.77; $P$ = .39) and subsequent infection of the biliary tree (OR, 0.34; $P$>.05). Procedure times were similar between the groups based on 2 studies that reported this outcome.[45] The literature on EPBD after EST suggests added value for extracting stones greater than 10 mm size in terms of need for mechanical lithotripsy, procedure expense, and complications.

## LITHOTRIPSY
### Mechanical Lithotripsy

The technique of mechanical fragmentation of common bile duct stones at the time of biliary endoscopy was first described more than 30 years ago. The design of biliary mechanical lithotripters universally includes a basket for stone capture, a metal sheath advanced over the traction wires that connect the basket, and finally a handle that enables the operator to retract the basket wires, impacting the stone against the metallic sheath causing fragmentation.[46]

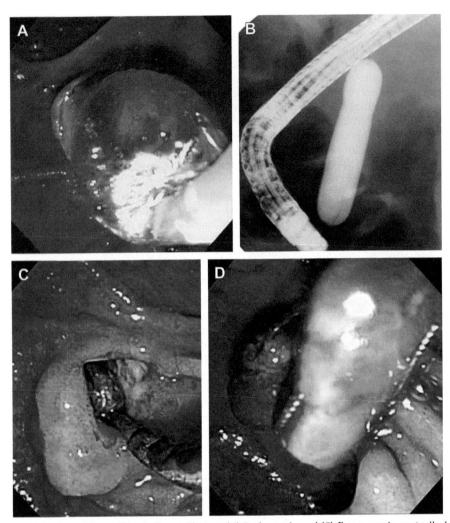

**Fig. 3.** Endoscopic papillary balloon dilation. (*A*) Endoscopic and (*B*) fluoroscopic controlled radial expansion balloon dilation of the biliary orifice. (*C*) Biliary orifice after balloon dilation (*D*) Subsequent stone extraction with retrieval basket.

There are 2 broad categories of device designs. Initial reports of mechanical lithotripsy involved per-oral systems that are operated outside the working channel of the duodenoscope. After capture of a stone using a basket, the handle of the basket is removed (cut) and the scope withdrawn from the patient. A metallic sheath is then advanced over the exposed basket (traction) wires under fluoroscopic guidance to a point of contact with the stone and the wires are retracted within a crank handle (**Fig. 4**). These early, single use systems ultimately evolved into crank devices (Soehendra lithotripter) now used for per-oral stone fragmentation and salvage lithotripsy.[47,48] Early systems reported rates of success of greater than 85% for large stones. The authors were ultimately able to fragment and extract the majority of stones greater than 24 mm in size. However, a distinct disadvantage of per-oral systems is

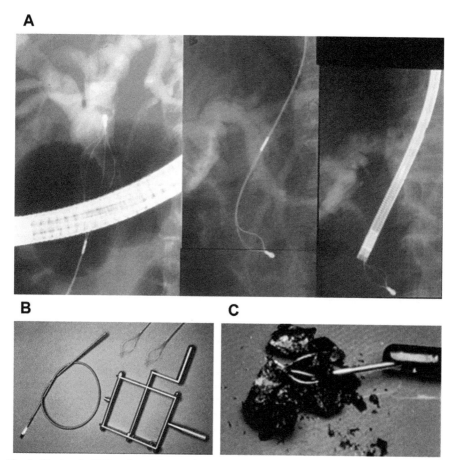

**Fig. 4.** Mechanical lithotripsy. (*A*) Intraductal lithotripsy. (*B*) Soehendra lithotripter. (*C*) Stone fragmentation, basket, and lithotriptor. ([*B*] *Courtesy of* Cook Medical, Bloomington, IN; with permission.)

the inability of a basket to repeatedly deploy within the bile duct to capture and fragment multiple stones in rapid succession.

The next generation of "through-the-scope," integrated basket and mechanical lithotriptor systems have a design that incorporates a basket positioned within layers of internal plastic and outer metallic sheaths. A reusable handle system interfaces with the sheath/basket systems allowing for repeated deployment of the basket (which may remain intact after stone fragmentation) for multiple stone fragmentation sessions during a single ERCP session. The lithotripter is detachable and can be recycled across patients.[46] A disadvantage of this newer generation systems is that the sheaths are longer and thinner to facilitate use through the working channel of the duodenoscope, which may limit the axial force transmitted to the stone. However, these systems can be converted to the per-oral (Soehendra) lithotripsy systems under circumstances of technical failure or wire fracture.[10]

Overall, success rates for mechanical lithotripsy are greater than 90% if a stone can be captured within the basket. One large, multicenter survey of complications related to mechanical lithotripsy encompassing experience across 7 expert centers reported an overall complication rate of 3.6%, (1 in 26 patient sessions). The majority of these patients (>65%) had multiple stones with a mean stone diameter of 2.2 cm. Entrapment of the basket within the common bile duct, traction wire fracture, and broken handle were the most frequent complications. Almost all complications were managed with nonoperative interventions, with only 1 patient requiring surgery.[10] Extension of the sphincterotomy to facilitate foreign body (basket) delivery, extracorporeal shock wave lithotripsy, electrohydraulic lithotripsy, and exchange to a per-oral Soehendra lithotripter were most often used to address successfully complications and obviate the need for surgery. Case reports and series continue to accumulate within the literature supporting an initial nonoperative approach to management of complications of mechanical lithotripsy.[49–51]

### Electrohydraulic Lithotripsy

The electrohydraulic lithotripsy (EHL) system consists of a bipolar probe and electrocautery generator. Together they generate a charge that travels across the tip of the catheter. This "spark" (75–90 V, 5–6 shocks per second) is generated within an aqueous media. Continuous irrigation of the bile duct is necessary to this purpose. The spark generates rapid expansion of surrounding fluid and the consequent shock-wave transmits energy to the target stone, causing fragmentation.[46] Direct visualization of the stone is necessary and the standard of care is to administer therapy using a cholangioscope system to avoid soft tissue trauma and perforation of the duct wall, and to provide continuous bile duct irrigation The EHL probe is optimally position within 2 mm of the stone and 5 mm from the tip of the cholangioscope (**Fig. 5**). A significant advantage of EHL is it is a mobile, compact unit that requires little formal training for use.

Literature supporting this technique exists is in the form of large case series.[52,53] Arya and colleagues[54] reported the largest, multicenter experience with this technique after at least 1 failed ERCP stone extraction (99%). Thirty-three percent of patients had proximal stones (common hepatic duct, intrahepatic ducts), 50% multiple stones, greater than 85% stones larger than 2 cm, with these factors accounting for most of the circumstances of failure of initial, standard ERCP extraction. Overall stone clearance was achieved in 90% of patients with EHL. The majority of patients (57%) required no further interventions after a single session of ERCP–EHL. Thirty-four percent of patients required only 1 additional ERCP. Failure of stone clearance by EHL was attributed to difficult stone location, stones proximal to biliary strictures, and poor patient health precluding further intervention. The complication rate was 18%, with cholangitis and jaundice being the most frequent. Hemobilia occurred in 1 patient. Significant bile duct injuries were not reported.

Overall, EHL has gained acceptance as an established technique for intracorporeal lithotripsy, reporting a high rate of technical success for extraction of large, complex common bile duct stones. EHL demonstrates a favorable safety profile and offers lower rates of complications when compared with such alternative approaches as biliary indwelling biliary prostheses. In this context, it may be a preferred intervention for managing complex stone burden in the frail and elderly.[13,55]

### Intracorporeal Laser Lithotripsy

Intracorporeal laser lithotripsy describes the use of a holmium or neodymium:yttrium–aluminum–garnet (YAG) fiber to focus a high-energy laser on a stone target. By generating an oscillating plasma bubble the laser tunnels into and shatters the stone. Multiple laser systems are approved by the US Food and Drug Administration for the management of choledocholithiasis. Parameters such as laser–pulse duration (microseconds), power settings (mJ), cycles (Hz), and wavelength (nm) must be considered

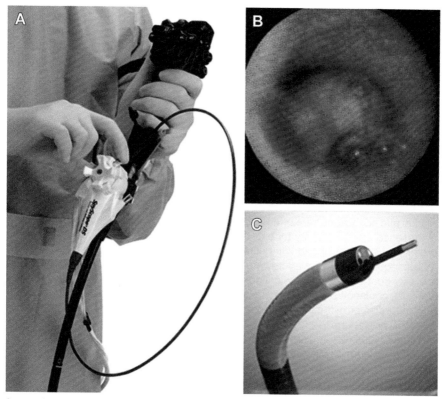

**Fig. 5.** Cholangioscopy. (*A*) SpyGlass DS system. (*B*) Impacted common bile duct stone on cholangioscopy. (*C*) SpyGlass DS catheter with electrohydraulic lithotripsy probe. Copyright © 2015 Boston Scientific Corporation. All rights reserved. Image provided courtesy of Boston Scientific.

when administering therapy and create a level of complexity beyond such techniques as EHL. Recommended settings vary by device and manufacturer, and dedicated training on laser equipment for both physicians and staff is mandatory.[46] The standard of care is to use this technique through a cholangioscope system; however, series describing therapy applied under fluoroscopic guidance, through the catheter of a novel basket design that captures and fixes the laser on a target stone, have been described.[56,57]

Case series evaluating the efficacy of intraductal laser lithotripsy (ILL) have demonstrated rates of common bile duct clearance of greater than 90% and rates of complications less than 10%. Prospective studies have demonstrated superiority over extracorporeal shockwave lithotripsy (ESWL) for first session stone clearance, need for subsequent treatment sessions, shorter procedure duration, and at a lesser expense to the patient.[57–60] However, the complexity of operating laser equipment dictates a large time commitment for formal training of the physician(s) and staff. Additionally, personal protection equipment and careful device calibration before each session are necessary. Also, a substantial upfront cost (laser unit >$50,000; fibers $250-$1000) has limited the wide dissemination of this technique, especially in the setting of less complex alternatives such as EHL and mechanical lithotripsy, which offer similar rates of efficacy.[46]

### Extracorporeal Shockwave Lithotripsy

ESWL should be mentioned as an option for complicated biliary stone disease. Described as a therapeutic option that follows failure of ERCP techniques to extract large, complicated stones, it is considered a second line therapy to mechanical lithotripsy (ML), EHL, and ILL. Much as with EHL, the mechanism involves stone fragmentation using a shockwave that is directed toward the common bile duct stone. However, the shockwave is generated by an underwater spark gap, piezoelectric crystals, or electromagnetic membrane generated outside of the patient (extracorporeal) and transmitted through an external liquid medium, tissues of the patient to the target the intraductal stone. This wave is focused through tissues toward the target stone using transducers with an intervening liquid media, compressible fluid-filled bags, and/or a gel. Performed under general anesthesia and fluoroscopic or ultrasound guidance, success is related to stone size, architecture, and microcrystalline content. The radio-opacity of the common bile stones can be limited, precluding direct fluoroscopic visualization and such stones are often not seen on ultrasound. Thus, ESWL often requires the presence of a nasobiliary tube or T-tube for contrast instillation during the procedure or precisely positioned biliary stent(s) for localization.[12,46] As such, antecedent and subsequent ERCP procedures are required for targeting and/or clearance of common bile duct stones. Complications are frequent (30%–40%), with biliary colic, hemobilia, cholangitis, perinephric hematomas, and hematuria being reported. Symptomatic cardiac arrhythmias have also been reported and telemetry is recommended during the procedure.[61]

This technique has largely been supplanted by EHL and ILL for removal of large, complicated common bile duct stones. Intraductal lithotripsy techniques demonstrate significantly greater rates of stone clearance (>90%) compared with ESWL (70%–90%) in comparative studies. Outcomes of these studies demonstrate shorter procedure times, need for fewer sessions, and lower complication rates with intracorporeal techniques of lithotripsy.[57,58,61,62] Subsequent ERCP procedures to extract stone fragments add substantially to the procedure burden inherent in an ESWL approach. Populations of patients for whom this technique may be advantageous are those with large, complex biliary stones in the setting of altered luminal anatomy (Billroth II anatomy with long afferent limbs, Roux-en-Y gastric bypass, pancreaticoduodenectomy) that limit the spectrum endoscopic accessories used for intracorporeal lithotripsy as they would need to be deployed through single or double balloon enteroscopes with lengths beyond that of these accessories.[12] A unique indication for ESWL stems from reports of its efficacy as a rescue intervention for stones impacted within the bile duct within basket devices ("impacted basket") after fragmentation of traction wires or failed lithotripsy; however, EHL has also been described for this purpose with case reports of technical success.[50,63]

## CHOLANGIOSCOPY

Per-oral cholangioscopy was first reported in 1977 and is now the preferred technique for therapy of complicated biliary stone disease that requires direct visualization of the biliary system (ie, EHL, ILL).[64] Cholangioscopy platforms have evolved through multiple iterations. Early systems included a mother–baby design, whereby a small diameter cholangioscope was positioned across the papilla through the channel of a duodenoscope. This format required 2 separate skilled operators for each of the components. Additional drawbacks of early systems included fragile cholangioscope systems, limited maneuverability within the bile duct, and the lack of dedicated irrigation channels. The most recent and widely used platform (Spyglass, 2006, Boston

Scientific, MA) is a single operator system with 4-way tip defection, 4 separate channels (2 for irrigation, 1 for an optical probe, and one 1.2-mm accessory channel) and addresses the limitations of early cholangioscope system designs[65] (see **Fig. 5**). Direct cholangioscopy has also been reported using stand alone ultraslim (15 Fr, 18 Fr) pediatric gastroscopes maneuvered across the papilla with or without the aid of an extraction balloon. Rates of biliary intubation in cases series with this technique are greater than 80% with a mean time required to position the scope within the bile duct of 9.3 minutes (range, 3–23). Advantages of the direct peroral technique include higher resolution images, a narrow band imaging option, a large diameter working channel, and a less complex, single operator approach.[66]

Cholangioscopy through direct visualization of the biliary tree is a reliable way to definitively clear the bile duct of stone burden. Interval detection of residual extrahepatic and intrahepatic stones in patients previously evaluated with occlusion cholangiography during conventional ERCP is reported to be as high as 20% to 30% in cholangioscopy series. As such, cholangioscopy may offer advantages for stone clearance in patients whom an end of procedure cholangiogram is at risk for failing to detect residual stone burden (ie, capacious, redundant, angulated extrahepatic common bile duct, distal strictures, morbidly obese patients, and when mechanical lithotripsy was done).[65,67,68]

Cholangioscopy directed lithotripsy offers greater than 80% stone clearance rates in patients with complicated stone disease (proximal stones, common bile duct strictures) when combined with intraductal lithotripsy devices (EHL, ILL). Recurrence rates of stone disease in cases series are low (18%).[67] However, cholangitis, postprocedure systemic inflammatory response syndrome and case reports of devastating air embolism remain an added concern with cholangioscopy. As such antibiotics prophylaxis, use of $CO_2$ insufflation when using direct per-oral cholangioscopy or mother–baby systems, and examination of the biliary system through an aqueous (Spyglass) medium using continuous water irrigation (Spyglass) may be preferable.[65,66]

## DISCUSSION: ALGORITHM FOR THE MANAGEMENT OF CHOLEDOCHOLITHIASIS

Patients with biliary pancreatitis should be assessed for concomitant clinical cholangitis and risk stratified for the presence of persistent biliary obstruction (**Fig. 6**). When choledocholithiasis is confirmed, management with ERCP is most often the most appropriate intervention. The majority of patients (>85%) with bile duct stones are managed successfully with conventional techniques for stone extraction (endoscopic biliary sphincterotomy with duct clearance using a stone extraction balloon and basket). Patients with an irreversible coagulopathy, on anti-platelet therapy or Billroth II anatomy may be appropriate populations to use EPBD without EST. Maximal post-ERCP prophylaxis should be undertaken under these circumstances (pancreatic stent, rectal indomethacin) to minimize life-altering complications (see **Fig. 6**). Patients with gastroenterostomy anatomy and in who a long afferent segment is anticipated to be traversed to achieve cannulation of either a native papilla or a choledochoenterostomy may benefit from an attempt at deep enteroscopy; however, endoscopic accessories in this context are limited and rates of technical success are lower than ERCP in conventional anatomy (60%–70%).[69–71] Of note, intracorporeal options for lithotripsy (ML, EHL, ILL) are not available within the context of deep endoscopy ERCP owing to limitations in catheter length. Laparoscopic assisted ERCP or surgical common bile duct exploration are interventions with high rates of therapeutic success and acceptable rates of complications in most patients, and are also appropriate first-line interventions in patients with gastroenterostomy anatomy.[8,69,70]

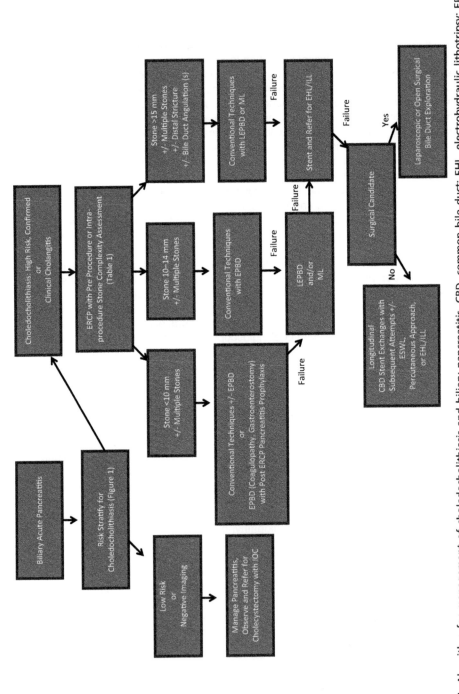

**Fig. 6.** Algorithm for management of choledocholithiasis and biliary pancreatitis. CBD, common bile duct; EHL, electrohydraulic lithotripsy; EPBD, endoscopic papillary balloon dilation; ERCP, endoscopic retrograde cholangiopancreatography; ESWL, extracorporeal shockwave lithotripsy; IOC, intra-operative cholangiography; ILL, intraductal laser lithotripsy; LEPBD, large endoscopic papillary balloon dilation; ML, mechanical lithotripsy.

When ERCP is elective, preprocedure risk assessment for factors associated with an elevated level of complexity for the ERCP stone extraction procedure should be undertaken to plan for advanced biliary endoscopic techniques, accessories and evaluate appropriateness of procedure within the context of personal skill level (see **Table 1**). At this point, referral to a tertiary care center, where advanced endoscopic techniques for management of choledocholithiasis are available such as EHL, may be most appropriate. Patients with clinical findings, and stone or bile duct morphology associated with high complexity procedures identified before or at the time of endoscopic cholangiography may benefit from early utilization of EPBD, balloon dilation of distal strictures after EST or ML to shorten procedure times and minimize complications associated with distal stone impaction or impaction of endoscopic accessories (see **Fig. 6**). Large balloon dilation of the biliary orifice, EHL, or ILL have high rates of described success after failure of conventional ERCP extraction techniques and mechanical lithotripsy. EHL or ILL may be more appropriate up-front interventions for large impacted common bile duct stones with or without distal strictures. Ultimately, if endoscopic techniques fail, surgery in patients fit for operative intervention should be considered because high rates of technical success and reasonable rates of complications can be anticipated[8] (see **Fig. 6**).

## REFERENCES

1. Fogel EL, Sherman S. ERCP for gallstone pancreatitis. N Engl J Med 2014; 370(20):1956.
2. van Geenen EJ, van Santvoort HC, Besselink MG, et al. Lack of consensus on the role of endoscopic retrograde cholangiography in acute biliary pancreatitis in published meta-analyses and guidelines: a systematic review. Pancreas 2013; 42(5):774–80.
3. Maple JT, Ben-Menachem T, Anderson MA, et al. The role of endoscopy in the evaluation of suspected choledocholithiasis. Gastrointest Endosc 2010;71(1):1–9.
4. Petrov MS. ERCP versus conservative treatment in acute pancreatitis: meta-analysis or meta-confusion? Dig Liver Dis 2008;40(9):800–1 [author reply: 801–2].
5. Folsch UR, Nitsche R, Ludtke R, et al. Early ERCP and papillotomy compared with conservative treatment for acute biliary pancreatitis. The German Study Group on Acute Biliary Pancreatitis. N Engl J Med 1997;336(4):237–42.
6. Tse F, Yuan Y. Early routine endoscopic retrograde cholangiopancreatography strategy versus early conservative management strategy in acute gallstone pancreatitis. Cochrane Database Syst Rev 2012;(5):CD009779.
7. Arendt T, Wendt M, Olszewski M, et al. Cerulein-induced acute pancreatitis in rats–does bacterial translocation occur via a transperitoneal pathway? Pancreas 1997;15(3):291–6.
8. Dasari BV, Tan CJ, Gurusamy KS, et al. Surgical versus endoscopic treatment of bile duct stones. Cochrane database Syst Rev 2013;(12):CD003327.
9. McHenry L, Lehman G. Difficult bile duct stones. Curr Treat Options Gastroenterol 2006;9(2):123–32.
10. Thomas M, Howell DA, Carr-Locke D, et al. Mechanical lithotripsy of pancreatic and biliary stones: complications and available treatment options collected from expert centers. Am J Gastroenterol 2007;102(9):1896–902.
11. Kim HJ, Choi HS, Park JH, et al. Factors influencing the technical difficulty of endoscopic clearance of bile duct stones. Gastrointest Endosc 2007;66(6):1154–60.
12. Trikudanathan G, Navaneethan U, Parsi MA. Endoscopic management of difficult common bile duct stones. World J Gastroenterol 2013;19(2):165–73.

13. Stefanidis G, Christodoulou C, Manolakopoulos S, et al. Endoscopic extraction of large common bile duct stones: a review article. World J Gastrointest Endosc 2012;4(5):167–79.

14. Horiuchi A, Nakayama Y, Kajiyama M, et al. Biliary stenting in the management of large or multiple common bile duct stones. Gastrointest Endosc 2010;71(7): 1200–3.e2.

15. Di Giorgio P, Manes G, Grimaldi E, et al. Endoscopic plastic stenting for bile duct stones: stent changing on demand or every 3 months. A prospective comparison study. Endoscopy 2013;45(12):1014–7.

16. Hong WD, Zhu QH, Huang QK. Endoscopic sphincterotomy plus endoprostheses in the treatment of large or multiple common bile duct stones. Dig Endosc 2011;23(3):240–3.

17. Chan AC, Ng EK, Chung SC, et al. Common bile duct stones become smaller after endoscopic biliary stenting. Endoscopy 1998;30(4):356–9.

18. Ang TL, Fock KM, Teo EK, et al. An audit of the outcome of long-term biliary stenting in the treatment of common bile duct stones in a general hospital. J Gastroenterol 2006;41(8):765–71.

19. Bergman JJ, Rauws EA, Tijssen JG, et al. Biliary endoprostheses in elderly patients with endoscopically irretrievable common bile duct stones: report on 117 patients. Gastrointest Endosc 1995;42(3):195–201.

20. Lee TH, Han JH, Kim HJ, et al. Is the addition of choleretic agents in multiple double-pigtail biliary stents effective for difficult common bile duct stones in elderly patients? A prospective, multicenter study. Gastrointest Endosc 2011;74(1):96–102.

21. Cai XB, Zhang WX, Wan XJ, et al. The effect of a novel drug-eluting plastic stent on biliary stone dissolution in an ex vivo bile perfusion model. Gastrointest Endosc 2014;79(1):156–62.

22. Cai XB, Zhang WX, Zhang RL, et al. Safety and efficacy of a novel plastic stent coated with stone-dissolving agents for the treatment of biliary stones in a porcine model. Endoscopy 2015;47(5):457–61.

23. Staritz M, Ewe K. Meyer zum Buschenfelde KH. Endoscopic papillary dilatation, a possible alternative to endoscopic papillotomy. Lancet 1982;1(8284):1306–7.

24. Arnold JC, Benz C, Martin WR, et al. Endoscopic papillary balloon dilation vs. sphincterotomy for removal of common bile duct stones: a prospective randomized pilot study. Endoscopy 2001;33(7):563–7.

25. Bergman JJ, van Berkel AM, Bruno MJ, et al. Is endoscopic balloon dilation for removal of bile duct stones associated with an increased risk for pancreatitis or a higher rate of hyperamylasemia? Endoscopy 2001;33(5):416–20.

26. Bergman JJ, Rauws EA, Fockens P, et al. Randomised trial of endoscopic balloon dilation versus endoscopic sphincterotomy for removal of bile duct stones. Lancet 1997;349(9059):1124–9.

27. Disario JA, Freeman ML, Bjorkman DJ, et al. Endoscopic balloon dilation compared with sphincterotomy for extraction of bile duct stones. Gastroenterology 2004;127(5):1291–9.

28. Minami A, Nakatsu T, Urchida N, et al. Papillary dilation vs sphincterotomy in endoscopic removal of bile duct stones. A randomized trial with manometric function. Dig Dis Sci 1995;40(12):2550–4.

29. Zhao HC, He L, Zhou DC, et al. Meta-analysis comparison of endoscopic papillary balloon dilatation and endoscopic sphincteropapillotomy. World J Gastroenterol 2013;19(24):3883–91.

30. Baron TH, Harewood GC. Endoscopic balloon dilation of the biliary sphincter compared to endoscopic biliary sphincterotomy for removal of common bile

duct stones during ERCP: a metaanalysis of randomized, controlled trials. Am J Gastroenterol 2004;99(8):1455–60.

31. Freeman ML, DiSario JA, Nelson DB, et al. Risk factors for post-ERCP pancreatitis: a prospective, multicenter study. Gastrointest Endosc 2001;54(4):425–34.

32. Weinberg BM, Shindy W, Lo S. Endoscopic balloon sphincter dilation (sphincteroplasty) versus sphincterotomy for common bile duct stones. Cochrane Database Syst Rev 2006;(4):CD004890.

33. Liao WC, Lee CT, Chang CY, et al. Randomized trial of 1-minute versus 5-minute endoscopic balloon dilation for extraction of bile duct stones. Gastrointest Endosc 2010;72(6):1154–62.

34. Lu Y, Wu JC, Liu L, et al. Short-term and long-term outcomes after endoscopic sphincterotomy versue endoscopic papillary balloon dilation for bile duct stones. Eur J Gastroenterol Hepatol 2014;(26):1367–73.

35. Jang SI, Yun GW, Lee DK. Balloon dilation itself may not be a major determinant of post-endoscopic retrograde cholangiopancreatography pancreatitis. World J Gastroenterol 2014;20(45):16913–24.

36. Bergman JJ, van Berkel AM, Bruno MJ, et al. A randomized trial of endoscopic balloon dilation and endoscopic sphincterotomy for removal of bile duct stones in patients with a prior Billroth II gastrectomy. Gastrointest Endosc 2001;53(1):19–26.

37. Jang HW, Lee KJ, Jung MJ, et al. Endoscopic papillary large balloon dilatation alone is safe and effective for the treatment of difficult choledocholithiasis in cases of Billroth II gastrectomy: a single center experience. Dig Dis Sci 2013; 58(6):1737–43.

38. Itoi T, Ishii K, Itokawa F, et al. Large balloon papillary dilation for removal of bile duct stones in patients who have undergone a Bilroth II gastrectomy. Dig Endosc 2010;22(Suppl 1):S98–102.

39. Park DH, Kim MH, Lee SK, et al. Endoscopic sphincterotomy vs. endoscopic papillary balloon dilation for choledocholithiasis in patients with liver cirrhosis and coagulopathy. Gastrointest Endosc 2004;60(2):180–5.

40. Aizawa T, Ueno N. Stent placement in the pancreatic duct prevents pancreatitis after endoscopic sphincter dilation for removal of bile duct stones. Gastrointest Endosc 2001;54(2):209–13.

41. Kim HG, Cheon YK, Cho YD, et al. Small sphincterotomy combined with endoscopic papillary large balloon dilation versus sphincterotomy. World J Gastroenterol 2009;15(34):4298–304.

42. Heo JH, Kang DH, Jung HJ, et al. Endoscopic sphincterotomy plus large-balloon dilation versus endoscopic sphincterotomy for removal of bile-duct stones. Gastrointest Endosc 2007;66(4):720–6 [quiz: 768, 771].

43. Stefanidis G, Viazis N, Pleskow D, et al. Large balloon dilation vs. mechanical lithotripsy for the management of large bile duct stones: a prospective randomized study. Am J Gastroenterol 2011;106(2):278–85.

44. Teoh AY, Cheung FK, Hu B, et al. Randomized trial of endoscopic sphincterotomy with balloon dilation versus endoscopic sphincterotomy alone for removal of bile duct stones. Gastroenterology 2013;144(2):341–5.e1.

45. Yang XM, Hu B. Endoscopic sphincterotomy plus large-balloon dilation vs endoscopic sphincterotomy for choledocholithiasis: a meta-analysis. World J Gastroenterol 2013;19(48):9453–60.

46. DiSario J, Chuttani R, Croffie J, et al. Biliary and pancreatic lithotripsy devices. Gastrointest Endosc 2007;65(6):750–6.

47. Riemann JF, Seuberth K, Demling L. Clinical application of a new mechanical lithotripter for smashing common bile duct stones. Endoscopy 1982;14(6):226–30.

48. Schneider MU, Matek W, Bauer R, et al. Mechanical lithotripsy of bile duct stones in 209 patients–effect of technical advances. Endoscopy 1988;20(5):248–53.

49. Merrett M, Desmond P. Removal of impacted endoscopic basket and stone from the common bile duct by extracorporeal shock waves. Endoscopy 1990;22(2):92.

50. Attila T, May GR, Kortan P. Nonsurgical management of an impacted mechanical lithotriptor with fractured traction wires: endoscopic intracorporeal electrohydraulic shock wave lithotripsy followed by extra-endoscopic mechanical lithotripsy. Can J Gastroenterol 2008;22(8):699–702.

51. Hintze RE, Adler A, Veltzke W, et al. Management of traction wire fracture complicating mechanical basket lithotripsy. Endoscopy 1997;29(9):883–5.

52. Swahn F, Edlund G, Enochsson L, et al. Ten years of Swedish experience with intraductal electrohydraulic lithotripsy and laser lithotripsy for the treatment of difficult bile duct stones: an effective and safe option for octogenarians. Surg Endosc 2010;24(5):1011–6.

53. Prachayakul V, Aswakul P, Kachintorn U. Electrohydraulic lithotripsy as an highly effective method for complete large common bile duct stone clearance. J Interv Gastroenterol 2013;3(2):59–63.

54. Arya N, Nelles SE, Haber GB, et al. Electrohydraulic lithotripsy in 111 patients: a safe and effective therapy for difficult bile duct stones. Am J Gastroenterol 2004; 99(12):2330–4.

55. Hui CK, Lai KC, Ng M, et al. Retained common bile duct stones: a comparison between biliary stenting and complete clearance of stones by electrohydraulic lithotripsy. Aliment Pharmacol Ther 2003;17(2):289–96.

56. Lee JE, Moon JH, Choi HJ, et al. Endoscopic treatment of difficult bile duct stones by using a double-lumen basket for laser lithotripsy–a case series. Endoscopy 2010;42(2):169–72.

57. Jakobs R, Adamek HE, Maier M, et al. Fluoroscopically guided laser lithotripsy versus extracorporeal shock wave lithotripsy for retained bile duct stones: a prospective randomised study. Gut 1997;40(5):678–82.

58. Neuhaus H, Zillinger C, Born P, et al. Randomized study of intracorporeal laser lithotripsy versus extracorporeal shock-wave lithotripsy for difficult bile duct stones. Gastrointest Endosc 1998;47(5):327–34.

59. Schreiber F, Gurakuqi GC, Trauner M. Endoscopic intracorporeal laser lithotripsy of difficult common bile duct stones with a stone-recognition pulsed dye laser system. Gastrointest Endosc 1995;42(5):416–9.

60. Hochberger J, Bayer J, May A, et al. Laser lithotripsy of difficult bile duct stones: results in 60 patients using a rhodamine 6G dye laser with optical stone tissue detection system. Gut 1998;43(6):823–9.

61. Amplatz S, Piazzi L, Felder M, et al. Extracorporeal shock wave lithotripsy for clearance of refractory bile duct stones. Dig Liver Dis 2007;39(3):267–72.

62. Sackmann M, Holl J, Sauter GH, et al. Extracorporeal shock wave lithotripsy for clearance of bile duct stones resistant to endoscopic extraction. Gastrointest Endosc 2001;53(1):27–32.

63. Sauter G, Sackmann M, Holl J, et al. Dormia baskets impacted in the bile duct: release by extracorporeal shock-wave lithotripsy. Endoscopy 1995;27(5):384–7.

64. Urakami Y, Seifert E, Butke H. Peroral direct cholangioscopy (PDCS) using routine straight-view endoscope: first report. Endoscopy 1977;9(1):27–30.

65. Gabbert C, Warndorf M, Easler J, et al. Advanced techniques for endoscopic biliary imaging: cholangioscopy, endoscopic ultrasonography, confocal, and beyond. Gastrointest Endosc Clin N Am 2013;23(3):625–46.

66. Weigt J, Kandulski A, Malfertheiner P. Technical improvement using ultra-slim gastroscopes for direct peroral cholangioscopy: analysis of the initial learning phase. J Hepatobiliary Pancreat Sci 2015;22(1):74–8.

67. Piraka C, Shah RJ, Awadallah NS, et al. Transpapillary cholangioscopy-directed lithotripsy in patients with difficult bile duct stones. Clin Gastroenterol Hepatol 2007;5(11):1333–8.

68. Huang SW, Lin CH, Lee MS, et al. Residual common bile duct stones on direct peroral cholangioscopy using ultraslim endoscope. World J Gastroenterol 2013;19(30):4966–72.

69. Schreiner MA, Chang L, Gluck M, et al. Laparoscopy-assisted versus balloon enteroscopy-assisted ERCP in bariatric post-Roux-en-Y gastric bypass patients. Gastrointest Endosc 2012;75(4):748–56.

70. Choi EK, Chiorean MV, Cote GA, et al. ERCP via gastrostomy vs. double balloon enteroscopy in patients with prior bariatric Roux-en-Y gastric bypass surgery. Surg Endosc 2013;27(8):2894–9.

71. Skinner M, Popa D, Neumann H, et al. ERCP with the overtube-assisted enteroscopy technique: a systematic review. Endoscopy 2014;46(7):560–72.

# Diagnosing Biliary Malignancy

Ming-ming Xu, MD, Amrita Sethi, MD*

## KEYWORDS

- Cholangiocarcinoma (CCA) • Endoscopic ultrasonography (EUS)
- Fluorescence in situ hybridization (FISH) • Intraductal ultrasonography (IDUS)
- Indeterminate biliary stricture • Pancreatic cancer
- Primary sclerosing cholangitis (PSC)
- Probe-based confocal endomicroscopy (pCLE)

## KEY POINTS

- Approximately 15% to 24% of biliary strictures are considered indeterminate after standard endoscopic retrograde cholangiopancreatography with sampling and are found to be benign at the time of surgery.
- Combining sampling techniques, including cytology, directed biopsies, and advanced molecular analysis, with fluorescence-in situ hybridization can significantly improve the yield of tissue diagnosis of malignant biliary strictures.
- Advanced imaging techniques such as cholangioscopy and confocal endomicroscopy may assist in improving the diagnosis of biliary strictures and help determine targeted areas for biopsy.

## INTRODUCTION

The diagnosis of malignant biliary obstruction remains a significant clinical challenge. Accurately differentiating benign from malignant causes of a bile duct stricture is of obvious clinical importance for therapeutic planning and prognosis. The 2 most common causes of malignant strictures are cholangiocarcinoma (CCA) and pancreatic cancer. Diagnosis of these malignancies at an early stage can allow curative surgical resection or even liver transplantation for early-stage CCA. Tissue diagnosis of pancreaticobiliary malignancies via endoscopic approaches is well known to be limited by poor cellular yield and often requires surgical exploration for definite diagnosis. For cases of suspected pancreatic cancer, in which an extrinsic pancreatic mass is seen on cross-sectional imaging, or a double-duct sign (dilatation of both bile duct and pancreatic duct), endoscopic ultrasonography (EUS) should be the primary

Division of Digestive and Liver Diseases, Columbia University Medical Center, New York, NY, USA
* Corresponding author.
*E-mail address:* amrita72@hotmail.com

Gastrointest Endoscopy Clin N Am 25 (2015) 677–690
http://dx.doi.org/10.1016/j.giec.2015.06.011
1052-5157/15/$ – see front matter © 2015 Elsevier Inc. All rights reserved.

form of diagnosis and tissue should be sampled with fine-needle aspiration (FNA). This challenge in the evaluation of biliary strictures is made even more difficult in the case of an indeterminate stricture in which preprocedural cross-sectional imaging does not show an overt mass that would be highly suggestive of malignancy. Furthermore, surgical series show that 15% to 24% of patients who undergo resection for suspected malignant strictures based on preoperative imaging or endoscopic retrograde cholangiopancreatography (ERCP) ultimately have a benign diagnosis on pathology.[1,2] This small but significant cohort of patients with benign strictures highlights the importance of accurate preoperative tissue diagnosis to avoid the morbidity and mortality of hepatobiliary surgery. This article reviews the causes of biliary strictures, the initial clinical evaluation of biliary obstruction, the diagnostic yield of ERCP-based sampling methods, the role of newer tools in the approach to evaluating strictures, and ways to address the ongoing challenge of stricture evaluation in patients with primary sclerosing cholangitis (PSC).

## CAUSES OF BILIARY STRICTURES

The leading causes of malignant biliary obstruction are pancreatic cancer and CCA.[3] Cholangiocarcinoma is a primary malignancy of the bile duct epithelium, and as such can involve both the intrahepatic and extrahepatic bile ducts. Worldwide, CCA accounts for 3% of all gastrointestinal malignancies and is the second most common primary liver malignancy after hepatocellular carcinoma.[4] When CCA is diagnosed at an early T1 stage, surgical resection can have an excellent prognosis.[5] The difficulty in the diagnosis of CCA is the poor cellular yield from the current first-line method of ERCP with brush cytology and/or biopsy. In addition, there is a known spectrum of benign causes of biliary strictures that can radiographically mimic CCA, making the exclusion of malignancy in these benign disorders clinically challenging.

Pancreatic cancer most often presents as a distal common bile duct stricture caused by extrinsic compression of the extrahepatic duct from a pancreatic head mass. This is in contrast with CCA, which often develops along the length of the bile duct, making its early detection particularly difficult because of the lack of a visible growth or tumor on imaging. Other less common malignant causes of biliary strictures include intraductal hepatocellular carcinoma, metastatic lesion, and extrinsic compression of the biliary tree from an associated visible mass or lymphadenopathy (**Table 1**).

Benign biliary strictures can develop from a variety of causes ranging from recurrent cholangitis, iatrogenic causes (most commonly after cholecystectomy or liver transplantation), to cholangiopathy from autoimmune disease, human immunodeficiency virus, and PSC. One of the least understood mimickers of a malignant process is autoimmune or immunoglobulin G4 (IgG4)–associated sclerosing cholangitis (IgG4-SC). The prevalence and pathogenesis of this disease remains largely unknown but more than 80% of patients have increases of serum IgG4 levels to more than the upper limit of normal and a similar percentage of patients have an associated autoimmune pancreatitis.[6,7] On cholangiogram, hilar IgG4-SC strictures are often indistinguishable from CCA; however, histology can be diagnostic, showing massive infiltration of IgG4-positive plasma cells with fibroinflammatory involvement of the submucosa of the bile duct wall.[6]

## LABORATORY EVALUATION

The most common laboratory abnormality seen in patients with malignant biliary stricture is obstructive cholestasis. Direct hyperbilirubinemia is seen more commonly in

| Table 1 Causes of biliary strictures | |
| --- | --- |
| **Malignant** | **Benign** |
| Cholangiocarcinoma | Chronic pancreatitis |
| Pancreatic adenocarcinoma | PSC |
| Ampullary adenocarcinoma | IgG4 (autoimmune) sclerosing cholangitis |
| Gallbladder cancer | Postsurgical, anastomotic stricture |
| Hepatocellular carcinoma | Mirizzi syndrome |
| Metastatic disease | Fibrostenotic benign stricture |
| Lymphoma | Ischemic stricture Radiation-induced stricture Infectious (HIV associated, parasitic cholangiopathy, tuberculosis) Vasculitis |

*Abbreviations:* HIV, human immunodeficiency virus; Ig4, immunoglobulin 4.

patients with malignant obstruction than in those with a benign cause such as choledocholithiasis.[8] Hyperbilirubinemia also has a higher likelihood of being associated with malignancy than increases in alkaline phosphatase level.[9,10] Serum CA 19-9 (carbohydrate antigen 19-9) has been reported to have a sensitivity of 70% to 80% in the diagnosis of malignant strictures, with a specificity of 80% to 90%.[11,12] The major limitation of CA 19-9 as a diagnostic tool of malignancy is its low specificity because its level can be increased in benign causes of cholestasis.[12,13] In addition, the diagnostic accuracy of CA 19-9 in CCA is significantly lower than in pancreatic cancer, even when the cutoff values of CA 19-9 are increased.[12] The interpretation of CA 19-9 as a diagnostic marker of bile duct cancer should be made in the context of the overall clinical impression, particularly when there is an acute cholangitis or cholestasis, which can cause false increases.

## IMAGING EVALUATION

MRI and magnetic resonance cholangiopancreatography (MRCP) have become essential parts of the baseline evaluation of patients presenting with biliary obstruction. MRCP has a very high sensitivity (96%–99%) for identifying the presence and anatomic location of a biliary obstruction but is primarily limited by poorer specificity (85%) in differentiating benign from malignant causes of obstruction.[14] Cross-sectional imaging such as computed tomography (CT) can provide staging information such as nodal, vascular, and metastatic involvement in the presence of an overt mass but has poorer overall sensitivity for detection of CCA (only 40%–63%).[15] Although no tissue diagnosis can be obtained from any imaging modality, they play an important role in providing the anatomic details needed for planning of ERCP-related interventions and preoperative staging before surgical resection.

## ENDOSCOPIC RETROGRADE CHOLANGIOPANCREATOGRAPHY

The goals of endoscopic evaluation of a suspected malignant biliary stricture are to, first, obtain definite tissue diagnosis to obviate exploratory surgery and, second, to provide palliation of biliary obstruction with stent placement. The current first-line approach to endoscopic evaluation of biliary stricture remains ERCP with brush cytology and/or biliary biopsy. Although cholangiography provides clues to malignancy, such as complete obstruction, surface irregularity, location, and stricture length, these features cannot reliably distinguish the stricture's cause and thus obtaining tissue for histopathology remains the gold standard.[10,16] Routine brush cytology is known to have low sensitivity for diagnosing malignancy (23%–56%) despite a specificity of greater than 95%.[17–20] There are a multitude of factors that contribute to the poor cytologic yield of ERCP, including tumor characteristics (submucosal growth pattern of CCA, malignant extrinsic compression), the anatomic location of the stricture (yield of biliary biopsy is higher in distal compared with proximal strictures), and the number of and processing of specimens.[21] Several methods designed to improve the sensitivity of brush cytology have been studied with varying degrees of improvement. Fogel and colleagues[22] reported on the use of a longer cytology brush with no significant improvement in the cancer detection rate. Attempts at stricture dilation with subsequent brush cytology sampling only marginally improved malignancy detection rate, from 27% to 34%.[21] Endobiliary biopsy has a higher diagnostic yield compared with cytology alone (**Table 2**), and when both modalities are combined sensitivity can be increased to 70% with preserved specificity of 100%.[23] The addition of endoluminal FNA to the other 2 modalities, or triple tissue sampling, has the highest sensitivity at 77%.[20] Wright and colleagues[24] developed the so-called smash protocol for tissue sampling at ERCP to achieve a 72% on-site pathologic diagnosis for suspected biliary malignancy by changing the processing protocol for biopsies. The biliary biopsy tissue is smashed between 2 slides, stained by the Papanicolaou method with immediate on-site cytopathology review, and repeated sampling was obtained until a diagnosis was reached.[24] This technique provides several distinct advantages, including its relative cost-effectiveness, on-site diagnosis, ease of performance, and low rate of complications despite multiple samplings, and it should be considered as a preferred method for biliary biopsy sampling in cases with high pretest suspicion for malignancy.

## FLUORESCENCE IN SITU HYBRIDIZATION

A promising tissue-based diagnostic tool that has recently been helping to improve the diagnostic yield of ERCP is fluorescence in situ hybridization (FISH) for detecting chromosomal aneuploidy or polysomy. These changes are thought to be present in an estimated 80% of pancreatobiliary malignancies.[28] FISH uses fluorescently labeled DNA probes to detect cells with an abnormal number of chromosomes or mutations in a specific locus of a chromosome. There are 4 commercially available FISH probes, which bind to chromosomes 3 (CEP3), 7 (CEP7), 17 (CEP17), and the 9p21 locus of chromosome 9. The main advantage of FISH lies in its ease of use, because it can be performed on cells obtained from routine brush cytology samples during ERCP.

**Table 2**
Diagnostic yield of techniques for evaluation of suspected malignant biliary strictures

| Diagnostic Method | Sensitivity (%) | Specificity (%) |
|---|---|---|
| MRCP[14,25,26] | 80 | 70–85 |
| ERCP brush cytology[17–20] | 23–56 | 95–100 |
| ERCP with long brush[22] | 27 | 100 |
| ERCP biliary biopsy[27] | 44–89 CCA<br>33–71 pancreatic CA | 97–100 |
| Brush cytology plus biopsy[23] | 70 | 100 |

The earliest prospective data on the diagnostic yield of FISH in indeterminate strictures by Levy and colleagues[28] using CEP3, CEP7, and CEP 17 probes found that, in previously cytology-negative strictures, the sensitivity of FISH was 62% with specificity of 79% for malignancy. When trisomy 7 was considered a marker of malignancy in the combined cohort of patients both with and without PSC the overall sensitivity for diagnosing malignancy was 64%, specificity 82%, and diagnostic accuracy 72%. The main limitation of FISH is its reduced specificity in the setting of chronic inflammatory conditions such as PSC, in which polysomy can occur in the absence of CCA.[29] Trisomy 7 in particular can be found in benign strictures of patients with PSC and decreases the specificity of FISH for malignancy in that challenging cohort. When a fourth FISH probe to the 9p21 locus of chromosome 9 (associated with mutation of the p16 tumor suppressor gene) is added to the repertoire the sensitivity of FISH can be improved significantly from 47% to 84% with preserved specificity of 97%.[30] Other molecular-based techniques that have been examined to improve the diagnostic yield include bile aspirate analysis for p53 and KRAS mutations, but these are not currently considered part of the routine work-up and are still in the early phases of investigation.[31]

## ENDOSCOPIC ULTRASONOGRAPHY: FINE-NEEDLE ASPIRATION

EUS with FNA has increasingly become part of the standard first-line evaluation of pancreatobiliary lesions as a complementary tool to ERCP for tissue sampling, tumor staging, and the exclusion of benign causes of biliary obstruction, such as stone disease. It has a reported overall sensitivity of between 43% and 86% for the diagnosis of all malignant strictures, but seems to be more sensitive in the evaluation of distal strictures, which are more often caused by pancreatic adenocarcinoma and more easily accessible for FNA sampling.[32–35] EUS-FNA is generally less reliable in the evaluation of proximal CCA because its sensitivity decreases to 59% compared with 81% in distal CCA.[36] The presence of a previously placed biliary stent can also decrease its sensitivity for malignancy detection because of a combination of stent-related acoustic shadowing, image degradation, and difficult needle access.

Perhaps the most concerning issue in the use of EUS-FNA in suspected CCA is the theoretic potential for malignant peritoneal seeding via the needle access pathway. This concern arises from a small number of case series of patients who underwent percutaneous biliary biopsies for CCA and developed carcinomatosis, with rates as alarmingly high as 83% in one series.[37,38] Although there have been no cases reported of peritoneal carcinomatosis from EUS-FNA sampling of CCA, these concerns have led some transplant centers to consider tissue sampling via this method to be a contraindication for liver transplantation of hilar CCA.[39] EUS-FNA remains an important complementary tool to ERCP in the evaluation of biliary strictures and can be particularly helpful in distal biliary strictures from pancreatic cancer, in cases of a suspected mass that may have been missed on other imaging techniques, or when ERCP-based tissue sampling techniques have been nondiagnostic.

## INTRADUCTAL ULTRASONOGRAPHY

Along with the evolution of EUS-FNA, intraductal ultrasonography (IDUS) was developed as a tool to enhance endobiliary imaging by the wire-guided placement of a high-frequency probe directly into the bile ducts. The main advantage of IDUS is its ease of use, because it can be done as part of routine ERCP without any need for biliary sphincterotomy or significantly prolonging the procedure. It can provide high-quality imaging of the periductal tissue along with limited tumor staging such as mass size and periportal vascular invasion (full lymph node staging still requires EUS).[40] IDUS criteria for differentiating benign from malignant strictures have been established (**Box 1**).[41] Multiple studies show the sensitivity of IDUS to be 80% to 90%, specificity 83%, and it can improve the accuracy of ERCP from 58% to 83%.[42,43] Note that IDUS ultimately does not provide histopathology but is another adjunctive tool to ERCP to help direct further work-up of these strictures.

## CHOLANGIOSCOPY

The initial idea for direct bile duct visualization, or cholangioscopy, emerged in the 1970s but the widespread adoption of the first-generation so-called mother-baby cholangioscope was limited by the need for 2 operators, scope fragility, limited tip maneuverability, and prolonged procedures.[44] The development of single-operator cholangioscopy (SOC), or the SpyGlass Direct Visualization System (Boston Scientific, Marlborough, MA) has provided increased diagnostic outcomes for cholangioscopic evaluation of biliary strictures.

The SpyGlass system consists of a 10-Fr access catheter (SpyScope) that can be inserted through the standard 4.2-mm working channel of a therapeutic duodeno-scope, a reusable optical probe (SpyGlass) that fits through the SpyScope catheter, and disposable 3-Fr biliary biopsy forceps to allow visually directed biopsies (SpyBite) (**Fig. 1**). The optical catheter provides 6000 pixel images and has tip maneuverability to allow 30° views in 4 directions.[45] Despite limitations with video cholangioscopy, this modality has provided excellent images of intraductal epithelium (**Fig. 2**A) and has led to considerations for imaging criteria that have been proposed for the diagnosis of malignancy (**Box 2**). The strongest feature suggestive of malignancy is the presence of dilated and tortuous vessels, with a reported specificity and positive predictive value of 100% (see **Box 2**).[46–48] The high predictive value of this finding is thought to be caused by the underlying neovascularization of the malignant tumor. Although video cholangioscopy can allow for addition of modalities, such as narrow band imaging, that can improve vessel visualization, there has been no demonstration that this improves the diagnosis of malignancy. A new digital cholangioscope using the same platform (SpyScope DS, Boston Scientific, Marlborough, MA) has recently been introduced that provides higher resolution imaging than its predecessor (see **Fig. 2**B, C).

---

**Box 1**
**Malignant stricture criteria using IDUS**

Disruption of 3-layer architecture of normal bile duct

Eccentric wall thickening

Hypoechoic mass with irregular margins

Hypoechoic mass with invasion of adjacent structures

Area with heterogeneous echo patterns

Papillary surface

Malignant-appearing periductal lymph nodes (hypoechoic, round shape, large size)

Periportal vascular invasion

*Adapted from* Farrell RJ, Agarwal B, Brandwein SL, et al. Intraductal US is a useful adjunct to ERCP for distinguishing malignant from benign biliary strictures. Gastrointest Endosc 2002;56:681–7.

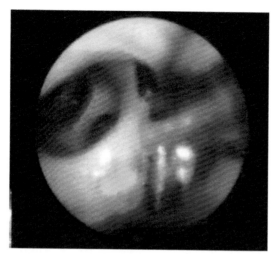

**Fig. 1.** SpyBite forceps under direct visualization.

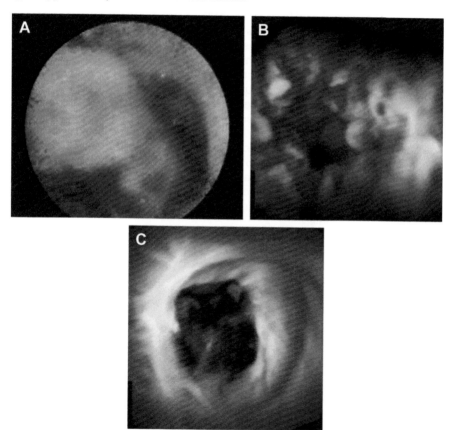

**Fig. 2.** (*A*) Inflammatory mass in patient with PSC using SpyScope Legacy. (*B*) Cholangiocarcinoma in a patient without PSC using SpyScope DS (Boston Scientific). (*C*) Anastomotic stricture with cast debris in a patient status post–liver transplant using SpyScope DS. (*Courtesy of* Amrita Sethi, MD, New York, NY.)

---

**Box 2**
**Malignant stricture criteria for SOC cholangioscopy**

Dilated, tortuous blood vessels

Intraductal nodules or mass

Infiltrative or ulcerated stricture

Papillary or villous mucosal projections

*Adapted from* Seo DW, Lee SK, Yoo KS, et al. Cholangioscopic findings in bile duct tumors. Gastrointest Endosc 2000;52:630–4.

---

The largest prospective, multicenter, observational study of the operating characteristics of the SOC system, by Chen and colleagues,[49] included 226 patients with biliary strictures (not all were cytology negative) with a sensitivity, specificity, positive predictive value, and negative predictive value for malignancy of 78%, 82%, 80%, and 80% respectively based on the visual impression criteria.[49,50] Visual impression had a higher sensitivity than visually targeted biopsy, which was only 47%, although biopsy specificity was much higher at 98% with a positive predictive value of 100%. A smaller prospective series from Ramchandani and colleagues[51] involving 36 patients with indeterminate strictures also found the sensitivity of the SOC visual impression to be higher (95%; specificity, 79%) than biopsies (sensitivity, 82%; specificity, 82%). The poorer yield from visually targeted samples may be attributable to a combination of early phases of learning the technique for targeted visual biopsy and the small size of the acquired biopsy samples from the SpyBite forceps.[51] Although results regarding diagnostic accuracies of cholangioscopy-based diagnosis are consistent among various studies, a validated criteria system has not been established and raises questions as to the absolute value of intraductal visualization without corresponding clinical data. In 2 consecutive studies, interobserver agreement of SOC visual findings and final diagnosis were only slight to fair and the accuracy was less than 50% on diagnosing malignancy.[52,53] With the forthcoming availability of digital SOC and its suspected increased utility, the development of a reliable, validated set of visual criteria will be even more valuable.

The major limitations to consider when using cholangioscopy are the need for biliary sphincterotomy to advance the system into the biliary tree and higher rates of complications caused by sphincterotomy and cholangitis. Chen and colleagues[49] reported serious procedural complication rates of 7.5%; a later study by Sethi and colleagues[54] confirmed a complication rate of 7.0% versus the routine ERCP rate of 2.9%, with the difference attributed to higher incidence of cholangitis in the cholangioscopy group.

## CONFOCAL LASER ENDOMICROSCOPY

Probe-based confocal laser endomicroscopy (pCLE) uses an optical probe during ERCP to allow real-time, microscopic-level examination of the bile ducts.[55] The CholangioFlex probe (Maunakea Tech, Paris, France) fits into multiple ERCP accessory devices or the 1.2-mm diameter working channel of a SpyGlass (Boston Scientific, Natick, MA) cholangioscope. This probe provides images with a field of view of 325 μm and depth of view 40 to 70 μm below the tissue surface. An intravenous contrast agent, usually fluorescein, is used to enhance optical visualization of vascular formations and varying degrees of contrast uptake within the biliary epithelium and subepithelium, which helps to determine the likelihood of malignancy in vivo.

An initial feasibility study of 14 patients with indeterminate stricture showed the potential for pCLE to predict malignancy, with an overall diagnostic accuracy of 86%, sensitivity of 83%, and specificity of 88%.[56] Subsequently, formal classification criteria for malignancy, the Miami classification, were developed and prospectively studied in a multicenter, larger cohort of 89 patients with indeterminate pancreatobiliary strictures by 8 investigators (**Fig. 3**A) (**Table 3**).[57,58] The sensitivity, specificity, positive predictive value, and negative predictive value of pCLE using the Miami criteria were 98%, 67%, 71%, and 97%; the accuracy of a combination ERCP with pCLE was significantly higher than ERCP with tissue sampling alone (90% vs 73%).[57] Notably, the learning curve for interpreting pCLE in this study was fairly short, with training modules of about 50 procedures thought to be adequate for procedural competence of investigators with no prior experience with pCLE.[57] The high false-positive rate of pCLE was attributed to difficulty discerning inflammatory changes seen in benign conditions such as PSC from true malignant features. This finding led to attempts at refining the Miami classification with more specific criteria for benign chronic inflammatory changes. The Paris classification added more specific criteria for inflammatory stenosis, such as vascular congestion, thickened reticular structures, dark granularity, and increased interglandular space, to decrease false-positive confocal interpretations[59] (see **Fig. 3**B). By applying these new criteria, the investigators were able to improve the specificity and accuracy of diagnosing malignancy to 88%, albeit at the cost of a decreased sensitivity. Analysis of the performance of a subgroup of patients in which sampling remained inconclusive after the procedure showed a negative predictive value of 88%.[60] Prospective validation of the Paris classification is still needed to clarify its applicability to the difficult problem of indeterminate strictures.

In practice, the low specificity of pCLE and the dedicated operator training needed for accurate interpretation of confocal images remain the major limiting factors of its widespread use as a routine tool in the evaluation of indeterminate strictures. However, in expert centers with pCLE experience it has become a valuable tool in the multimodality approach to the management of difficult cases of biliary stricture.

## CHOLANGIOCARCINOMA IN PRIMARY SCLEROSING CHOLANGITIS

PSC is a chronic, progressive inflammatory condition of the intrahepatic and extrahepatic bile ducts that can lead to biliary cirrhosis and increases patients' risk for CCA

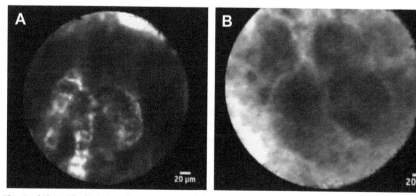

**Fig. 3.** (*A*) Epithelial structure as seen with pCLE of a malignant lesion. (*B*) Increased intraglandular space, which is an inflammatory criterion as described by the Paris classification.

**Table 3**
**Miami classification of pCLE for predicting malignant biliary stricture**

| Criteria Suggestive of Malignancy | Criteria Suggestive of Benign Disease |
| --- | --- |
| Thick, dark bands (>40 μm) | Thin, dark bands |
| Thick, white bands (>20 μm) | Thin, white bands |
| Dark clumps | — |
| Villous glands | — |
| Fluorescein leakage | — |

*Adapted from* Meining A, Shah RJ, Slivka A, et al. Classification of probe-based confocal laser endomicroscopy findings in pancreaticobiliary strictures. Endoscopy 2012;3:251–7.

and colorectal cancer.[61,62] Natural history studies show that 10% to 30% of patients with PSC develop CCA; that incidence is even higher in autopsy series of patients with PSC.[63] Liver transplantation is the only curative treatment of both end-stage biliary cirrhosis and early-stage hilar CCA, with a posttransplantation 5-year survival of 65% to 88% when performed in expert centers under rigorous protocols.[64,65] However, because of the chronic stricturing nature of the disease, differentiating between benign and malignant strictures in this population is particularly difficult. There have been conflicting data on the value of serum markers such as CA 19-9 and carcinoembryonic antigen in the evaluation of CCA in PSC. One suggested cutoff value for CA 19-9 of greater than 100 U/mL was based on a retrospective study showing a sensitivity and specificity for detection of CCA of 89% and 86%.[66] However, prospective studies of tumor markers have largely been unable to confirm a significant role for their use in distinguishing the causes of PSC strictures.[67,68] On cholangiogram, the presence of a dominant stricture is thought to be suggestive of malignancy but tissue diagnosis can be elusive. The newer modalities for tissue acquisition during ERCP generally all perform poorly in patients with PSC. A recent meta-analysis showed that FISH sensitivity for CCA in PSC is only 51%, although specificity is preserved at 93%.[69] Similarly, the main drawback of confocal microscopy is its lower reliability in distinguishing chronic inflammatory benign changes from malignant transformation. Cholangioscopy may be the most promising, with some prospective studies suggesting sensitivity for CCA in patients with PSC of 92%, specificity 93%, and overall accuracy of 93%, but in half of the patients a second cholangioscopy was needed for tissue diagnosis.[44]

Taken together, the literature suggests a multimodality approach in any patient with PSC in whom there is a high clinical suspicion for malignancy, such as a persistently, markedly increased CA 19-9 level despite biliary decompression, or new or symptomatic dominant stricture. First-line approach should include routine ERCP with brushings and FISH, and if nondiagnostic despite high clinical concern to consider an adjunct endobiliary imaging study, depending on local expertise and availability, to either confirm clinical suspicions or to use for continued close surveillance. Proximal biliary strictures may be best imaged by IDUS, whereas EUS can evaluate for suspicious periductal lymph nodes. Practices in the use of cholangioscopy and confocal endomicroscopy will vary more widely depending on its availability, operator experience, and further definition of diagnostic criteria.

## SUMMARY

The diagnosis of indeterminate biliary strictures remains an ongoing challenge for biliary endoscopists. It is clear that standard ERCP and conventional sampling methods need to be combined with advanced molecular testing and imaging modalities, the diagnostic accuracies of which are currently being investigated. In future, endoscopic evaluation of biliary strictures will need to move toward developing a diagnostic algorithm that reconciles the cost-effectiveness of extensive and repeated evaluations for stable-appearing strictures with the potential for a missed malignancy and/or unnecessary surgical exploration. This topic has the potential to be a rich area for research and to change paradigms of practice as clinicians become more familiar with the new tools in their expanding arsenal.

## REFERENCES

1. Clayton RA, Clarke DL, Currie EJ, et al. Incidence of benign pathology in patients undergoing hepatic resection for suspected malignancy. Surgeon 2003;1:32–8.
2. Gerhards MF, Vos P, van Gulik TM, et al. Incidence of benign lesions in patients resected for suspicious hilar obstruction. Br J Surg 2001;88:48–51.
3. Ustundag Y, Bayraktar Y. Cholangiocarcinoma: a compact review of the literature. World J Gastroenterol 2008;14:6458–66.
4. Vauthey JN, Blumgart LH. Recent advances in the management of cholangiocarcinomas. Semin Liver Dis 1994;14:109–14.
5. Mizumoto R, Ogura Y, Kusuda T. Definition and diagnosis of early cancer of the biliary tract. Hepatogastroenterology 1993;40:69–77.
6. Ohara H, Okazaki K, Tsubouchi H, et al. Clinical diagnostic criteria of IgG4-related sclerosing cholangitis 2012. J Hepatobiliary Pancreat Sci 2012;19: 536–42.
7. Okazaki K, Uchida K, Koyabu M, et al. IgG4 cholangiopathy-current concept, diagnosis, and pathogenesis. J Hepatol 2014;61:690–5.
8. Hayat JO, Loew CJ, Asrress KN, et al. Contrasting liver function test patterns in obstructive jaundice due to biliary strictures and stones. QJM 2005;98:35–40.
9. Greca GL, Sofia M, Lombardo R, et al. Adjusting CA19-9 values to predict malignancy in obstructive jaundice: influence of bilirubin and C-reactive protein. World J Gastroenterol 2012;18(31):4150–5.
10. Bain VG, Abraham N, Jhangri GS, et al. Prospective study of biliary strictures to determine the predictors of malignancy. Can J Gastroenterol 2000;14(5): 397–402.
11. Goonetilleke KS, Siriwardena AK. Systematic review of carbohydrate antigen (CA 19–9) as a biochemical marker in the diagnosis of pancreatic cancer. Eur J Surg Oncol 2007;33:266–70.
12. Kim HJ, Kim MH, Myung SJ, et al. A new strategy for the application of CA 19-9 in the differentiation of pancreatobiliary cancer: analysis using a receiver operating characteristic curve. Am J Gastroenterol 1999;94:1941–6.
13. Steinberg W. The clinical utility of the CA19-9 tumor-associated antigen. Am J Gastroenterol 1990;85:350–5.
14. Romagnuolo J. Magnetic resonance cholangiopancreatography: a meta-analysis of test performance in suspected biliary disease. Ann Intern Med 2003;139: 547–57.
15. Tillich M, Mischinger HJ, Preisegger KH, et al. Multiphasic helical CT in diagnosis and staging of hilar cholangiocarcinoma. Am J Roentgenol 1998;171:651–8.
16. Pasanen PA, Partanen KP, Pikkarainen PH, et al. A comparison of ultrasound, computed tomography and endoscopic retrograde cholangiopancreatography in the differential diagnosis of benign and malignant jaundice and cholestasis. Eur J Surg 1993;159:23–9.

17. Burnett AS, Calvert TJ, Chokshi RJ. Sensitivity of endoscopic retrograde cholangiopancreatography standard cytology: 10-y review of the literature. J Surg Res 2013;184:304–11.

18. Ponchon T, Gagnon P, Berger F, et al. Value of endobiliary brush cytology and biopsies for the diagnosis of malignant bile duct stenosis: results of a prospective study. Gastrointest Endosc 1995;42:565–72.

19. Glasbrenner B, Ardan M, Boeck W, et al. Prospective evaluation of brush cytology of biliary strictures during endoscopic retrograde cholangiopancreatography. Endoscopy 1999;31:712–7.

20. Jailwala J, Fogel EL, Sherman S, et al. Triple-tissue sampling at ERCP in malignant biliary obstruction. Gastrointest Endosc 2000;51:383–90.

21. de Bellis M, Fogel EL, Sherman S, et al. Influence of stricture dilation and repeat brushing on the cancer detection rate of brush cytology in the evaluation of malignant biliary obstruction. Gastrointest Endosc 2003;58:176–82.

22. Fogel EL, deBellis M, McHenry L, et al. Effectiveness of a new long cytology brush in the evaluation of malignant biliary obstruction: a prospective study. Gastrointest Endosc 2006;63:71–7.

23. Schoefl R, Haefner M, Wriba F, et al. Forceps biopsy and brush cytology during endoscopic retrograde cholangiopancreatography for the diagnosis of biliary stenosis. Scand J Gastroenterol 1997;32:363–8.

24. Wright ER, Bakis G, Srinivasan R, et al. Intraprocedural tissue diagnosis during ERCP employing a new cytology preparation of forceps biopsy (Smash protocol). Am J Gastroenterol 2011;106:294–9.

25. Park MS, Kim TK, Kim KW, et al. Differentiation of extrahepatic bile duct cholangiocarcinoma from benign stricture: findings at MRCP versus ERCP. Radiology 2004;233:234–40.

26. Kim MJ, Mitchell DG, Ito K, et al. Biliary dilatation: differentiation of benign from malignant causes–value of adding conventional MR imaging to MR cholangiopancreatography. Radiology 2000;214:173–81.

27. Higashizawa T, Tamada K, Tomiyama T, et al. Biliary guide-wire facilitates bile duct biopsy and endoscopic drainage. J Gastroenterol Hepatol 2002;17:332–6.

28. Levy MJ, Baron TH, Clayton AC, et al. Prospective evaluation of advanced molecular markers and imaging techniques in patients with indeterminate bile duct strictures. Am J Gastroenterol 2008;103:1263–73.

29. Bangarulingam SY, Bjornsson E, Enders F, et al. Long-term outcomes of positive fluorescence in situ hybridization tests in primary sclerosing cholangitis. Hepatology 2010;51:174–80.

30. Gonda TA, Glick MP, Sethi A, et al. Polysomy and p16 deletion by fluorescence in situ hybridization in the diagnosis of indeterminate biliary strictures. Gastrointest Endosc 2012;75:74–9.

31. Naut JC, Zucman-Rossi J. Genetics of hepatobiliary carcinogenesis. Semin Liver Dis 2011;31:173–87.

32. Rosch T, Hofrichter K, Frimberger E, et al. ERCP or EUS for tissue diagnosis of biliary strictures? A prospective comparative study. Gastrointest Endosc 2004; 60:390–6.

33. Lee JH, Salem R, Aslanian H, et al. Endoscopic ultrasound and fine-needle aspiration of unexplained bile duct strictures. Am J Gastroenterol 2004;99: 1069–73.

34. Eloubeidi MA, Chen VK, Jhala NC, et al. Endoscopic ultrasound-guided fine needle aspiration biopsy of suspected cholangiocarcinoma. Clin Gastroenterol Hepatol 2004;2:209–13.

35. Fritscher-Ravens A, Broering DC, Sriram PV, et al. EUS-guided fine-needle aspiration cytodiagnosis of hilar cholangiocarcinoma: a case series. Gastrointest Endosc 2000;52:534–40.
36. Mohamadnejad M, DeWitt JM, Sherman S, et al. Role of EUS for preoperative evaluation of cholangiocarcinoma: a large single center experience. Gastrointest Endosc 2011;73:71–8.
37. Heimbach JK, Sanchez W, Rosen CB, et al. Trans-peritoneal fine needle aspiration biopsy of hilar cholangiocarcinoma is associated with disease dissemination. HPB (Oxford) 2011;13:356–60.
38. Nakamuta M, Tanabe Y, Ohashi M, et al. Transabdominal seeding of hepatocellular carcinoma after fine-needle aspiration biopsy. J Clin Ultrasound 1993;21:551–6.
39. Rosen CB, Heimbach JK, Gores GJ. Liver transplantation for cholangiocarcinoma. Transpl Int 2010;23:692–7.
40. Tamada K, Ueno N, Tomiyama T, et al. Characterization of biliary strictures using intraductal ultrasonography: comparison with percutaneous cholangioscopic biopsy. Gastrointest Endosc 1998;47:341–9.
41. Farrell RJ, Agarwal B, Brandwein SL, et al. Intraductal US is a useful adjunct to ERCP for distinguishing malignant from benign biliary strictures. Gastrointest Endosc 2002;56:681–7.
42. Stavropoulos S, Larghi A, Verna E, et al. Intraductal ultrasound for the evaluation of patients with biliary strictures and no abdominal mass on computed tomography. Endoscopy 2005;37:715–21.
43. Vazquez-Sequeiros E, Baron TH, Clain JE, et al. Evaluation of indeterminate bile duct strictures by intraductal US. Gastrointest Endosc 2002;56:372–9.
44. Tischendorf JJ, Krüger M, Trautwein C, et al. Cholangioscopic characterization of dominant bile duct stenoses in patients with primary sclerosing cholangitis. Endoscopy 2006;38:665–9.
45. Chen YK, Pleskow DK. SpyGlass single-operator peroral cholangiopancreatoscopy system for the diagnosis and therapy of bile-duct disorders: a clinical feasibility study (with video). Gastrointest Endosc 2007;65:832–41.
46. Itoi T, Neuhaus H, Chen YK. Diagnostic value of image-enhanced video cholangiopancreatoscopy. Gastrointest Endosc Clin North Am 2009;19(4):557–66.
47. Nimura Y, Kamiya J. Cholangioscopy. Endoscopy 1998;30:182–8.
48. Kim HJ, Kim MH, Lee SK, et al. Tumor vessel: a valuable cholangioscopic clue of malignant biliary stricture. Gastrointest Endosc 2000;52:635–8.
49. Chen YK, Parsi MA, Binmoeller KF, et al. Single-operator cholangioscopy in patients requiring evaluation of bile duct disease or therapy of biliary stones (with videos). Gastrointest Endosc 2011;74:805–14.
50. Nishikawa T, Tsuyuguchi T, Sakai Y, et al. Comparison of the diagnostic accuracy of peroral video-cholangioscopic visual findings and cholangioscopy guided forceps biopsy findings for indeterminate biliary lesions: a prospective study. Gastrointest Endosc 2013;77:219–26.
51. Ramchandani M, Reddy DN, Gupta R, et al. Role of single-operator peroral cholangioscopy in the diagnosis of indeterminate biliary lesions: a single-center, prospective study. Gastrointest Endosc 2011;74:511–9.
52. Sethi A, Widmer J, Shah NL, et al. Interobserver agreement for evaluation of imaging with single operator choledochoscopy: what are we looking at? Dig Liver Dis 2014;46:518–22.
53. Sethi A, Doukides T, Sejpal DV, et al. Interobserver agreement for single operator choledochoscopy imaging: can we do better? Diagn Ther Endosc 2014;2014:730731.

54. Sethi A, Chen YK, Austin GL, et al. ERCP with cholangiopancreatoscopy may be associated with higher rates of complications than ERCP alone: a single-center experience. Gastrointest Endosc 2011;73:251–6.

55. Meining A, Saur D, Bajbouj M, et al. In vivo histopathology for detection of gastro-intestinal neoplasia with a portable, confocal miniprobe: an examiner blinded analysis. Clin Gastroenterol Hepatol 2007;5:1261–7.

56. Meining A, Frimberger E, Becker V, et al. Detection of cholangiocarcinoma in vivo using miniprobe-based confocal fluorescence microscopy. Clin Gastroenterol Hepatol 2008;6:1057–60.

57. Meining A, Chen YK, Pleskow D, et al. Direct visualization of indeterminate pan-creaticobiliary strictures with probe-based confocal laser endomicroscopy: a multicenter experience. Gastrointest Endosc 2011;74:961–8.

58. Meining A, Shah RJ, Slivka A, et al. Classification of probe-based confocal laser endomicroscopy findings in pancreaticobiliary strictures. Endoscopy 2012;3: 251–7.

59. Caillol F, Filoche B, Gaidhane M, et al. Refined probe-based confocal laser endo-microscopy classification for biliary strictures: the Paris classification. Dig Dis Sci 2013;58:1784–9.

60. Slivka A, Gan I, Jamidar P, et al. Validation of the diagnostic accuracy of probe-based confocal laser endomicroscopy for the characterization of indeterminate biliary strictures: results of a prospective multicenter international study. Gastro-intest Endosc 2015;81(2):282–90.

61. La Russo NF, Wiesner RH, Ludwig J, et al. Primary sclerosing cholangitis. N Engl J Med 1984;310:899–903.

62. Farrant JM, Hayllar KM, Wilkinson ML, et al. Natural history and prognostic vari-ables in primary sclerosing cholangitis. Gastroenterology 1991;100:1710–7.

63. MacFaul GR, Chapman RW. Sclerosing cholangitis. Curr Opin Gastroenterol 2006;22:288–93.

64. Heimbach JK, Gores GJ, Haddock MG, et al. Liver transplantation for unresect-able perihilar cholangiocarcinoma. Semin Liver Dis 2004;24:201–7.

65. Murad DS, Kim WR, Harnois DM, et al. Efficacy of neoadjuvant chemoradiation followed by liver transplantation, for perihilar cholangiocarcinoma at 12 US cen-ters. Gastroenterology 2012;143:88–98.

66. Ramage JK, Donaghy A, Farrant JM, et al. Serum tumor markers for the diagnosis of cholangiocarcinoma in primary sclerosing cholangitis. Gastroenterology 1995; 108:865–9.

67. Bjornsson E, Kilander A, Olsson R. CA19-9 and CEA are unreliable markers for cholangiocarcinoma in patients with primary sclerosing cholangitis. Liver 1999; 19:501–8.

68. Hultcrantz R, Olsson R, Danielsson A, et al. A 3-year prospective study on serum tumor markers used for detecting cholangiocarcinoma in patients with primary sclerosing cholangitis. J Hepatol 1999;30:669–73.

69. Navaneethan U, Njei B, Venkatesh P, et al. Fluorescence in situ hybridization for diagnosis of cholangiocarcinoma in primary sclerosing cholangitis:a systematic review and meta-analysis. Gastrointest Endosc 2014;79:943–50.

# Stenting in Malignant Biliary Obstruction

Majid A. Almadi, MBBS, FRCPC, MSc (Clinical Epidemiology)[a,b],
Jeffrey S. Barkun, MD, CM, FRCS, MSc[c],
Alan N. Barkun, MD, CM, FRCPC, MSc (Clinical Epidemiology)[b,d,*]

## KEYWORDS

- Malignant • Stents • Bile duct malignancy • Pancreas malignancy
- Gallbladder malignancy • Jaundice • Palliative care

## KEY POINTS

- Routine preoperative biliary drainage is associated with negative outcomes.
- Endoscopic palliative biliary drainage has been associated with an improvement in quality of life.
- Antibiotic administration is prudent in patients in whom there is failure or suspicion of failure to drain the targeted biliary system.
- It is unnecessary to perform a sphincterotomy in patients with pancreatic cancer requiring biliary stenting.
- In patients with short survival, there is no significant difference in the total cost per patient between plastic stents and self-expandable metal stents (SEMSs).

## INTRODUCTION

It is estimated that in 2014, a total of 46,420 cases of pancreatic cancer were diagnosed in the United States,[1] as well as 10,650 cases of gallbladder and other biliary tumors with a trend toward a higher incidence of intrahepatic compared with extrahepatic cholangiocarcinomas.[2–8] The median survival of all patients with biliary tract cancers is 4.8 months with 1-year and 5-year survival rates of 31% and 10%, respectively.[3]

   Given this poor prognosis, in a significant proportion of these patients biliary drainage is required because a palliative approach is indicated.

[a] Division of Gastroenterology, King Khalid University Hospital, King Saud University Medical City, King Saud University, Riyadh 11461, Saudi Arabia; [b] Division of Gastroenterology, The McGill University Health Center, Montreal General Hospital, McGill University, 1650 Cedar Avenue, Montréal, Quebec H3G 1A4, Canada; [c] Division of General Surgery, The McGill University Health Centre, McGill University, 1650 Cedar Avenue, Montréal, Quebec H3G 1A4, Canada; [d] Division of Clinical Epidemiology, The McGill University Health Center, Montreal General Hospital, McGill University, 1650 Cedar Avenue, Montréal, Quebec H3G 1A4, Canada
* Corresponding author. Montreal General Hospital, 1650 Cedar Avenue, #D7-148, Montréal, Quebec H3G 1A4, Canada.
E-mail address: alan.barkun@muhc.mcgill.ca

Gastrointest Endoscopy Clin N Am 25 (2015) 691–711
http://dx.doi.org/10.1016/j.giec.2015.06.002
1052-5157/15/$ – see front matter © 2015 Elsevier Inc. All rights reserved.

This review covers stenting of the biliary system in different clinical scenarios: patients with either palliative or resectable malignant biliary obstruction located either proximally or in the distal biliary tree. After a succinct discussion on drainage strategy, the authors focus on comparative data available to address technical and periprocedural considerations. This article does not cover issues pertaining to the evaluation, diagnosis, or treatment other than stenting or treatments incorporated within stents even if they are performed endoscopically (eg, photodynamic therapy or radiofrequency ablation).

## WHO SHOULD UNDERGO BILIARY DRAINAGE?

Any biliary drainage is associated with possible complications, the risk of which has to be weighed against benefits in any given clinical situation (**Table 1**). Meta-analyses have suggested more frequent negative outcomes in patients undergoing routine preoperative biliary drainage[9–11] before surgery for potentially resectable distal malignant biliary obstruction. Therefore, biliary drainage is usually performed only in surgical patients who are candidates for neoadjuvant therapies, in patients with acute cholangitis, or in patients with intense pruritus or in whom surgery will be delayed.[12]

When drainage is attempted for patients scheduled to receive neoadjuvant therapies, a plastic or short intrapancreatic covered SEMS is preferred,[12] with recent data favoring SEMS insertion in this clinical situation because of premature plastic stent clogging[13–15] in the face of a paucity of adequately controlled data for this clinical situation. In the case of hilar cholangiocarcinoma, a meta-analysis of observational studies has noted that in those with resectable tumors, the use of preoperative biliary drainage was also associated with greater overall postoperative complication and infectious rates[9]; the investigators did not differentiate between percutaneous and endoscopic approaches. Endoscopic palliative biliary drainage has also been associated with an improved quality of life as demonstrated in a randomized controlled trial (RCT)[16] and in a real-life setting.[17]

## BILIARY DRAINAGE FOR UNRESECTABLE DISTAL BILIARY LESIONS

In the case of unresectable pancreatic and peripancreatic tumors in which palliation is the goal, a meta-analysis of RCTs comparing surgical drainage procedures with an endoscopic approach has demonstrated a lower rate of recurrent biliary obstruction (relative risk [RR], 0.14; 95% confidence interval [CI], 0.03–0.63) with surgery and no difference in major complications or mortality, but endoscopy was associated with a shorter hospital stay.[18] Of note, 4 of the 5 studies in this meta-analysis used plastic stents as definitive endoscopic drainage method, limiting the contemporary interpretation of these results[18] in the era of metal stents. Issues related to actual patient resectability in an unselected group, coupled with the availability of timely surgery and the recent encouraging responses to preoperative neoadjuvant therapies for locally advanced tumors that become resectable, are perhaps the principal reasons why an endoscopic approach is currently the preferred method of drainage in the palliative setting in spite of these data. A more recent factor is the increasing effectiveness of triple chemotherapy for pancreatic cancer, which has introduced the possibility of downstaging of the tumor in several patients initially deemed unresectable and palliative.

## BILIARY DRAINAGE OF HILAR LESIONS: MAPPING AND MINIMIZING RISK OF ENDOSCOPIC DRAINAGE

The optimal strategy involved in the biliary drainage of patients who present with hilar lesions is particularly complex owing to 3 main factors: the possible contamination of

**Table 1**
Severity grading of complications other than recurrent biliary obstruction after stent placement as per Tokyo 2014 criteria

| Complication | Mild | Moderate | Severe |
|---|---|---|---|
| Pancreatitis | Requirement of admission or prolongation of hospitalization for 3 d | Hospitalization of 4–10 d or at least 1 of the following:<br>1. Requirement for stent removal<br>2. Organ failure that resolves within 48 h<br>3. Local or systemic complications without persistent organ failure | Hospitalization for ≥10 d |
| Cholangitis | Antibiotics only | Febrile or septic illness requiring >3 d of hospitalization or endoscopic or percutaneous intervention | Hospitalization for ≥10 d, septic shock, or organ failure |
| Cholecystitis | Conservative treatment only (antibiotics and/ or no oral intake) | Hospitalization >3 d or requiring any intervention; percutaneous, endoscopic drainage, stent removal, or surgery | Hospitalization for ≥10 d, septic shock, or organ failure |
| Bleeding | No requirement for transfusion | Transfusion of ≤4 units without angiographic intervention and surgery | Requirement for transfusion of ≥5 units or intervention (angiographic or surgical) |
| Perforation | Possible or only very slight leak of fluid or contrast, treated medically for ≤3 d | Any definite perforation treated medically for 4–10 d or endoscopic/ percutaneous intervention | Hospitalization >10 d or surgery |
| Other complications associated with stent placement procedure | Conservative treatment only | Prolonged hospitalization >3 d | Requirement for intervention or surgery |

bile in sequestered biliary segments, the potential for resection with curative intent, and the need to optimize the preservation of liver function.

A new classification system for the prediction of survival in patients with perihilar cholangiocarcinoma, defined as tumors extending from the secondary branches of the right and left hepatic ducts to just above the site of cystic duct origin, has been found to exhibit better performance in predicting survival than the conventional TNM system.[19] This categorization is useful when planning the best method of intervention.

To reduce the incidence of cholangitis, which is a serious complication attributable to undrained ducts after contrast injection, it has been advocated to plan in advance which duct to drain and to avoid unnecessary and possibly damaging use of contrast during endoscopic retrograde cholangiopancreatography (ERCP) as discussed further on.

Preprocedural planning and assessment of the site and extent of biliary obstruction, as well as the presence of lobar atrophy, should precede the insertion of any stent or percutaneous drain.[20] This procedure includes imaging with a view to resectability (including appropriate identification of the hilar vascular anatomy and possible vascular invasion) and early surgical consultation.[12] Preprocedural imaging also assesses the size of the liver segments and the possibility of preoperative segmental portal vein embolization to promote preoperative growth of residual liver volume when radical liver surgery is being considered. When a lobe is atrophied, suggesting vascular tumoral hilar involvement, there is little if any rationale to support stenting of that lobe. Draining 50% of the liver volume is associated with better drainage effectiveness and survival compared with draining less than 50% of the liver volume.[12] Indeed, a study by Vienne and colleagues[21] demonstrated that draining more than 50% of the liver volume produced the best results in terms of drainage effectiveness (odds ratio [OR], 4.5; 95% CI, 1.07–6.46) as well as patient survival (OR, 0.56; 95% CI, 0.32–0.82). Furthermore, intubating an atrophic sector resulting in less than 30% of the total liver volume was unhelpful and increased the risk of cholangitis (OR, 3.04; 95% CI, 1.24–7.48).[21] A similar finding was demonstrated in a study by Chang and colleagues.[22] The choice of liver segment or segments to be drained must also take into account any embolization and anticipated regional postembolization hypertrophy. Patient-related factors that have been associated with failure of resolution of jaundice include a high baseline bilirubin level, diffuse liver metastases, and an international normalized ratio greater than 1.5.[12] Technical considerations in the biliary drainage of hilar lesions are described in later sections.

## PROPHYLACTIC ANTIBIOTICS

A meta-analysis that included 7 RCTs with 1389 cases did not find a reduction in routine post-ERCP cholangitis among unselected cases (RR, 0.58; 95% CI, 0.22–1.55).[23] In a large population-based registry that included 31,188 ERCPs for a variety of indications, the postprocedure adverse event rate was 11.6% in patients who received prophylactic antibiotics compared with 14.2% in those who did not receive them (OR, 0.74; 95% CI, 0.69–0.79).[24] This effect was also present in the subgroup of patients with obstructive jaundice, in whom a resultant reduction in septic complications was observed (OR, 0.76; 95% CI, 0.58–0.97).[24] In contrast, a recent meta-analysis of 9 RCTs and 1573 patients showed a generalized reduction in cholangitis (RR, 0.54; 95% CI, 0.33–0.91), septicemia (RR, 0.35; 95% CI, 0.11–1.11), and bacteremia (RR, 0.50; 95% CI, 0.33–0.78), but no reduction in complications among patients undergoing a successful initial ERCP drainage (RR, 0.98; 95% CI, 0.35–2.69).[25] The investigators of this Cochrane review concluded that further research was required to determine whether antibiotics should be given during or after an ERCP if it becomes apparent that biliary obstruction cannot be relieved during that procedure.

The authors thus suggest that in cases in which technical success is achieved by inserting the stent or stents in the desired segment or segments of the biliary tree (and a clinical success is anticipated with all opacified segments adequately drained), there is likely no need for antibiotic administration; in contradistinction, antibiotic administration is prudent in patients in whom there is failure or suspicion of failure to drain the targeted biliary system.

## AVAILABLE TECHNOLOGIES FOR BILIARY DRAINAGE
### Plastic Stents

Plastic stents are made from different materials such as polyethylene, Teflon, or polyurethane.[26] Polyethylene stents have the advantage of being softer than Teflon stents and possibly change their shape, to a certain extent, in the bile duct (**Fig. 1**). These stents also come in different designs, some with a slightly curved shape to adapt to the common bile duct (CBD) contour and to decrease migration. S-shaped stents are used for draining the left biliary system. Stents with single or double pigtail ends are also available for anchoring these stents. Tannenbaum stents with multiple side flaps, to prevent stent migration, but without side holes are also available, and they may adopt a double-layer design. Plastic stents with an antireflux valve have also been developed.[26]

The size of plastic stents is limited by the size of the accessory channel of the scope, with 14F stents being the largest insertable,[27] but these are difficult to deliver. Among plastic stents, those with 10F diameter have the longest demonstrated patency.[12] However, the average plastic stent patency does not exceed 3 to 4 months,[28] with as mentioned earlier, more recent data suggesting shorter actual patency times in real life (**Fig. 2**).[15]

### Self-Expandable Metal Stents

SEMSs have been developed to overcome the limitations of plastic stents (early obstruction due to small caliber),[27] but these stents can still occlude (**Box 1**). Covered SEMSs are available for distal malignant biliary obstruction; their use in hilar tumors is not indicated because they would block the contralateral hepatic duct as well as intrahepatic side branches and potentially cause cholangitis. Two meta-analyses comparing covered with uncovered SEMSs have been published.[29,30] Each analysis drew different conclusions but differed as to the included studies. The meta-analysis by Saleem and colleagues[30] included 5 RCTs involving 781 patients. The use of covered SEMSs resulted in a longer median stent patency time with a weighted mean difference of 60.6 days (95% CI, 26.0–95.2); however, there were also greater associated rates of stent migration (RR, 8.11; 95% CI, 1.47–44.76), tumor overgrowth (RR, 2.02; 95% CI, 1.08–3.78), and sludge formation (RR, 2.89; 95% CI, 1.27–6.55). In contradistinction, the meta-analysis by Almadi and colleagues[29] included 4 abstract publications in addition to the 5 fully published RCTs, totaling 1061 patients. The weighted mean difference in stent patency was 67.9 days, favoring covered SEMSs over uncovered SEMSs (95% CI, 60.3–75.5), but this conclusion was based on only 2 trials.[29] There existed no difference in patency rates when comparing both stents at 6 months (OR, 1.82; 95% CI, 0.62–5.25) or 12 months (OR, 1.25; 95% CI, 0.65–2.39).[29] These analyses are limited by marked variability in the adopted definitions of stent patency, patient selection, presence of metastasis, type of tumors, as well as the route of insertion across studies (**Figs. 3 and 4**).[31,32]

Furthermore, there exist differences across commercially available SEMS types in axial and radial forces, extent of covering (whether partial or complete), smoothness of the inner surface, as well as the presence of antimigration systems (flared ends, flanges, anchoring fins, flaps, etc).[33] Two more recent RCTs have since assessed partially or completely covered SEMS with antimigration systems. Both demonstrated increased duration of stent patency for the covered SEMS with disparate conclusions about migration rates.[34,35]

In a small study, the use of SEMSs with an antireflux system was studied in 13 patients with distal malignant biliary obstruction that had already occluded because of

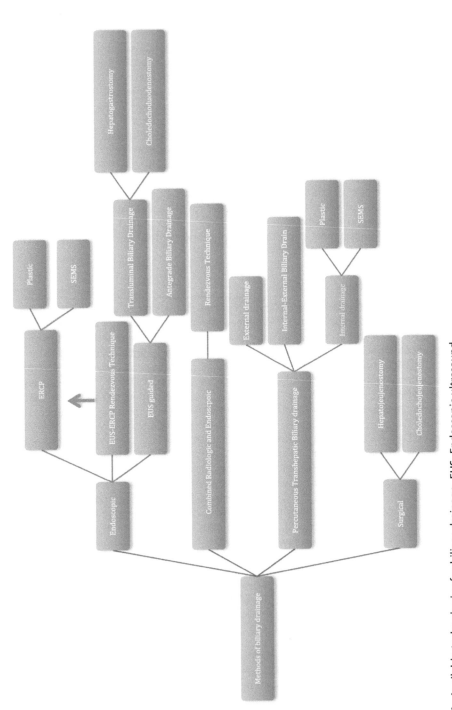

**Fig. 1.** Available technologies for biliary drainage. EUS, Endoscopic ultrasound.

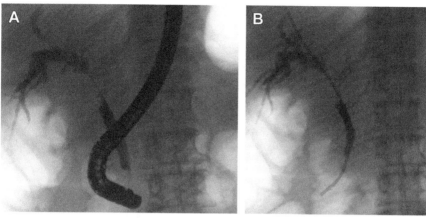

**Fig. 2.** A 64-year-old woman with metastatic adenocarcinoma of unknown origin and poor functional status developed biliary obstruction due to liver metastasis. (*A*) There is external compression of the common hepatic duct with dilatation of the right biliary system; selective cannulation of the duct is achieved. (*B*) A plastic biliary stent is inserted with satisfactory position.

food debris. Although this technology was effective in this small sample and resulted in a longer patency time compared with the initial conventional SEMS use, the novel stent design carried a high migration rate (31%).[36]

An RCT noted a survival advantage for the use of percutaneously placed covered Viabil SEMS (Conmed) compared with uncovered Wallstents (Boston Scientific) (243.5 vs 180.5 days, respectively; *P* value = .04) in palliating extrahepatic cholangiocarcinomas[37]; another RCT by the same group comparing covered with uncovered SEMS for patients with pancreatic head cancers did not show any difference in clinical outcomes.[38]

## THE USE OF SPHINCTEROTOMY

In a meta-analysis that included 3 RCTs, the use of sphincterotomy before stent insertion was associated with a lower rate of pancreatitis (OR, 0.34; 95% CI, 0.12–0.93) but a higher rate of bleeding (OR, 9.70; 95% CI, 1.21–77.75).[39] Of note, a different type of

---

**Box 1**
**Causes of stent occlusion**

Tumor ingrowth/mucosal hyperplasia

Tumor overgrowth

Sludge with/without stones

Hemobilia

Food impaction

Bile duct kinking

Others

*Adapted from* the Isayama H, Hamada T, Yasuda I, et al. TOKYO criteria 2014 for transpapillary biliary stenting. Dig Endosc 2015;27:259–64.

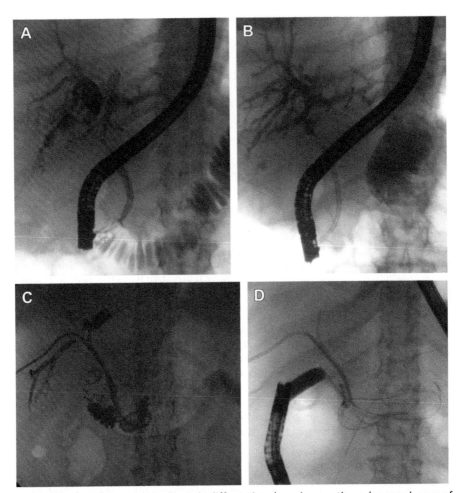

**Fig. 3.** A 58-year-old woman had poorly differentiated mucin-secreting adenocarcinoma of the gallbladder. (A) Initial ERCP was performed when the patient had cholangitis, and no clear diagnosis was reached. A long stricture is seen involving the common hepatic duct and extending into the right and left hepatic ducts. (B) A plastic biliary stent was inserted. (C) The patient developed cholangitis, and an internal/external percutaneous biliary drain was inserted through interventional radiology. (D) She subsequently developed signs of gastric outlet obstruction and did not want percutaneous drains, so an ERCP was performed and the duodenum was dilated to facilitate insertion of the duodenoscope. (E) Both the right and left biliary systems were cannulated with a wire, and an uncovered SEMS was inserted in to the left system. (F) Then, a second uncovered SEMS was inserted into the right biliary system. (G) Next, a duodenal stent was inserted. (H) Final image after removal of the percutaneous drain.

stent was used in each of these studies including plastic,[40] uncovered,[41] and covered[42] SEMSs. Furthermore, most of the cases of pancreatitis originated from the study by Zhou and colleagues[41] that had an unusually high rate of post-ERCP pancreatitis (31.7%) in the nonsphincterotomy group. A recent RCT found no added benefit in performing a sphincterotomy in cases with nonresectable pancreatic cancer.[43] Whether these considerations apply to perihilar tumor strictures when more

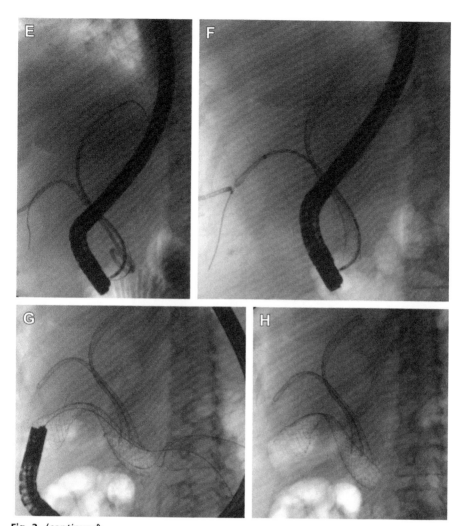

**Fig. 3.** (*continued*).

than 1 stent may be needed, and in which the geometric forces exerted onto the pancreatic opening, is unclear.[12]

The Otaru consensus[44] has recently stated that it is unnecessary to perform a sphincterotomy in patients with pancreatic cancer requiring biliary stenting, although there were reservations in generalizing this statement to patients with all causes of distal malignant biliary obstruction.

## INSERTION OF STENTS ABOVE VERSUS ACROSS THE SPHINCTER OF ODDI

It has been postulated that stent insertion where the distal tip remains above the papilla could prevent the reflux of bacteria and undigested materials into the biliary system as well as the stent and thus contribute to prolonged patency. In an RCT of patients with malignant biliary obstruction, there was no difference according to where the lower extremity of a plastic stent was placed with regard to its impact on stent patency duration,

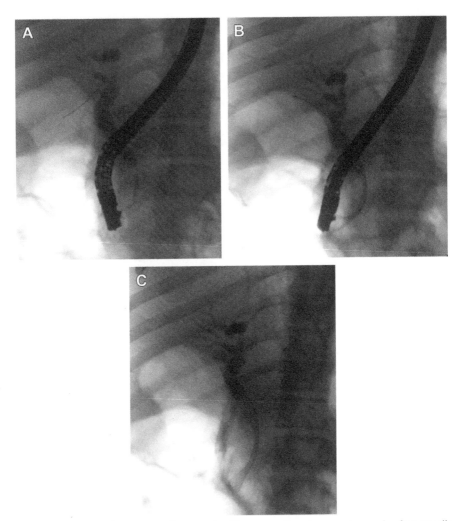

**Fig. 4.** A 50-year-old man was diagnosed with pancreatic adenocarcinoma by fine-needle aspiration via endoscopic ultrasound that was deemed to be unresectable. (*A*) ERCP shows a distal common bile duct stricture. (*B*) A single uncovered SEMS was inserted. (*C*) Final image after deployment of the stent.

but the study might have been underpowered.[45] A retrospective cohort study suggested that the most significant risk factor for the development of cholangitis was a transpapillary position of the SEMS[46] but that the corresponding CI on multivariable modeling was extremely wide,[46] whereas a second study found that inserting the SEMS across the sphincter was associated with developing pancreatitis (4.1% vs 25.0%, *P* value <.01) but that there was no effect on cumulative stent patency or patient survival.[47] An international RCT of 84 patients with unresectable malignant biliary obstruction randomized subjects to either insertion of a fully covered SEMS above the sphincter of Oddi without a sphincterotomy versus insertion of the same SEMS across the sphincter of Oddi after a sphincterotomy. Placement of the SEMS above the sphincter of Oddi did not prolong SEMS patency and did not reduce the incidence of cholangitis without occlusion, whereas placement across the sphincter of Oddi resulted in more external migration.[48] SEMS occlusion was also more frequent in those with pancreatic cancer if the SEMS was inserted above the sphincter of Oddi.[48]

## PLASTIC STENTS VERSUS SELF-EXPANDABLE METAL STENTS

A meta-analysis of 7 trials (724 patients) suggested that SEMS were associated with greater patency rates when compared with plastic stents for malignant biliary obstruction with an RR of stent occlusion of 0.44 (95% CI, 0.3–0.63).[49] In a meta-analysis comparing SEMSs to plastic stents in hilar malignant strictures, SEMSs were associated with a higher successful drainage rate (OR, 0.26; 95% CI, 0.16–0.42), lower early complication rate (OR, 2.92; 95% CI, 1.65–5.17), longer stent patency (hazard ratio [HR], 0.43; 95% CI, 0.30–0.61), and a patient survival advantage (HR, 0.73; 95% CI, 0.56–0.96).[50] This result was emphasized in the Otaru consensus.[51]

It has been suggested that it is cost effective to insert plastic stents if the patient's survival is expected to be less than 4 months, whereas insertion of an SEMS is favored[12] if anticipated survival is greater or if the cost of the SEMS is less than 50% of the cost of the ERCP. SEMS were recently found to be more cost effective in settings not only in which ERCP costs are high but also in which these are lower than the cost of SEMS.[49,52] Most recently, a cost analysis in an RCT determined an average cost of US $6541 when an SEMS was inserted initially compared with US $19,054 when a plastic stent was first used.[53,54] Furthermore, the chance of experiencing no occlusion over the 12 months was 65% for the SEMS group, whereas it was only 13.85% for the plastic stent group.[53] A second very recent cost-effectiveness analysis of an RCT from the Netherlands confirmed no significant difference in the total cost per patient between plastic stent and SEMS in patients with short survival (€6555 vs €5719, respectively; $P = .4$) or metastatic disease (€6593 vs €6179, respectively; $P = .69$).[55]

## HILAR NEOPLASMS: SPECIAL CONSIDERATIONS

Numerous devices have been used in the management of patients with hilar tumors requiring bilateral biliary drainage including parallel placement of 2 SEMSs, that is, stent-by-stent,[56,57] a partial stent-in-stent using large-cell-width stents or open-cell stents,[58,59] or inserting a plastic stent initially to facilitate insertion of SEMS at a later time.[60] Note that any SEMS used in the proximal biliary tree should be uncovered because of the risk of blocking side branch biliary radicals and developing cholangitis.[12]

A retrospective cohort study demonstrated decreased survival when both lobes were opacified but only 1 lobe was drained. Indeed, the investigators reported a median patient survival of 46 days in such patients versus 131 days in those in whom both lobes were opacified and drained versus 160 days in whom only the targeted lobe was opacified and drained.[22]

A meta-analysis[61] assessed the use of bilateral stents in the drainage of hilar biliary neoplasms. In the case of SEMS, the insertion of bilateral SEMS was less successful when compared with unilateral drainage (OR, 0.33; 95% CI, 0.16–0.69) but resulted in a greater decrease in serum bilirubin level (OR, 2.25; 95% CI, 1.29–3.90) and less-frequent early complications (OR, 0.11; 95% CI, 0.04–0.28), late complications (OR, 0.23; 95% CI, 0.07–0.75), and overall complications (OR, 0.53; 95% CI, 0.32–0.86). However, there was no difference in the incidence of cholangitis (OR, 0.90; 95% CI, 0.59–1.38) or 30-day mortality (OR, 4.34; 95% CI, 0.74–25.56). For plastic stenting, when comparing bilateral to unilateral stenting, there was no difference in the success of placement (OR, 0.94; 95% CI, 0.64–1.38), decrease in bilirubin levels (OR, 2.29; 95% CI, 0.67–7.81), overall complications (OR, 1.42; 95% CI, 0.21–9.33), overall cholangitis (OR, 1.46; 95% CI, 0. 68–3.16), or 30-day mortality (OR, 0.78; 95% CI, 0.38–1.61).[61] A limitation of this meta-analysis is that it could not evaluate the effect of stents in subgroups of patients afflicted with different stages of hilar tumors.[61]

A second meta-analysis comparing multiple strategies of unilateral to bilateral stenting in malignant hilar obstruction found that unilateral drainage had a higher success in stent insertion (OR, 3.44; 95% CI, 1.91–6.19) but that there was no difference in drainage success (OR, 1.73; 95% CI, 0.89–3.37), early complications (OR, 0.96; 95% CI, 0.18–5.13), late complications (OR, 1.41; 95% CI, 0.54–3.67), stent patency (HR, 0.57; 95% CI, 0.19–1.73), or patient survival (HR, 0.75; 95 %CI, 0.31–1.80).[50] This meta-analysis has multiple limitations including incorporating together retrospective studies as well as RCTs.[50]

In a large retrospective study of 480 patients with hilar cholangiocarcinoma, the independent prognostic factors associated with prolonged stent patency on multivariate analysis was the use of SEMS ($P<.01$) and bilateral stenting ($P<.01$).[62]

Although most of the literature has centered on the use of different types or numbers of stents, an RCT that used carbon dioxide to perform a cholangiogram as opposed to standard contrast showed a reduction in the rate of cholangitis (5.6% vs 33.3%, $P = .04$) as well as mean hospital stay ($P<.05$) in the carbon dioxide group[63]; similar findings were seen in another RCT using air cholangiography.[64]

In light of these summary data, the authors recommend that in experienced centers, after appropriate pre-ERCP mapping of the site of obstruction, at the very least, a unilateral drainage procedure should be performed if only 1 side is opacified, ideally with an uncovered SEMS. If the endoscopist has confidence in its success or if both sides have been injected with contrast, bilateral biliary drainage should be performed.

## SIDE-BY-SIDE METHOD VERSUS STENT-IN-STENT METHOD

After cannulation of the CBD, a sphincterotomy is usually performed to allow manipulation of the SEMS and instrument in the biliary system. Stricture dilation is performed if necessary to facilitate SEMS insertion. When using the side-by-side method for SEMS, both the right and left biliary systems are cannulated and the wires are inserted and kept in place in a sequential manner; SEMSs are inserted and then deployed in either a simultaneous or a sequential manner after which the wires and the delivery systems are removed.[56] In the stent-in-stent technique, the first SEMS is inserted over the guidewire into the more acutely angulated left hepatic duct and the SEMS is deployed; the wire and deployment system are then removed. A wire is then introduced and redirected through the interstices of the first SEMS wall into the contralateral intrahepatic ductal system, dilatation of the intersects could be performed if needed, and the second SEMS is inserted over the wire and then deployed in a Y-shaped configuration.[56]

In a Korean study, both techniques were associated with similar success of drainage (78.9% vs 81.8%), early complications (31.6% vs 22.7%), late complications (36.8% vs 50.0%), or death (47.4% vs 54.5%).[65] A second study demonstrated 100% technical success but with a need for reintervention in 50% of cases after a median of 98 days.[56] There was no difference in the need for reintervention, successful reintervention, or procedural length between both techniques. Of note, the sample sizes of both studies[56] were small and these might have been underpowered. A study by Naitoh and colleagues[66] found that the complication rate for the side-by-side technique was greater and the cumulative patency was longer when compared with that of the stent-in-stent method.

Also, the management of an occluded SEMS is challenging when a stent-in-stent method is used because access to the later inserted SEMS would be easy but access to the first SEMS could be problematic.

## PERCUTANEOUS DRAINAGE AND THE CHOICE OF APPROACH: ENDOSCOPIC VERSUS RADIOLOGICAL

Percutaneous interventions into the biliary system in the context of malignant biliary obstruction can be performed to provide biliary drainage in the case of proximal or distal biliary obstruction, either as a temporary method or to palliate the patient by placing either plastic stents or long-term SEMSs.[67] From a technical point of view, percutaneous drainage is performed through accessing the peripheral biliary tree through insertion of a needle under imaging guidance followed by obtaining a cholangiogram and subsequently insertion of guidewires and catheters with manipulation under imaging and then insertion of a tube or stent for external and/or internal drainage. These interventions usually are performed in multiple sessions to achieve the intended result.[67] The success rate for the cannulation of a dilated biliary tree is around 95%.[67] Potential complications include sepsis, cholangitis, bile leaks, hemorrhage, or pneumothorax in about 2% of procedures, while mortality is reported in 1.7% of cases. Also, inadvertent catheter dislodgement requiring a repeated percutaneous intervention is well recognized.[67]

A rendezvous procedure refers to the situation when a percutaneous transhepatic cholangiographic approach is used to facilitate stent insertion at ERCP. This procedure involves advancing a wire through the puncture created for access in an antegrade manner through the papilla and then retrieving the wire with a snare through the duodenoscope. The ERCP procedure is then completed in a regular manner.

Although the choice of an endoscopic versus a percutaneous approach is influenced by available expertise (that also affects the generalizability of published data), this decision is an important one. The aforementioned clinical effectiveness data on biliary drainage often have mixed both approaches, especially with regard to hilar tumors. In the following discussion, the authors attempt to tease out the information that can guide clinicians in deciding on the best route of drainage, endoscopic versus percutaneous, in specific situations.

In the case of distal biliary obstruction, endoscopic approaches for biliary stenting are usually less technically challenging and are the preferred guidelines-based approach[68] given some of the limitations of the percutaneous approach including portal vein injury, peritoneal dissemination, and tract recurrence.

When compared with the endoscopic approach, the main advantages of percutaneous drainage relate to drainage in cases of hilar lesions especially with respect to drainage of the intended lobe of the liver. This comes at the cost of the need for repeated procedures because it is a multistep process and is uncomfortable for the patient at the percutaneous site of the catheter insertion, especially on the right side. There also exists the risk of catheter dislodgement, infection, and bile leaks around the catheter.[69] In cases with perihilar tumors and a Bismuth-Corlette type 2 or greater, a percutaneous approach might achieve better biliary drainage with fewer infectious complications.[12] If an ERCP is performed and an injected biliary system cannot be drained, there is a high probability of cholangitis, whereas if a percutaneous drainage procedure fails and a stricture cannot be passed, an external drain can still be left in place with a lower probability of cholangitis.[12,69,70] Furthermore, low-volume centers tend to have a lower success rate of endoscopic drainage, thus the decision to perform endoscopic versus percutaneous drainage procedure depends on the available expertise as well as the presence of multidisciplinary teams.[12,70] A meta-analysis of 5 retrospective studies and 3 RCTs (2 performed in 1987 and 2002) comparing percutaneous with endoscopic drainage showed no difference in therapeutic success between the 2 approaches.[69] Furthermore, 1 of the 3 RCTs compared percutaneously inserted SEMS with endoscopically inserted plastic stents,[71] whereas the remaining 2 studied exclusively plastic stent insertion.[72,73] A second meta-analysis on the topic demonstrated no difference between the percutaneous and endoscopic approaches (OR 2.34; 95% CI, 0.32–17.16).[74] Paik and colleagues[75] compared percutaneously inserted SEMSs to those inserted endoscopically in a retrospective study and found the technical success to be higher in the percutaneous group (92% vs 77.3%). The endoscopic success rate in the study by Paik and colleagues[75] was much lower compared with that reported in experienced centers where initial and final technical success rates were 96% and 100%, respectively, for malignant perihilar biliary obstruction, with a functional success rate of 89%.[76] The finding in the study by Paik and colleagues[75,77] may be explained by the higher percentage of patients who had 2 stents inserted in the percutaneous intervention group (54%) compared with only 16% of patients in the endoscopy group.

Another concern relates to the possibility of peritoneal seeding in those undergoing percutaneous drainage followed by radical surgery for hilar cholangiocarcinoma.[78] A retrospective study found that survival was compromised because of tumor seeding in those undergoing percutaneous as opposed to endoscopic drainage (HR, 2.08; 95% CI, 1.21–3.07).[78]

In summary, there is a paucity of evidence to favor either a percutaneous or an endoscopic drainage approach in patients with hilar tumors because of the limitations of the studies conducted. At present, and till further studies clarify the optimal method of drainage,[79] the preferred choice may depend mainly on local experience and available resources; when endoscopic expertise is limited, percutaneous biliary drainage in perihilar tumors is favored.[80]

## RECURRENT BILIARY OBSTRUCTION AFTER INITIAL DRAINAGE

When a plastic stent gets obstructed, it should be exchanged for an SEMS, whereas if an SEMS is occluded, a second SEMS should be inserted within the older one unless the expected survival is less than 3 months, in which case a plastic stent can be used.[12] A systematic review of 10 retrospective studies demonstrated that there existed no differences between the insertion of a plastic stent or an SEMS when the initial SEMS gets occluded (RR, 1.24; 95% CI, 0.92–1.67) and that the weighted mean RR difference for the duration of patency of the second stent was 0.46 (95% CI, −0.30 to 1.23); the investigators noted no difference in survival with a weighted mean RR difference of −1.13 (95% CI, −2.33 to 0.07),[81] neither being significant.

## CHOLYCYSTITIS AND CHOLANGITIS

Although it is perceived that cholecystitis would occur more often in patients drained with a covered versus an uncovered SEMS, it has not been confirmed in RCTs. In RCTs, the rates of cholecystitis in those randomized to SEMS versus plastic stents ranged from 5% to 7%.[82,83] In retrospective studies, cholecystitis developed after insertion of SEMSs for malignant biliary obstruction from 1% to 9.7% of all cases.[47,84,85] Factors associated with this complication included location of the tumor across the cystic duct (OR, 12.7; 95% CI, 3.2–49.8) and the presence of gallstones (OR, 6.6; 95% CI, 1.5–29.3).[84] A retrospective study of 376 patients who underwent SEMS insertion for distal malignant biliary obstruction found on multivariable analysis that cholecystitis was associated with tumor involvement of the origin of the cystic duct (OR, 5.40; 95% CI, 2.32–13.14) if the axial force of the SEMS was greater than or equal to 4 N (OR, 5.33; 95% CI, 1.74–23.27) or if the length of the SEMS was less than or equal to 6 cm (OR, 3.19; 95% CI, 1.30–8.62).[85] The highest rate of incidence of cholecystitis was in patients with involvement of the origin of the cystic duct by the tumor and with an SEMS less than or equal to 6 cm in length (27.3% vs 7.8%) or a high axial force (25.0% vs 5.2%).[85]

Covered SEMSs were not found to be associated with cholecystitis when compared with uncovered SEMSs (8.0 vs 2.6%, $P = .129$),[85] thus this complication seems, at least significantly, inherent to the underlying tumor mainly and may be compounded by changes in the orientation of the cystic duct in relation to the common bile duct induced by the stent.

If cholangitis does develop, then biliary drainage should be attempted endoscopically, or if difficult, a percutaneous transhepatic biliary drain may be considered as an alternative.[86] Furthermore, the proper antimicrobial agent should be prescribed based on the severity of the cholangitis as well as the local antimicrobial susceptibility patterns as per health care institution and whether the infection is health care related or the patient presented from the community.[87]

## RECENT INNOVATIONS
### Nonconventional Approaches to Malignant Biliary Drainage

Endoscopic ultrasound (EUS)-guided biliary drainage is starting to be used outside tertiary referral centers and is an alternative to percutaneous drainage when conventional ERCP has failed.[88,89] Usually before pursuing drainage procedures with EUS, a trial of EUS-facilitated biliary cannulation is attempted whereby, after an intrahepatic or extrahepatic biliary duct is punctured, a guidewire is advanced from the dilated proximal biliary system through the stricture and out through the papilla. The EUS scope is then withdrawn while keeping the guidewire in place, a duodenoscope is introduced, and the guidewire is retrieved with the procedure completed as a regular ERCP. In EUS-guided biliary drainage, after the introduction of the guidewire into the proximal dilated biliary system, a SEMS is introduced with its proximal end into the biliary system and its distal end either in the stomach or in the duodenal lumen. In a small RCT[90] comparing EUS-guided choledochoduodenostomy to percutaneous drainage, there was no difference noted in the technical as well as clinical success and no difference in complication rates. Also, the use of an EUS-guided rendezvous procedure or the insertion of stents in an antegrade manner have been found to be associated with similar success and complication rates,[91] with only needle-knife use as a factor significantly associated with adverse events.[92]

### Radioactive Stents

Data for the use of stents that provide radiation have been encouraging; an RCT for percutaneously inserted SEMS that contained $^{125}$I radioactive seeds of CIAE-6711 demonstrated that the overall survivals in the irradiation stent group were higher than those in the conventional SEMS group, median being 7.40 versus 2.50 months, respectively.[93]

### Three-Dimensional Endoscopic Retrograde Cholangiopancreatography

This new technology using cone beam computed tomography has recently been used in ERCP with the aim of better spatial resolution of the biliary tree.[94] Although this application has not been used in cases with malignant biliary obstruction requiring stenting, it does seem to be of potential use in this patient population.

## SUMMARY

The approach to malignant biliary drainage has evolved significantly over the past decade with improvements in endoscopic technologies and drainage devices. The strategy differs when assessing distal versus proximal sites of obstruction. Regardless, the choice of optimal stent remains unclear, even though more recent data favor SEMS for distal tumors. In hilar obstruction, a percutaneous approach may be more effective, especially if endoscopic expertise is lacking. As a rule, preprocedural imaging should identify the optimal drainage strategy, with an attempt at draining all opacified segments at the time of the procedure. In all cases, an integrated multidisciplinary approach should help determine the best approach based on local expertise and technological availabilities.

## REFERENCES

1. Siegel R, Ma J, Zou Z, et al. Cancer statistics, 2014. CA Cancer J Clin 2014;64: 9–29.
2. Alvaro D, Crocetti E, Ferretti S, et al, AISF Cholangiocarcinoma committee. Descriptive epidemiology of cholangiocarcinoma in Italy. Dig Liver Dis 2010;42:490–5.
3. Pinter M, Hucke F, Zielonke N, et al. Incidence and mortality trends for biliary tract cancers in Austria. Liver Int 2014;34:1102–8.
4. Coupland VH, Kocher HM, Berry DP, et al. Incidence and survival for hepatic, pancreatic and biliary cancers in England between 1998 and 2007. Cancer Epidemiol 2012;36:e207–14.
5. Jepsen P, Vilstrup H, Tarone RE, et al. Incidence rates of intra- and extrahepatic cholangiocarcinomas in Denmark from 1978 through 2002. J Natl Cancer Inst 2007;99:895–7.
6. Patel T. Worldwide trends in mortality from biliary tract malignancies. BMC Cancer 2002;2:10.
7. Shaib YH, Davila JA, McGlynn K, et al. Rising incidence of intrahepatic cholangiocarcinoma in the United States: a true increase? J Hepatol 2004;40:472–7.
8. von Hahn T, Ciesek S, Wegener G, et al. Epidemiological trends in incidence and mortality of hepatobiliary cancers in Germany. Scand J Gastroenterol 2011;46: 1092–8.
9. Liu F, Li Y, Wei Y, et al. Preoperative biliary drainage before resection for hilar cholangiocarcinoma: whether or not? A systematic review. Dig Dis Sci 2011;56:663–72.
10. Sun C, Yan G, Li Z, et al. A meta-analysis of the effect of preoperative biliary stenting on patients with obstructive jaundice. Medicine 2014;93:e189.
11. Fang Y, Gurusamy KS, Wang Q, et al. Pre-operative biliary drainage for obstructive jaundice. Cochrane Database Syst Rev 2012;(9):CD005444.
12. Dumonceau JM, Tringali A, Blero D, et al. Biliary stenting: indications, choice of stents and results: European Society of Gastrointestinal Endoscopy (ESGE) clinical guideline. Endoscopy 2012;44:277–98.
13. Baron TH, Kozarek RA. Preoperative biliary stents in pancreatic cancer–proceed with caution. N Engl J Med 2010;362:170–2.
14. Bonin EA, Baron TH. Preoperative biliary stents in pancreatic cancer. J Hepatobiliary Pancreat Sci 2011;18:621–9.
15. Ge PS, Hamerski CM, Watson RR, et al. Plastic biliary stent patency in patients with locally advanced pancreatic adenocarcinoma receiving downstaging chemotherapy. Gastrointest Endosc 2015;81:360–6.
16. Barkay O, Mosler P, Schmitt CM, et al. Effect of endoscopic stenting of malignant bile duct obstruction on quality of life. J Clin Gastroenterol 2013;47:526–31.

17. Abraham NS, Barkun JS, Barkun AN. Palliation of malignant biliary obstruction: a prospective trial examining impact on quality of life. Gastrointest Endosc 2002; 56:835–41.
18. Glazer ES, Hornbrook MC, Krouse RS. A meta-analysis of randomized trials: immediate stent placement vs surgical bypass in the palliative management of malignant biliary obstruction. J Pain Symptom Manage 2014;47:307–14.
19. Chaiteerakij R, Harmsen WS, Marrero CR, et al. A new clinically based staging system for perihilar cholangiocarcinoma. Am J Gastroenterol 2014;109:1881–90.
20. Kozarek RA. Malignant hilar strictures: one stent or two? Plastic versus self-expanding metal stents? The role of liver atrophy and volume assessment as a predictor of survival in patients undergoing endoscopic stent placement. Gastrointest Endosc 2010;72:736–8.
21. Vienne A, Hobeika E, Gouya H, et al. Prediction of drainage effectiveness during endoscopic stenting of malignant hilar strictures: the role of liver volume assessment. Gastrointest Endosc 2010;72:728–35.
22. Chang WH, Kortan P, Haber GB. Outcome in patients with bifurcation tumors who undergo unilateral versus bilateral hepatic duct drainage. Gastrointest Endosc 1998;47:354–62.
23. Bai Y, Gao F, Gao J, et al. Prophylactic antibiotics cannot prevent endoscopic retrograde cholangiopancreatography-induced cholangitis: a meta-analysis. Pancreas 2009;38:126–30.
24. Olsson G, Arnelo U, Lundell L, et al. The role of antibiotic prophylaxis in routine endoscopic retrograde cholangiopancreatography investigations as assessed prospectively in a nationwide study cohort. Scand J Gastroenterol 2015;50: 924–31.
25. Brand M, Bizos D, O'Farrell P Jr. Antibiotic prophylaxis for patients undergoing elective endoscopic retrograde cholangiopancreatography. Cochrane Database Syst Rev 2010;(10):CD007345.
26. Dumonceau JM, Heresbach D, Deviere J, et al. Biliary stents: models and methods for endoscopic stenting. Endoscopy 2011;43:617–26.
27. Isayama H, Nakai Y, Kogure H, et al. Biliary self-expandable metallic stent for unresectable malignant distal biliary obstruction: which is better: covered or uncovered? Dig Endosc 2013;25(Suppl 2):71–4.
28. Park YJ, Kang DH. Endoscopic drainage in patients with inoperable hilar cholangiocarcinoma. Korean J Intern Med 2013;28:8–18.
29. Almadi MA, Barkun AN, Martel M. No benefit of covered vs uncovered self-expandable metal stents in patients with malignant distal biliary obstruction: a meta-analysis. Clin Gastroenterol Hepatol 2013;11:27–37.e1.
30. Saleem A, Leggett CL, Murad MH, et al. Meta-analysis of randomized trials comparing the patency of covered and uncovered self-expandable metal stents for palliation of distal malignant bile duct obstruction. Gastrointest Endosc 2011; 74:321–7.e1–3.
31. Almadi MA, Barkun AN, Martel M. Two meta-analyses with different conclusions: stent outcomes should be standardized before their integration–reply. Clin Gastroenterol Hepatol 2013;11:748–9.
32. Hamada T, Nakai Y, Isayama H. Two meta-analyses with different conclusions: stent outcomes should be standardized before their integration. Clin Gastroenterol Hepatol 2013;11:748.
33. Isayama H, Nakai Y, Kawakubo K, et al. Covered metallic stenting for malignant distal biliary obstruction: clinical results according to stent type. J Hepatobiliary Pancreat Sci 2011;18:673–7.

34. Kitano M, Yamashita Y, Tanaka K, et al. Covered self-expandable metal stents with an anti-migration system improve patency duration without increased complications compared with uncovered stents for distal biliary obstruction caused by pancreatic carcinoma: a randomized multicenter trial. Am J Gastroenterol 2013;108:1713–22.

35. Hu B, Wang TT, Wu J, et al. Antireflux stents to reduce the risk of cholangitis in patients with malignant biliary strictures: a randomized trial. Endoscopy 2014; 46:120–6.

36. Hamada T, Isayama H, Nakai Y, et al. Novel antireflux covered metal stent for recurrent occlusion of biliary metal stents: a pilot study. Dig Endosc 2014;26: 264–9.

37. Krokidis M, Fanelli F, Orgera G, et al. Percutaneous treatment of malignant jaundice due to extrahepatic cholangiocarcinoma: covered Viabil stent versus uncovered Wallstents. Cardiovasc Intervent Radiol 2010;33:97–106.

38. Krokidis M, Fanelli F, Orgera G, et al. Percutaneous palliation of pancreatic head cancer: randomized comparison of ePTFE/FEP-covered versus uncovered nitinol biliary stents. Cardiovasc Intervent Radiol 2011;34:352–61.

39. Cui PJ, Yao J, Zhao YJ, et al. Biliary stenting with or without sphincterotomy for malignant biliary obstruction: a meta-analysis. World J Gastroenterol 2014;20: 14033–9.

40. Giorgio PD, Luca LD. Comparison of treatment outcomes between biliary plastic stent placements with and without endoscopic sphincterotomy for inoperable malignant common bile duct obstruction. World J Gastroenterol 2004;10:1212–4.

41. Zhou H, Li L, Zhu F, et al. Endoscopic sphincterotomy associated cholangitis in patients receiving proximal biliary self-expanding metal stents. Hepatobiliary Pancreat Dis Int 2012;11:643–9.

42. Artifon EL, Sakai P, Ishioka S, et al. Endoscopic sphincterotomy before deployment of covered metal stent is associated with greater complication rate: a prospective randomized control trial. J Clin Gastroenterol 2008;42:815–9.

43. Hayashi T, Kawakami H, Osanai M, et al. No Benefit of Endoscopic Sphincterotomy Before Biliary Placement of Self-expandable Metal Stents for Unresectable Pancreatic Cancer. Clin Gastroenterol Hepatol 2015;13(6):1151–8.e2.

44. Irisawa A, Katanuma A, Itoi T. Otaru consensus on biliary stenting for unresectable distal malignant biliary obstruction. Dig Endosc 2013;25(Suppl 2):52–7.

45. Pedersen FM, Lassen AT, Schaffalitzky de Muckadell OB. Randomized trial of stent placed above and across the sphincter of Oddi in malignant bile duct obstruction. Gastrointest Endosc 1998;48:574–9.

46. Okamoto T, Fujioka S, Yanagisawa S, et al. Placement of a metallic stent across the main duodenal papilla may predispose to cholangitis. Gastrointest Endosc 2006;63:792–6.

47. Jo JH, Park BH. Suprapapillary versus transpapillary stent placement for malignant biliary obstruction: which is better? J Vasc Interv Radiol 2015;26:573–82.

48. Cho JN, Han J, Kim HG, et al. Prospective randomized trial comparing covered metal stent placed above and across the sphincter of Oddi in malignant biliary obstruction. Gastrointest Endosc 2013;77:AB139–40.

49. Moss AC, Morris E, Leyden J, et al. Do the benefits of metal stents justify the costs? A systematic review and meta-analysis of trials comparing endoscopic stents for malignant biliary obstruction. Eur J Gastroenterol Hepatol 2007;19:1119–24.

50. Hong W, Sun X, Zhu Q. Endoscopic stenting for malignant hilar biliary obstruction: should it be metal or plastic and unilateral or bilateral? Eur J Gastroenterol Hepatol 2013;25:1105–12.

51. Katanuma A, Irisawa A, Itoi T. Otaru consensus on biliary stenting for unresectable malignant hilar biliary obstruction. Dig Endosc 2013;25(Suppl 2): 58–62.
52. Yoon WJ, Ryu JK, Yang KY, et al. A comparison of metal and plastic stents for the relief of jaundice in unresectable malignant biliary obstruction in Korea: an emphasis on cost-effectiveness in a country with a low ERCP cost. Gastrointest Endosc 2009;70:284–9.
53. Barkun AN, Adam V, Martel M. Cost effectiveness analysis of partially covered self expandable metal versus polyethylene stent for patients with malignant biliary obstruction. Gastrointest Endosc 2013;77:AB241.
54. Wang AY. Is plastic stenting for pancreatic cancer still relevant or obsolete in 2015? Gastrointest Endosc 2015;81:367–9.
55. Walter D, van Boeckel PG, Groenen MJ, et al. Cost efficacy of metal stents for palliation of extrahepatic bile duct obstruction in a randomized controlled trial. Gastroenterology 2015;149:130–8.
56. Law R, Baron TH. Bilateral metal stents for hilar biliary obstruction using a 6Fr delivery system: outcomes following bilateral and side-by-side stent deployment. Dig Dis Sci 2013;58:2667–72.
57. Lee TH, Park do H, Lee SS, et al. Technical feasibility and revision efficacy of the sequential deployment of endoscopic bilateral side-by-side metal stents for malignant hilar biliary strictures: a multicenter prospective study. Dig Dis Sci 2013; 58:547–55.
58. Kogure H, Isayama H, Nakai Y, et al. Newly designed large cell Niti-S stent for malignant hilar biliary obstruction: a pilot study. Surg Endosc 2011;25: 463–7.
59. Kim DU, Kang DH, Kim GH, et al. Bilateral biliary drainage for malignant hilar obstruction using the 'stent-in-stent' method with a Y-stent: efficacy and complications. Eur J Gastroenterol Hepatol 2013;25:99–106.
60. Hookey LC, Le Moine O, Deviere J. Use of a temporary plastic stent to facilitate the placement of multiple self-expanding metal stents in malignant biliary hilar strictures. Gastrointest Endosc 2005;62:605–9.
61. Puli SR, Kalva N, Pamulaparthy SR, et al. Bilateral and unilateral stenting for malignant hilar obstruction: a systematic review and meta-analysis. Indian J Gastroenterol 2013;32:355–62.
62. Liberato MJ, Canena JM. Endoscopic stenting for hilar cholangiocarcinoma: efficacy of unilateral and bilateral placement of plastic and metal stents in a retrospective review of 480 patients. BMC Gastroenterol 2012;12:103.
63. Zhang R, Zhao L, Liu Z, et al. Effect of CO2 cholangiography on post-ERCP cholangitis in patients with unresectable malignant hilar obstruction - a prospective, randomized controlled study. Scand J Gastroenterol 2013;48:758–63.
64. Sud R, Puri R, Choudhary NS, et al. Air cholangiogram is not inferior to dye cholangiogram for malignant hilar biliary obstruction: a randomized study of efficacy and safety. Indian J Gastroenterol 2014;33:537–42.
65. Kim KM, Lee KH, Chung YH, et al. A comparison of bilateral stenting methods for malignant hilar biliary obstruction. Hepatogastroenterology 2012;59:341–6.
66. Naitoh I, Hayashi K, Nakazawa T, et al. Side-by-side versus stent-in-stent deployment in bilateral endoscopic metal stenting for malignant hilar biliary obstruction. Dig Dis Sci 2012;57:3279–85.
67. Saad WE, Wallace MJ, Wojak JC, et al. Quality improvement guidelines for percutaneous transhepatic cholangiography, biliary drainage, and percutaneous cholecystostomy. J Vasc Interv Radiol 2010;21:789–95.

68. Yoshitomi H, Miyakawa S, Nagino M, et al. Updated clinical practice guidelines for the management of biliary tract cancers: revision concepts and major revised points. J Hepatobiliary Pancreat Sci 2015;22:274–8.

69. Zhao XQ, Dong JH, Jiang K, et al. Comparison of percutaneous transhepatic biliary drainage and endoscopic biliary drainage in the management of malignant biliary tract obstruction: a meta-analysis. Dig Endosc 2015;27:137–45.

70. Kloek JJ, van der Gaag NA, Aziz Y, et al. Endoscopic and percutaneous preoperative biliary drainage in patients with suspected hilar cholangiocarcinoma. J Gastrointest Surg 2010;14:119–25.

71. Pinol V, Castells A, Bordas JM, et al. Percutaneous self-expanding metal stents versus endoscopic polyethylene endoprostheses for treating malignant biliary obstruction: randomized clinical trial. Radiology 2002;225:27–34.

72. Saluja SS, Gulati M, Garg PK, et al. Endoscopic or percutaneous biliary drainage for gallbladder cancer: a randomized trial and quality of life assessment. Clin Gastroenterol Hepatol 2008;6:944–50.e3.

73. Speer AG, Cotton PB, Russell RC, et al. Randomised trial of endoscopic versus percutaneous stent insertion in malignant obstructive jaundice. Lancet 1987;2: 57–62.

74. Leng JJ, Zhang N, Dong JH. Percutaneous transhepatic and endoscopic biliary drainage for malignant biliary tract obstruction: a meta-analysis. World J Surg Oncol 2014;12:272.

75. Paik WH, Park YS, Hwang JH, et al. Palliative treatment with self-expandable metallic stents in patients with advanced type III or IV hilar cholangiocarcinoma: a percutaneous versus endoscopic approach. Gastrointest Endosc 2009;69: 55–62.

76. Kogure H, Isayama H, Nakai Y, et al. High single-session success rate of endoscopic bilateral stent-in-stent placement with modified large cell Niti-S stents for malignant hilar biliary obstruction. Dig Endosc 2014;26:93–9.

77. Geller A. Klatskin tumor–palliative therapy: the jury is still out or may be not yet in. Gastrointest Endosc 2009;69:63–5.

78. Hirano S, Tanaka E, Tsuchikawa T, et al. Oncological benefit of preoperative endoscopic biliary drainage in patients with hilar cholangiocarcinoma. J Hepatobiliary Pancreat Sci 2014;21:533–40.

79. Wiggers JK, Coelen RJ, Rauws EA, et al. Preoperative endoscopic versus percutaneous transhepatic biliary drainage in potentially resectable perihilar cholangiocarcinoma (DRAINAGE trial): design and rationale of a randomized controlled trial. BMC Gastroenterol 2015;15:20.

80. Ho CS, Warkentin AE. Evidence-based decompression in malignant biliary obstruction. Korean J Radiol 2012;13(Suppl 1):S56–61.

81. Shah T, Desai S, Haque M, et al. Management of occluded metal stents in malignant biliary obstruction: similar outcomes with second metal stents compared to plastic stents. Dig Dis Sci 2012;57:2765–73.

82. Moses PL, Alnaamani KM, Barkun AN, et al. Randomized trial in malignant biliary obstruction: plastic vs partially covered metal stents. World J Gastroenterol 2013; 19:8638–46.

83. Isayama H, Yasuda I, Ryozawa S, et al. Results of a Japanese multicenter, randomized trial of endoscopic stenting for non-resectable pancreatic head cancer (JM-test): Covered Wallstent versus DoubleLayer stent. Dig Endosc 2011;23: 310–5.

84. Suk KT, Kim HS, Kim JW, et al. Risk factors for cholecystitis after metal stent placement in malignant biliary obstruction. Gastrointest Endosc 2006;64:522–9.

85. Nakai Y, Isayama H, Kawakubo K, et al. Metallic stent with high axial force as a risk factor for cholecystitis in distal malignant biliary obstruction. J Gastroenterol Hepatol 2014;29:1557–62.

86. Itoi T, Tsuyuguchi T, Takada T, et al. TG13 indications and techniques for biliary drainage in acute cholangitis (with videos). J Hepatobiliary Pancreat Sci 2013; 20:71–80.

87. Gomi H, Solomkin JS, Takada T, et al. TG13 antimicrobial therapy for acute cholangitis and cholecystitis. J Hepatobiliary Pancreat Sci 2013;20:60–70.

88. Khashab MA, Dewitt J. EUS-guided biliary drainage: is it ready for prime time? Yes! Gastrointest Endosc 2013;78:102–5.

89. Vila JJ, Perez-Miranda M, Vazquez-Sequeiros E, et al. Initial experience with EUS-guided cholangiopancreatography for biliary and pancreatic duct drainage: a Spanish national survey. Gastrointest Endosc 2012;76:1133–41.

90. Artifon EL, Aparicio D, Paione JB, et al. Biliary drainage in patients with unresectable, malignant obstruction where ERCP fails: endoscopic ultrasonography-guided choledochoduodenostomy versus percutaneous drainage. J Clin Gastroenterol 2012;46:768–74.

91. Khashab MA, Valeshabad AK, Modayil R, et al. EUS-guided biliary drainage by using a standardized approach for malignant biliary obstruction: rendezvous versus direct transluminal techniques (with videos). Gastrointest Endosc 2013; 78:734–41.

92. Park do H, Jang JW, Lee SS, et al. EUS-guided biliary drainage with transluminal stenting after failed ERCP: predictors of adverse events and long-term results. Gastrointest Endosc 2011;74:1276–84.

93. Zhu HD, Guo JH, Zhu GY, et al. A novel biliary stent loaded with (125)I seeds in patients with malignant biliary obstruction: preliminary results versus a conventional biliary stent. J Hepatol 2012;56:1104–11.

94. Weigt J, Pech M, Kandulski A, et al. Cone-beam computed tomography - adding a new dimension to ERCP. Endoscopy 2015;47:654–7.

# Benign Biliary Strictures and Leaks

Jacques Devière, MD, PhD

## KEYWORDS

- Bile leaks • Biliary stenosis • ERCP • Biliary stents • Cholangioscopy

## KEY POINTS

- Endoscopic approach plays a major role in the management of a vast majority of bile duct injuries (BDIs), including the most severe ones.
- These patients should be managed in highly specialized centers with a multidisciplinary environment and availability of multitechnical approaches.
- Biliary stricture calibration is successfully obtained with multiple plastic stents placement and serial exchanges for 1 year.
- Fully covered self-expandable metal stents (FCSEMS) represent a reasonable alternative to multiple plastic stents, particularly for biliary stenosis associated with chronic pancreatitis. Uncovered self-expandable metal stents (SEMS) are strictly contraindicated for any benign biliary stenosis.
- Autoimmune cholangiopathy (AIC) and primary sclerosing cholangitis (PSC) represent major diagnostic challenges whereby endoscopic retrograde cholangiopancreatography (ERCP) and cholangioscopy play a pivotal role.

## INTRODUCTION

Benign biliary strictures are secondary to surgery, chronic pancreatitis (CP), PSC, or autoimmune cholangitis. Biliary leaks mainly occur after surgery and, rarely, abdominal trauma.

BDIs occurring during surgery represent a major clinical problem associated with significant morbidity and mortality. Laparoscopic cholecystectomy is the leading cause of iatrogenic BDIs occurring in 0.3% to 0.5% of the cases.[1,2] They can also develop after hepatic surgery, such as hepatic resection and liver transplant, or follow nonbiliary surgery or nonoperative procedures in areas located close to the biliary tract.[3,4] Less frequently, abdominal trauma can also result in BDIs.[5]

BDIs can range from nonsevere bile duct leaks or strictures to more severe injuries including complete transection or occlusion of the main ducts. Different classifications

Department of Gastroenterology, Hepatopancreatology and Digestive Oncology, Erasme University Hospital, Université Libre de Bruxelles, 808 Route de Lennik, Brussels B 1070, Belgium
E-mail address: jacques.deviere@erasme.ulb.ac.be

Gastrointest Endoscopy Clin N Am 25 (2015) 713–723
http://dx.doi.org/10.1016/j.giec.2015.06.004                                giendo.theclinics.com

described in this article have been developed to evaluate their severity[6,7] and guide physicians in planning the most appropriate medical or surgical therapeutic intervention for each patient. ERCP and associated nonsurgical techniques play a pivotal and still growing role in their management.

Benign strictures due to CP may also benefit from endoscopic therapy, whereas those associated with PSC or AIC represent, in addition to potential therapy,[8] one of the few diagnostic indications of ERCP (and cholangioscopy) for characterization of undetermined strictures and differential diagnosis from malignancy.

This article covers the current indications and capabilities of ERCP (and associated nonsurgical techniques) for the management of benign biliary strictures and leaks.

## POSTOPERATIVE BILIARY STRICTURES AND LEAKS

Although most BDIs occur after cholecystectomy, other liver surgeries such as hepatectomies and liver transplant represent sources of major injuries. The early injury often results from complex dissection, poorly defined anatomy, or management of preoperative bleeding by clipping or diathermy.[1,3,5,7]

Delayed injury may arise from ischemia of the bile ducts, and stenoses may develop clinically up to decades after the original insult. Whatever their cause and timing and even if endoscopy has become pivotal in their management, these patients should be initially managed in tertiary referral centers and referred to multidisciplinary teams of endoscopists, radiologists, and surgeons having extensive experience. "Don't further mess the biliary system" by inappropriate attempts to repair should be the rule, keeping in mind that these complications often occur in young patients undergoing a minor surgery and that inappropriate management may affect at long term their quality of life.[9,10]

Even if multiple classifications have been published,[2,6,7] the most useful for endoscopists is the one described by the group of Amsterdam,[7] which is particularly relevant for postcholecystectomy injuries. BDIs were classified into 4 groups defined as follows:

Type A: Cystic duct leaks or leakages from aberrant or peripheral hepatic radicles
Type B: Major bile duct leaks with or without concomitant biliary stricture
Type C: Bile duct strictures without leakage
Type D: Complete transection of the duct with or without excision of a portion of the biliary tree

Type A leaks arise from the cystic duct and the ducts of Luschka after cholecystectomy. They are usually associated with low output and may require complete filling of the biliary tree with contrast to be demonstrated.

They respond favorably to biliary decompression achieved (and preferably) by transient stent placement (4–8 weeks), endoscopic sphincterotomy (recommended in case of associated common bile duct [CBD] stones), or placement of a nasobiliary catheter, often associated with an endoscopic sphincterotomy (ES).[10,11] The last is less comfortable for the patient but may be useful, particularly when leaks occur from peripheral radicles, the nasobiliary catheter (NBC) being inserted into the segment from which the leak originates. As for any leak, percutaneous drainage of biloma may be required in addition to endoscopic therapy. These treatments, combining biliary decompression and removal of a persisting obstacle or drainage of a biloma in selected cases, allow resolution of the leak in more than 90% of the cases.[12]

Leakages from major bile ducts (type B), at the level of the CBD after cholecystectomy or choledocal anastomosis or of the intrahepatic ducts after liver surgery, trauma, or in case of anatomic variants, are more challenging to treat endoscopically. They usually are high-output leaks, readily visible at opacification and associated with a biloma in most of the cases when not recognized or suspected and drained preoperatively. These leaks should always benefit from a multidisciplinary therapeutic plan before starting any treatment (mainly attempts at surgical repair), which may further compromise the chances of success.[7,10,13] Drainage of collection comes first, usually followed, after proper imaging (preferably with MRI to delineate biliary anatomy), by an ERCP during which the first goal is to reach the intrahepatic ducts proximal to the leak and to evaluate the integrity of all hepatic segments. An ES is always performed in these cases, and stents and/or NBCs are inserted to bypass the leak. At the level of the hilum, multiple stents, usually longer, are implanted in both liver lobes to bypass the leak and ensure stability. In some cases, this endoscopic drainage of the biliary tree can be associated with drainage of the leak itself using transpapillary pigtail stent or NBC to accelerate closure of the external fistula. Another feature of these major leaks is their propensity to be associated with the development of a biliary stricture after healing, another reason why stenting is important not only to favor closure but also to prevent the development of strictures (**Fig. 1**).

Unlike in minor leaks, stents should be left in place for 6 to 12 months, with exchange when appropriate, similar to what is done for postoperative strictures.

Postoperative biliary strictures (type C) may follow any surgery affecting the biliary system and may also occur at the level of an anastomosis after liver resection or liver transplant (OLTx).[14–16] When secondary to a direct trauma, they are usually recognized early in the postoperative period and respond more favorably to endoscopic treatment. Delayed presentation may occur up to years (or even decades) after surgery. In this case, their cause most probably involves ischemia and resulting fibrosis. Their

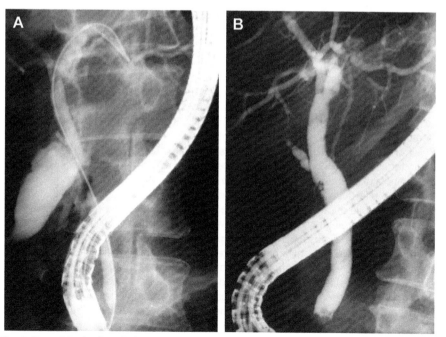

**Fig. 1.** Type B leak after cholecystectomy (A). Endoscopic sphincterotomy and placement of 2 plastic stents for 6 months allowed resolution without stricture formation (B).

treatment usually involves serial placement of multiple stents over a 1-year period. It is now widely accepted that a more aggressive approach including the placement of increasing number of stents over a 6- to 12-month period, with the aim to obtain an anatomic resolution of the stricture, yields more durable results with a success rate more than 80% and an incidence of relapse within 10 years after removal less than 12%.[17] A similar approach is also recommended for choledococholedocal anastomotic strictures after OLTx.[18] Strictures located at the level of the hilum are more difficult to calibrate and technically more demanding because the stents have to be implanted in both lobes or even segmental branches to ensure their stability and allow proper calibration[14,15,19]; this is also true for strictures affecting the upper third of the CBD.

Nonanastomotic strictures occurring after OLTx result from ischemia and are often associated with hepatic artery thrombosis. They are much less responsive to endoscopic therapy with long-term response rate equal to or less than 50%, and a significant proportion of patients may ultimately require transplant. These strictures are often located at the hilum, and their treatment includes placement of multiple plastic stents with serial exchanges. In addition, they are often associated with the formation of bile duct casts or mucocele, which must be repeatedly cleared endoscopically or by combined endoscopic-percutaneous approaches.[16,20,21]

ERCP can also be effective for calibration of bilioenteric anastomoses after duodenopancreatectomy or hepaticojejunostomy. Access to the anastomosis in these cases may require the use of device-assisted enteroscopes,[22] and the alternative percutaneous approach should always be considered because it may be less invasive when using dedicated percutaneous (Yamakawa/Munchener) stents.[23]

Whatever the approach, endoscopic or percutaneous, uncovered SEMS are strictly contraindicated for management of benign strictures.[24] Not only is their long-term patency, due to tissue hyperplasia, almost nil but also they cannot be removed in most cases and would compromise any further treatment and chance for cure.

FCSEMS are increasingly being investigated as a treatment option in benign strictures. They could provide more ample and prompt dilation than plastic stents and eliminate the need for multiple sequential ERCP stent exchanges and their attendant costs.[25,26] A recent multicentric study[27] confirmed the primary requisite of these stents, that is, removability in all cases (with, however, the need for more than 1 procedure in 5%), and showed that a 6-month indwell was able to provide stricture resolution in approximately 70% of patients with postcholecystectomy or anastomotic post-OLTx strictures. These results are surely not better than those reported with multiple plastic stents in these indications, a feature probably related to the high spontaneous migration rate of FCSEMS (around 17% in both groups). Even if technically easier to insert than multiple plastic stents and safe in terms of removability, FCSEMS have not been proved to have a similar efficacy than multiple plastic stents in postoperative and anastomotic strictures.

Complex bile duct injuries, with complete transection and possible excision of a portion of the bile ducts (type D), have been considered not amenable to endoscopic therapy.[7] These are highly complex cases where multidisciplinarity is the rule. Surgical reconstruction may be associated with high morbidity, and percutaneous drainage is usually performed to allow biliary decompression and symptomatic relief while waiting for a surgical procedure performed in stable conditions.

However, successful nonsurgical management of these patients with complex BDI using combined endoscopic/percutaneous or endoscopic ultrasound (EUS)-guided approaches has been described.[28–31] They consist in rendezvous technique with recanalization through a biloma (**Fig. 2**) or percutaneous puncture of a distal transected segment using a transjugular intrahepatic portosystemic shuntset (usually used for performing transjugular intrahepatic shunts and puncturing the portal branch

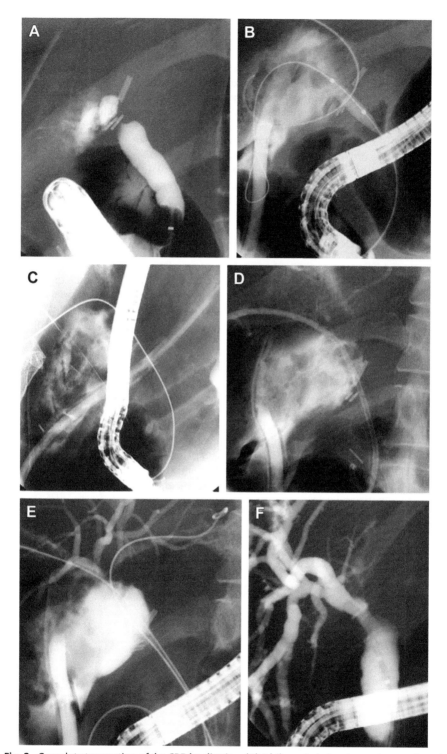

**Fig. 2.** Complete transection of the CBD by clipping. (*A*) A biloma is drained percutaneously and combined transhepatic/endoscopic approach with dilation of the communication to the biloma is performed. (*B*) Intrahepatic ducts are reconnected to CBD by a guidewire (*C*) and a Ring catheter (*D*) during the same session. A few days later, 2 stents are placed in the left and right lobes (*E*) and left in place for 12 months (with 2 exchanges). At 1 year, no residual stricture is observed (*F*).

through the liver, from a sus-hepatic vein).[31,32] What has been reported to date is that if stenting can be performed through an excised virtual segment, it effectively results in biliary recanalization and reepithelialization and can offer long-term outcomes similar to those obtained after calibration of a postoperative stricture. Another approach is the EUS-guided drainage of a biloma, which may restore the biliary drainage of a transected part of the bile duct to the gastrointestinal tract[33] or the direct EUS-guided drainage of the proximal transected part of the biliary system through a hepaticogastrostomy or (preferably if feasible) a hepaticobulbostomy (**Fig. 3**).[34] The place of these techniques in the armamentarium for managing these complex cases still has to be defined, but they represent an option not to be neglected when dealing with patients for whom surgical repair encompasses major surgery with high morbidity.

## BILIARY STRICTURES SECONDARY TO CHRONIC PANCREATITIS

In advanced CP, 10% to 30% of patients may develop a symptomatic biliary stricture.[12] The term symptomatic means persistent cholestasis in the absence of an acute pancreatitis, with risk for developing a secondary biliary cirrhosis. Most biliary stenoses (observed at imaging) associated with severe CP are asymptomatic and do not require treatment. In early series, the results of single plastic stent placement was disappointing, with long-term success rates of endoscopic therapy ranging between 10% and 30%.[35]

Uncovered metallic stents have shown promising midterm results,[36] but this was not confirmed at long-term and have been abandoned for this indication. Studies using multiple plastic stents have yielded better results, with long-term success rates around 65%, although these stenoses are still less responsive to endoscopic therapy and showed a higher recurrence rate than postoperative strictures with this management.[12] FCSEMS might find an interesting indication as shown in a large multicentric study in which 137 patients with CP undergoing placement of FCSEMS for 1 year had a resolution of the stricture in 83% of the cases with a relapse rate of only 11%.[27] This result suggests that, in this indication, FCSEMS offer at least similar results to multiple plastic stents, being easier to implant and avoiding risk and cost of serial ERCPs. On the opposite of what was previously observed with plastic stents, in this study, the migration rate of FCSEMS was also significantly lower than the one observed in

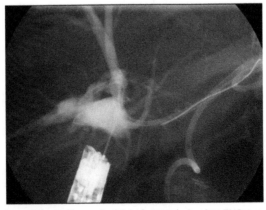

**Fig. 3.** Hepaticobulbostomy performed with a forward-viewing EUS scope in a patient with transection of the posterolateral segments (VI and VII) during cholecystectomy, restoring drainage to the duodenum.

postoperative strictures. These results are similar to those of a single-center study in which a stricture resolution rate of 84% was reported for the 44 patients with FCSEMS inserted for CP-associated biliary strictures.[25] Up to recently, CP-associated persistent symptomatic strictures were considered as a surgical indication. The recent data, first with multiple plastic stents and then with FCSEMS, strongly suggest that these patients should be offered appropriate endoscopic stenting, preferably with FCSEMS, for a period of 1 year, before considering those who would have relapse of symptoms for a surgical option.

## BILIARY STRICTURES DUE TO PRIMARY SCLEROSING CHOLANGITIS

For many years, ERCP was considered as one of the major diagnostic tool for PSC, an indication that has almost disappeared with the availability of magnetic resonance cholangiopancreatography. The use of ERCP to obtain a cholangiogram in these patients has become obsolete and should be strictly contraindicated because of a risk of cholangitis that may reach 10% with no additional value in terms of diagnostic accuracy. The diagnostic role of ERCP has become limited to the characterization of dominant strictures[37,38] in patients suspected to have a cholangiocarcinoma or manifesting a clinical deterioration.

If endoscopic brushing was the most frequently used mode of tissue acquisition in this instance, transpapillary cholangioscopy emerged as a useful tool to distinguish between malignant and benign dominant strictures, with reported sensitivity and specificity of 92% and 93%, respectively.[38] The availability of cholangioscopic devices that allow accurate visualization and effective targeted biopsies might further enhance the role of cholangioscopy in selected cases of PSC.[39]

Benign strictures in PSC respond well to endoscopic dilation, and it is widely accepted that stenting should be avoided in most cases.[37] The author's policy is to perform balloon dilation and leave an NBC for 24 hours, stenting being considered only in dominant strictures affecting the CBD and usually limited to a few weeks. Endoscopic therapy for PSC stricture should be considered for patients with deteriorating cholestasis, in association with endoscopic characterization of dominant stricture and in patients having stenoses affecting the CBD.

## AUTOIMMUNE CHOLANGIOPATHY

Immunoglobulin G 4 (IgG4)-associated cholangiopathy is an entity that has been characterized and better recognized over the last 15 years and probably accounted (and still do) for many unuseful surgical resections. It may affect any part of the biliary tree, mimicking PSC, hilum tumors (**Fig. 4**), or CBD tumors. IGg4-associated pancreatitis can also mimic pancreatic cancer when presenting with jaundice and inducing a distal CBD stenosis.[8,40] Cholangiopathy is often associated with autoimmune pancreatitis but can also occur as an isolated biliary disease. Serum IGg4 levels are a useful diagnostic tool in autoimmune pancreatitis (AIP) (and their treatment monitoring), but their sensitivity is low and they can be normal in many cases of cholangiopathy. The criteria for diagnosis are based on histology with IgG4 immunostaining. Tissue acquisition is better performed by biopsies than by brushing, and the role of cholangioscopy is obvious in this indication.[41] Biopsies of the ampulla of Vater have been reported helpful when showing infiltration by IgG4-positive plasma cells,[8] a feature that was never confirmed in the author's experience. IgG4 cholangiopathy respond extremely well and quickly (within 1 or 2 weeks) to steroid therapy.

For this reason, a trial treatment with steroids may be indicated in some cases. Besides this major role for tissue acquisition, the therapeutic role of ERCP in this disease

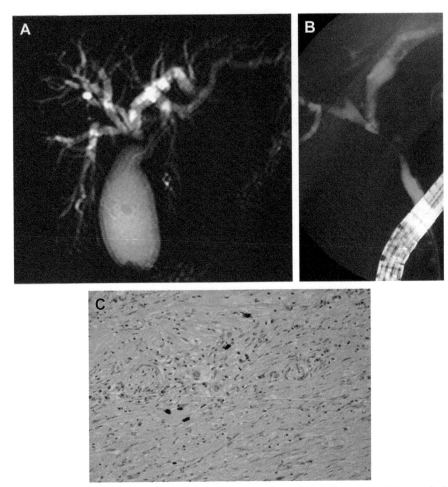

**Fig. 4.** A 50-year-old man with silent jaundice. Bismuth 1 hilum stricture mimicking a chol-angiocarcinoma at MRCP (*A*) and ERCP (*B*). Intrabiliary biopsies (*C*) at the level of the stricture reveal typical IgG4 immunostaining (*black spots*).

is limited to temporary stenting with plastic stents.[12] The major role of the endoscopist in this disease is to suspect it and do all the necessary diagnostic procedures (including PET-computed tomographic scan and MRI with diffusion imaging followed by a therapeutic trial with steroids) when a decision for extensive surgical resection has to be made without obvious histologic diagnosis of malignancy. This disease is the paramount illustration of the caution that should be taken before placing potentially nonremovable stents in a patient for whom the palliative indication and/or the histologic diagnosis has not been established.

## SUMMARY

Benign biliary strictures and leaks represent a peculiar indication for ERCP, which can offer a curative treatment in most cases. There has been development of strategies for the management of postoperative and CP-associated strictures, and the role of FCSEMS, even if still in need for evidence, becomes better defined. Uncovered SEMS have no role in this indication, whatever the route of introduction (endoscopic or percutaneous).

Endoscopic management of leaks after surgery or trauma has been one of the major achievements of ERCP, avoiding many risky and often difficult reinterventions and dramatically reducing the duration of hospitalization of these patients. The multitechnical approach, including percutaneous and EUS-guided procedures, allows one to consider nonsurgical approaches for almost any complication occurring after surgery; this also implies that those patients with severe complications should be systematically referred to tertiary (or quaternary) centers where a real multidisciplinary management of these rare cases can be organized.

Finally, ERCP has been abandoned for black and white pictures of the biliary tree, but its diagnostic role has been rejuvenated in some niche indications for tissue acquisition, including cholangioscopy, which has now improved visualization and sampling capabilities for undeterminate strictures. This being said, a technique is only an opportunity to review the clinical history of the patient, to integrate endoscopy in the other diagnostic and therapeutic procedures, to avoid misdiagnosis and unappropriate therapeutic decisions, and to offer, in these patients with benign conditions, the best chance for cure, with lowest morbidity.

## REFERENCES

1. Flum DR, Cheadle A, Prela C, et al. Bile duct injury during cholecystectomy and survival in Medicare beneficiaries. JAMA 2003;290:2168–73.
2. Stewart L. Iatrogenic biliary injuries: identification, classification and management. Surg Clin North Am 2014;94:297–310.
3. Rerknimitr R, Sherman S, Fogel EL, et al. Biliary tract complications after liver transplantation with choledochocholedochostomy anastomosis: endoscopic findings and results of therapy. Gastrointest Endosc 2002;55:224–31.
4. Shah JN. Endoscopic treatment of bile leaks: current standards and recent innovations. Gastrointest Endosc 2007;65:1069–72.
5. Mandal N, Mandal R, Ranjan R. Complete transection of common bile duct after blunt trauma abdomen - a case report. J Indian Med Assoc 2013;111:560–1.
6. Lau WY, Lai EC. Classification of iatrogenic bile duct injury. Hepatobiliary Pancreat Dis Int 2007;6:459–63.
7. Bergman JJ, van den Brink GR, Rauws EA, et al. Treatment of bile duct lesions after laparoscopic cholecystectomy. Gut 1996;38:141–7.
8. ASGE Guideline. The role of ERCP in benign diseases of the biliary tree. Gastrointest Endosc 2015;81:795–803.
9. Boerma D, Rauws EA, Keulemans YC, et al. Impaired quality of life 5 years after bile duct injury during laparoscopic surgery: a prospective analysis. Ann Surg 2001;234:750–7.
10. Costamagna G, Shah SK, Tringali A. Current management of postoperative complications and benign biliary strictures. Gastrointest Endosc Clin N Am 2003;13: 635–48.
11. Sandha GS, Bourke MJ, Haber GB, et al. Endoscopic therapy for bile leaks based on a new classification: results in 207 patients. Gastrointest Endosc 2004;60:567–74.
12. Dumonceau JM, Tringali A, Blero D, et al. European Society of Gastrointestinal Endoscopy. Biliary stenting: indications, choice of stents and results: European Society of Gastrointestinal Endoscopy (ESGE) clinical guideline. Endoscopy 2012;44:277–98.

13. Bhattacharjya S, Puleston J, Davidson BR, et al. Outcome of early endoscopic biliary drainage in the management of bile leaks after hepatic resection. Gastrointest Endosc 2003;57:526–31.
14. Baron TH Sr, Davee T. Endoscopic management of benign bile duct strictures. Gastrointest Endosc Clin N Am 2013;23:295–311.
15. Costamagna G, Boskoski I. Current treatment of benign biliary strictures. Ann Gastroenterol 2013;26:1–4.
16. Ayoub WS, Esquivel CO, Martin P. Biliary complications following liver transplantation. Dig Dis Sci 2010;55:1540–6.
17. Costamagna G, Tringali A, Mutignani M, et al. Endotherapy of postoperative biliary strictures with multiple stents: results after more than 10 years of follow-up. Gastrointest Endosc 2010;72:551–7.
18. Poley JW, Lekkerkerker MN, Metselaar HJ, et al. Clinical outcome of progressive stenting in patients with anastomotic strictures after orthotopic liver transplantation. Endoscopy 2013;45:567–70.
19. Draganov P, Hoffman B, Marsh W, et al. Long-term outcome in patients with benign biliary strictures treated endoscopically with multiple stents. Gastrointest Endosc 2002;55:680–6.
20. Srinivasaiah N, Reddy MS, Balupuri S, et al. Biliary cast syndrome: literature review and a single centre experience in liver transplant recipients. Hepatobiliary Pancreat Dis Int 2008;7:300–3.
21. Tarantino I, Barresi L, Petridis I, et al. Endoscopic treatment of biliary complications after liver transplantation. World J Gastroenterol 2008;14:4185–9.
22. Zepeda-Gómez S, Baron TH. Benign biliary strictures: current endoscopic management. Nat Rev Gastroenterol Hepatol 2011;8:573–81.
23. Giampalma E, Renzulli M, Mosconi C, et al. Outcome of post-liver transplant ischemic and nonischemic biliary stenoses treated with percutaneous interventions: the Bologna experience. Liver Transpl 2012;18:177–87.
24. Dumonceau JM, Devière J, Delhaye M, et al. Plastic and metal stents for postoperative benign bile duct strictures: the best and the worst. Gastrointest Endosc 1998;47:8–17.
25. Kahaleh M, Brijbassie A, Sethi A, et al. Multicenter trial evaluating the use of covered self-expanding metal stents in benign biliary strictures: time to revisit our therapeutic options? J Clin Gastroenterol 2013;47:695–9.
26. Tarantino I, Traina M, Mocciaro F, et al. Fully covered metallic stents in biliary stenosis after orthotopic liver transplantation. Endoscopy 2012;44:246–50.
27. Devière J, Reddy DN, Püspök A, et al, Benign Biliary Stenoses Working Group. Successful management of benign biliary strictures with fully covered self-expanding metal stents. Gastroenterology 2014;147:385–95.
28. Donatelli G, Bertrand MV, Derhy S, et al. Combined endoscopic and radiological approach for complete bile duct injuries (with video). Gastrointest Endosc 2014;79:855–64.
29. Fiocca F, Salvatori FM, Fanelli F, et al. Complete transection of the main bile duct: minimally invasive treatment with an endoscopic-radiologic rendezvous. Gastrointest Endosc 2011;74:1393–8.
30. Nasr JY, Hashash JG, Orons P, et al. Rendezvous procedure for the treatment of bile leaks and injury following segmental hepatectomy. Dig Liver Dis 2013;45:433–6.
31. Dumonceau JM, Baize M, Devière J. Endoscopic transhepatic repair of the common hepatic duct after excision during cholecystectomy. Gastrointest Endosc 2000;52:540–3.

32. Arvanitakis M, Delhaye M, Bali MA, et al. Endoscopic treatment of external pancreatic fistulas: when draining the main pancreatic duct is not enough. Am J Gastroenterol 2007;102:516–27.

33. Shami VM, Talreja JP, Mahajan A, et al. EUS-guided drainage of bilomas: a new alternative? Gastrointest Endosc 2008;67:136–40.

34. Park SJ, Choi JH, Park do H, et al. Expanding indication: EUS-guided hepatico-duodenostomy for isolated right intrahepatic duct obstruction (with video). Gastrointest Endosc 2013;78:374–80.

35. Devière J, Devaere S, Baize M, et al. Endoscopic biliary drainage in chronic pancreatitis. Gastrointest Endosc 1990;36:96–100.

36. Deviere J, Cremer M, Baize M, et al. Management of common bile duct stricture caused by chronic pancreatitis with metal mesh self expandable stents. Gut 1994;35(1):122–6.

37. Singh S, Talwalkar JA. Primary sclerosing cholangitis: diagnosis, prognosis and management. Clin Gastroenterol Hepatol 2013;11:898–907.

38. Tischendorf JJ, Krüger M, Trautwein C, et al. Cholangioscopic characterization of dominant bile duct stenoses in patients with primary sclerosing cholangitis. Endoscopy 2006;38:665–9.

39. Arnelo U, von Seth E, Bergquist A. Prospective evaluation of the clinical utility of single-operator peroral cholangioscopy in patients with primary sclerosing cholangitis. Endoscopy 2015. [Epub ahead of print].

40. Maillette de Buy Wenniger LJ, Beuers U. Immunoglobulin G4-related cholangiopathy: clinical and experimental insights. Curr Opin Gastroenterol 2015;31:252–7.

41. Itoi T, Kamisawa T, Igarashi Y, et al. The role of peroral video cholangioscopy in patients with IgG4-related sclerosing cholangitis. J Gastroenterol 2013;48:504–14.

# Preventing Postendoscopic Retrograde Cholangiopancreatography Pancreatitis

B. Joseph Elmunzer, MD

## KEYWORDS

- Endoscopic retrograde cholangiopancreatography • Pancreatitis
- Post-ERCP pancreatitis • Complications

## KEY POINTS

- Risk stratification and thoughtful patient selection are critical in reducing post-ERCP pancreatitis; in this era of highly accurate diagnostic alternatives, ERCP should be a near-exclusively therapeutic procedure.
- In the case of difficult cannulation, alternate techniques, such as double-wire cannulation and precut sphincterotomy, should be implemented early.
- Contrast-facilitated cannulation, aggressive/repeated pancreatic injection, dilation of an intact biliary sphincter, and sphincter of Oddi manometry without aspiration should be avoided.
- Prophylactic pancreatic stents should be placed in all high-risk cases.
- Rectal NSAIDs should be administered in all high-risk cases, and based on a favorable risk-benefit ratio, should be considered in all patients undergoing ERCP.

## OVERVIEW

Postendoscopic retrograde cholangiopancreatography (ERCP) pancreatitis (PEP) is defined as new or increased abdominal pain that is clinically consistent with a syndrome of acute pancreatitis and associated pancreatic enzyme elevation at least three times the upper limit of normal 24 hours after the procedure and resultant hospitalization (or prolongation of existing hospitalization) of at least 2 nights.[1] Pancreatitis is still the most common complication of ERCP, occurring in 2% to 15% of cases, and accounting for substantial morbidity, occasional mortality, and health care expenditures in excess of $200 million annually in the United States.[2,3] Despite significant advances

The author has no conflicts of interest to disclose.
Division of Gastroenterology and Hepatology, Medical University of South Carolina, MSC 702, 114 Doughty Street, Suite 249, Charleston, SC 29425, USA
E-mail address: Elmunzer@musc.edu

Gastrointest Endoscopy Clin N Am 25 (2015) 725–736
http://dx.doi.org/10.1016/j.giec.2015.06.006
1052-5157/15/$ – see front matter © 2015 Elsevier Inc. All rights reserved.

over the last several decades in terms of patient selection, equipment, procedural technique, and prophylactic interventions, PEP remains a serious health problem and its prevention remains a major clinical and research priority. Strategies to prevent PEP are broadly divided into five areas: (1) appropriate patient selection, (2) risk stratification of patients undergoing ERCP and meaningful use of this information in clinical decision-making, (3) atraumatic and efficient procedural technique, (4) prophylactic pancreatic stent placement (PSP), and (5) pharmacoprevention. All five strategy areas should be considered in every case, and the latter two should be implemented when appropriate.

## PATIENT SELECTION

Thoughtful patient selection before ERCP remains the most important strategy for reducing the incidence of PEP. Endoscopic ultrasound and magnetic resonance cholangiopancreatography allow highly accurate pancreaticobiliary imaging while avoiding the significant risks of ERCP. Two large meta-analyses have demonstrated that endoscopic ultrasound is highly sensitive and specific in the detection of bile duct stones (sensitivity, 89%–94%; specificity, 94%–95%).[4] Similarly, magnetic resonance cholangiopancreatography has a sensitivity of 85% to 92% and a specificity of 93% to 97% for the same indication,[5] although MRI seems less sensitive than endoscopic ultrasound for stones smaller than 6 mm.[6] Additionally, endoscopic ultrasound, MRI, and other noninvasive modalities, such as radionucleotide-labeled scan and percutaneous drain fluid analysis, are very accurate in diagnosing a multitude of other pancreaticobiliary processes (eg, chronic pancreatitis, malignancy, and leaks), often obviating ERCP.

Indeed, the use of ERCP as a diagnostic procedure has steadily declined in favor of less invasive but equally accurate alternative tests, and ERCP has appropriately become a near-exclusively therapeutic procedure reserved for patients with a high pretest probability of intervention. This trend is consistent with recent clinical practice guidelines on the role of endoscopy in the evaluation of choledocholithiasis and the National Institutes of Health consensus statement on ERCP for diagnosis and therapy, both favoring less invasive tests over ERCP in the diagnosis of biliary disease.[7,8]

An exception to the widespread practice of reserving ERCP for patients with a high likelihood of therapeutic intervention has been the evaluation of patients with suspected sphincter of Oddi dysfunction (SOD), for which an accurate, less-invasive alternative to ERCP-guided sphincter of Oddi manometry (SOM) remains elusive. Even when considering patients for SOM, however, thoughtful clinical judgment is necessary to select those who are most likely to benefit from the procedure. A recent multicenter randomized trial (the EPISOD study) has demonstrated that there seems to be no role for ERCP in patients with suspected SOD but no laboratory or radiographic abnormalities (previously known as type 3 SOD).[9] Additional studies are necessary to determine whether diagnostic ERCP with SOM is truly beneficial in cases of suspected type 2 biliary SOD or recurrent unexplained pancreatitis. Pending such studies, many experts believe ERCP remains reasonable in these scenarios after careful assessment of the risk-benefit ratio and detailed informed consent. Another possible exception to the therapeutic ERCP trend may be the evaluation of biliary complications in liver transplant recipients, for whom a recent retrospective study suggested that diagnostic ERCP is a reasonable and efficient clinical approach in this patient population based on a high likelihood of therapeutic intervention and a very low rate of complications, in particular PEP.[10]

## RECOGNIZING PATIENTS AT INCREASED RISK FOR POSTENDOSCOPIC RETROGRADE CHOLANGIOPANCREATOGRAPHY PANCREATITIS

A high index of suspicion for, and early identification of, post-ERCP pancreatitis are critically important in ensuring favorable clinical outcomes. The ability to risk-stratify patients based on well-established clinical characteristics can inform the decision-making process that surrounds (1) proceeding with ERCP, (2) referral to a tertiary center, (3) fluid resuscitation, (4) prophylactic stent placement, (5) pharmacoprevention, and (6) postprocedural hospital observation.

A substantial amount of research over the last two decades has contributed to the understanding of the independent risk factors for post-ERCP pancreatitis. These risk factors, listed in **Table 1**, can be divided into patient-related and procedure-related characteristics. The definite and probable patient-related risk factors that predispose to PEP are a clinical suspicion of SOD (regardless of whether or not SOM is performed), a history of prior PEP, a history of recurrent pancreatitis, normal bilirubin, younger age, and female gender. The definite and probable procedure-related risk factors for PEP are difficult cannulation, precut (access) sphincterotomy (discussed later), pancreatic sphincterotomy, ampullectomy, repeated or aggressive pancreatography, and short-duration balloon dilation of an intact biliary sphincter. Two recent systematic reviews have affirmed the association of most of these factors with PEP.[11,12] Additional risk factors that have been implicated, but are not concretely accepted, as independent predictors of PEP are biliary sphincterotomy, pancreatic duct wire passage (see later), pancreatic acinarization, self-expanding metal stent placement, nondilated bile duct, intraductal papillary mucinous neoplasm, intraductal ultrasound, and Billroth 2 anatomy.

Operator (endoscopist)-dependent characteristics have also been implicated in the risk of PEP. Endoscopist procedure volume is suggested to be a risk factor for PEP, although multicenter studies have not confirmed this observation, presumably because low-volume endoscopists tend to perform lower-risk cases. Nevertheless, potentially dangerous cases (based on either patient-related factors or anticipated high-risk interventions) are best referred to expert medical centers where a high-volume endoscopist with expertise in prophylactic PSP can perform the case, and where more experience with rescue from serious complications may improve clinical outcomes.[13] Similarly, trainee involvement in ERCP is a possible independent risk factor for PEP, although results of existing multivariable analyses are conflicting.[14,15] Inexperienced trainees may augment procedure-related risk factors, such as prolonging a difficult cannulation or delivering excess electrosurgical current during an inefficient pancreatic sphicterotomy. Therefore, additional research focused on improving the process of ERCP training is necessary to minimize the contribution of trainee involvement to the development of PEP.

**Table 1**
**Independent risk factors for post-ERCP pancreatitis**

| Patient-Related Factors | Procedure-Related Factors |
| --- | --- |
| Suspected sphincter of Oddi dysfunction | Difficult cannulation |
| Prior post-ERCP pancreatitis | Precut (access) sphincterotomy |
| Normal bilirubin | Pancreatic sphincterotomy |
| Younger age | Ampullectomy |
| Female gender | Repeated or aggressive pancreatography |
| History of recurrent pancreatitis | Balloon dilation of an intact biliary sphincter |

Several additional points regarding clinical risk stratification are worth considering. First, predictors of PEP seem multiplicative in nature. For example, a widely referenced multicenter study by Freeman and colleagues[14] predating prophylactic PSP showed that a young woman with a clinical suspicion of SOD, normal bilirubin, and a difficult cannulation has a risk of PEP in excess of 40%. Second, patients with a clinical suspicion of SOD, particularly women, are not only at increased risk for PEP in general, but are also more likely to develop severe pancreatitis and death.[14,16] When considering the risk-benefit ratio of ERCP in this patient population, not only should the patient's overall risk of PEP be assessed, but their probability of experiencing a more dramatic clinical course should also be considered and discussed. Additionally, several clinical characteristics are thought to significantly reduce the risk of PEP. First, biliary interventions in patients with a pre-existing biliary sphincterotomy probably confer a very low risk of PEP. Prior sphincterotomy generally separates the biliary and pancreatic orifices, allowing avoidance of the pancreas, and making pancreatic sphincter or duct trauma unlikely. Furthermore, patients with chronic pancreatitis, in particular those with calcific pancreatitis, are at lower risk for PEP because of gland atrophy, fibrosis, and consequent decrease in exocrine enzymatic activity. Similarly, the progressive decline in pancreatic exocrine function associated with aging may protect older patients from pancreatic injury. Lastly, perhaps because of postobstructive parenchymal atrophy, patients with pancreatic head malignancy seem to be relatively protected.

## PROCEDURE TECHNIQUE

Efficient and atraumatic technical practices during ERCP are central to minimizing the risk of pancreatitis. Many of the procedure-related risk factors listed previously, although predisposing to PEP, are mandatory elements of a successful case. Even though these high-risk interventions are unavoidable for execution of the clinical objective, certain strategies can be used to minimize procedure-related risk.

Difficult cannulation and pancreatic duct injection are independent risk factors for PEP. As such, interventions that improve the efficiency of cannulation and limit injection of contrast into the pancreas are likely to decrease the risk of pancreatitis. Guidewire-assisted cannulation accomplishes both, representing a major paradigm shift in ERCP practice. In contrast to conventional contrast-assisted cannulation, which may lead to inadvertent injection of the pancreatic duct or contribute to papillary edema, guidewire-assisted cannulation uses a small-diameter wire with a hydrophilic tip that is initially advanced into the duct, subsequently guiding passage of the catheter. Because the wire is thinner and more maneuverable than the cannula, it is easier to advance across a potentially narrow and off-angle orifice. Moreover, this process limits the likelihood of an inadvertent pancreatic or intramural papillary injection. A recent Cochrane Collaboration meta-analysis, which included 12 randomized controlled trials (RCTs) involving 3450 subjects, indeed confirms that guidewire-assisted cannulation reduces the risk of PEP by approximately 50% (relative risk, 0.51; 95% confidence interval, 0.32–0.82).[17] When wire cannulation is used for biliary access, it is important to advance the guidewire cautiously in the event it is actually in the pancreatic duct where forceful advancement may result in sidebranch perforation.

When initial cannulation attempts are unsuccessful, several alternative techniques are available to facilitate biliary access. The double-wire technique is a common second-line approach when initial cannulation attempts result in repeated unintentional passage of the wire into the pancreas. The wire can be left in the pancreatic duct, thereby straightening the common channel and partially occluding the pancreatic orifice, allowing subsequent biliary cannulation alongside the existing pancreatic wire. The double-wire technique has been shown to improve cannulation success compared with standard methods, although some data suggest a higher incidence of PEP with this technique or when a wire is passed into the pancreatic duct.[18–20] Furthermore, a recent RCT of difficult cannulation cases requiring double-wire technique demonstrated that prophylactic PSP reduced the incidence of PEP in this patient population.[21] Based on this, some experts believe that a prophylactic pancreatic stent should be placed in all patients requiring double-wire cannulation. Others, including the author, however, believe that placement of a wire in the pancreas does not independently predispose to PEP, and that pancreatitis in this context is generally related to the preceding difficult cannulation. If double-wire technique is used early (within two to three cannulation attempts) in a low-risk patient, and the wire advances seamlessly into the pancreatic duct in a typical pancreatic trajectory, PSP may not be necessary if rectal indomethacin is given.

Additional alternative cannulation techniques include wire cannulation alongside a pancreatic stent, precut sphincterotomy, septomotomy, and needle-knife fistulotomy. Although these techniques can be helpful in gaining biliary access during challenging cases, some have been implicated as procedure-related risk factors for PEP. In many cases, however, the risk of PEP is actually driven by the preceding prolonged cannulation time that leads to increasing papillary trauma and edema. Therefore, implementing alternate cannulation techniques early in the case and in rapid succession is an important aspect of reducing PEP. This principle is best demonstrated by a meta-analysis of six randomized trials that showed that early precut sphincterotomy significantly reduced the risk of PEP when compared with repeated standard cannulation attempts (2.5% vs 5.3%; odds ratio, 0.47).[22] Importantly, however, the studies included in this meta-analysis were conducted in mostly low-risk patients, often with favorable anatomy for precut sphincterotomy. Additional observational and randomized data have also suggested that precut sphincterotomy, especially if successful, is not an independent risk factor for PEP.[23,24] Further studies are needed to help define the exact point at which the risk-benefit ratio favors precut sphincterotomy over repeated cannulation attempts, although the natural tendency to continue standard cannulation attempts beyond 5 to 10 minutes should be controlled, and alternative strategies should be attempted early in a difficult case.

Other technical strategies that reduce the risk of PEP include minimizing the frequency and vigor of pancreatic duct injection, performing SOM using the aspiration technique, and avoiding balloon dilation of an intact sphincter, especially without prophylactic PSP. In coagulopathic patients with choledocholithiasis and native papillae, balloon dilation can be avoided by providing real-time decompression with a bile duct stent and repeating the ERCP with sphincterotomy and stone extraction when coagulation parameters have been restored. If this is not possible, and balloon dilation is mandatory, longer duration dilation (2–5 minutes) seems to result in lower rates of pancreatitis compared with 1-minute dilation.[25] Of note, balloon dilation after biliary sphincterotomy to facilitate large stone extraction does not seem to increase the risk of PEP.[26] All these factors are modifiable and should be considered during every ERCP.

## PROPHYLACTIC PANCREATIC STENT PLACEMENT

One of many proposed mechanisms of PEP implicates impaired pancreatic ductal drainage caused by trauma-induced edema of the papilla. PSP is therefore thought to reduce the risk of PEP by relieving pancreatic ductal hypertension that develops as a result of transient procedure-induced stenosis of the pancreatic orifice. Twelve published RCTs and at least as many nonrandomized trials have consistently demonstrated that PSP reduces the risk of PEP by approximately 60%.[27,28] Equally importantly, prophylactic pancreatic stents seem to profoundly reduce the likelihood of severe and necrotizing pancreatitis.[27,28]

It is important to keep in mind that the demonstrated benefits of PSP must be weighed against several potential disadvantages. First, attempting to place a pancreatic duct stent with subsequent failure actually increases the risk of PEP above baseline by inducing injury to the pancreatic orifice, but providing no subsequent ductal decompression.[29] Second, significant nonpancreatitis complications induced by PSP, such as stent migration and duct perforation, occur in up to 5% of cases. Furthermore, prolonged stent retention may induce ductal changes that resemble chronic pancreatitis, although the long-term clinical relevance of these changes remains unclear. PSP is associated with some patient inconvenience and increased costs by mandating follow-up abdominal radiography to ensure spontaneous passage of the stent and additional upper endoscopy to retrieve retained stents in 5% to 10% of cases.

Despite these considerations, PSP is widely regarded as an effective means of preventing PEP, is commonly used in academic medical centers in the United States,[30] and is recommended by the European Society of Gastrointestinal Endoscopy.[31] In light of the aforementioned concerns and the associated costs, however, PSP should be reserved for high-risk cases.[31,32] Based on the known independent patient and procedure-related risk factors for PEP, experts have suggested that the following cases are appropriate for prophylactic pancreatic duct stent placement: (1) clinical suspicion of SOD (whether or not manometry or therapeutic intervention performed), (2) prior PEP, (3) difficult cannulation, (4) precut (access) sphincterotomy, (5) pancreatic sphincterotomy (major or minor papilla), (6) endoscopic ampullectomy, (7) aggressive instrumentation or injection of the pancreatic duct, and (8) short-duration balloon dilation of an intact biliary sphincter.[30,33] Furthermore, preliminary studies have suggested that "salvage" PSP may be beneficial early in the course of PEP for patients who did not originally receive a stent, or in the case of early stent dislodgement.[34,35] Additional studies including a control group are necessary to fully evaluate PSP for this indication.

## PHARMACOPREVENTION

Nonsteroidal anti-inflammatory drugs (NSAIDs) are potent inhibitors of phospholipase $A_2$, cyclooxygenase, and neutrophil–endothelial interactions, all believed to play an important role in the pathogenesis of acute pancreatitis. Between 2003 and 2008, four studies evaluating the protective effects of single-dose rectal indomethacin or diclofenac demonstrated conflicting, but generally encouraging results. A meta-analysis of these RCTs, involving 912 patients, showed a robust 64% reduction in PEP associated with rectal NSAIDs (relative risk, 0.36; 95% confidence interval, 0.22–0.60) and no increase in associated adverse events.[36] A subsequent large-scale, multicenter, methodologically rigorous RCT was conducted to definitively evaluate the efficacy of prophylactic rectal indomethacin for preventing PEP in high-risk cases.[37] In this study, rectal indomethacin was associated with a 7.7% absolute risk reduction (number needed to treat = 13) and a 46% relative risk reduction in PEP ($P = .005$). To date, eight RCTs of rectal NSAIDs have been published; recent meta-analyses have demonstrated an associated risk reduction in excess of 50%.[38,39] However, several remaining questions surrounding NSAID pharmacoprevention remain.

## Should Rectal Nonsteroidal Anti-Inflammatory Drugs Be Given Routinely in Low-Risk Endoscopic Retrograde Cholangiopancreatography Pancreatitis Cases?

Controversy remains within the advanced endoscopy community regarding the role of NSAIDs in low-risk cases. The aforementioned large-scale RCT, which represents the most definitive study of rectal NSAIDs to date, only enrolled subjects at elevated risk for pancreatitis, leading to the perception that these medications may only be effective in high-risk cases. A post hoc analysis of this RCT, however, demonstrated that the benefit associated with indomethacin was consistent across the entire spectrum of enrolled subjects' risk for PEP. Among study subjects, those at mildly elevated risk (eg, difficult cannulation) derived similar benefit to those at more substantially elevated risk (eg, suspicion of SOD and pancreatic sphincterotomy), suggesting that the relative risk reduction of indomethacin may be consistent across risk groups, including average risk cases (Elmunzer, unpublished data, 2012). This observation is corroborated by data from the other published RCTs, which have demonstrated that rectal NSAIDs are effective in high- and average-risk cases.[38,39] Given these data, the favorable safety profile of rectal NSAIDs, and the time and cost necessary to conduct an adequately powered RCT in low-risk cases, it is reasonable to consider the use rectal NSAIDs universally. The European Society of Gastrointestinal Endoscopy recommends rectal indomethacin or diclofenac for all patients undergoing ERCP as a grade A recommendation.[40]

## What Is the Optimal Dose and Timing of Administration of Rectal Nonsteroidal Anti-Inflammatory Drugs?

Seven of the eight rectal NSAID RCTs administered a 100-mg dose (of indomethacin or diclofenac), and one study administered a 50-mg dose of diclofenac. Five studies, comprising 1439 subjects, administered the medication preprocedurally and three studies, comprising 922 subjects, administered the medication after the ERCP. Subgroup meta-analysis has revealed that both timings of administration seem equally effective.[38,39] Therefore, based on these data, it is appropriate to administer a 100-mg dose of rectal indomethacin or diclofenac immediately before or after ERCP. Because the exact periprocedural timing of administration does not seem critical, it may be reasonable to administer the dose at the time of cannulation, ensuring that the dose is not delivered too late in the event of a very long case (if delivered after ERCP) or too early (if delivered before ERCP) if cannulation is delayed for technical reasons (eg, difficulty advancing scope to papilla).

## Can Nonsteroidal Anti-Inflammatory Drugs Be Effectively Administered via Other (Nonrectal) Routes?

RCTs evaluating NSAIDs administered via nonrectal routes have demonstrated lack of efficacy in preventing PEP. Specifically, RCTs of intravascular valdecoxib, oral diclofenac, and intramuscular diclofenac have all yielded negative results. Even though these studies were underpowered and prone to type II statistical error, there are no existing data to support administration of prophylactic NSAIDs via any nonrectal route.

In the United States, practitioners may be tempted to administer intravenous ketorolac because of its widespread availability on anesthesia carts, its relative ease of delivery compared with suppository insertion, and the perception that NSAID efficacy is a class effect. Endoscopists, however, should resist this temptation because of the previously mentioned data suggesting that intravenous NSAIDs are not effective, and the absence of proof of a class effect. Indeed, indomethacin and diclofenac are postulated to be specifically effective because they are particularly potent inhibitors of phospholipase $A_2$ compared with other NSAIDs. In sum, based on available evidence, only rectal indomethacin or diclofenac should be prescribed for PEP prevention, as recommended by existing guidelines.

A related important question is whether investigators should continue to devote time and resources toward studying nonrectal NSAIDs for PEP pharmacoprevention. Because rectal NSAIDs are highly effective, safe, widely available, and easy to administer, it seems unlikely in the absence of any compelling new preclinical evidence that another formulation would provide enough clinical, logistical, or economic advantage over rectal NSAIDs to justify the time and cost necessary for high-quality clinical trials. Considering that the risk of PEP remains 15% despite the combination of rectal NSAIDs and prophylactic stent placement, other more pressing research that aims to further reduce risk or substantially limit costs should take priority.

### Can Rectal Nonsteroidal Anti-Inflammatory Drugs Replace Prophylactic Pancreatic Stent Placement in High-Risk Cases?

Available data indicate that the most evidence-based approach for preventing PEP in high-risk cases remains the combination of rectal indomethacin and PSP. This approach is based in part on the previously cited rectal indomethacin RCT wherein subjects who received indomethacin and a pancreatic stent (n = 247) had a PEP rate of 9.7% compared with 16.1% in those who received a stent alone (n = 249; $P = .04$).[37] This trial is the first to show that indomethacin confers protection in addition to PSP, but to date, there are no clinical trial data examining whether indomethacin is effective when administered instead of PSP.

A hypothesis-generating, post hoc analysis of the same indomethacin RCT suggested that subjects who received indomethacin alone were less likely to develop PEP than those who received a pancreatic stent alone or the combination of indomethacin and stent, even after adjusting for imbalances in PEP risk between groups.[41] Additionally, a recent network meta-analysis comparing the data supporting PSP with those supporting prophylactic NSAIDs suggested that the combination of NSAIDs and PSP is not better than rectal NSAIDs alone.[42] This observation is biologically plausible because a strategy of indomethacin alone avoids manipulation of the pancreatic orifice and instrumentation of the pancreatic duct, interventions necessary to place a stent but also believed to contribute to pancreatitis.

Although indomethacin monoprevention may offer clinical, logistical, and financial advantages, additional research is necessary to determine whether PSP remains necessary in the era of indomethacin prophylaxis is critical. To this end, a multicenter randomized noninferiority trial comparing rectal indomethacin alone with the combination of indomethacin and prophylactic stent placement is in its final planning phases, should begin enrolling subjects late 2015, and will hopefully provide concrete guidance for this critical management issue. Until the results of this trial are available, however, the combination of PSP and rectal indomethacin should remain the standard approach to preventing PEP in high-risk patients.

Despite extensive research over three decades, no other pharmacologic agent has been adopted into widespread clinical use. A recent systematic review aiming to inform future research in PEP pharmacoprevention identified sublingual nitroglycerin, bolus-administration somatostatin, and nafamostat as promising agents for which there is a high priority of definitive studies. Additionally, topical epinephrine, aggressive intravenous administration of lactated Ringer's solution, gabexate, ulinastatin, secretin, and antibiotics were considered appropriate for additional exploratory research before confirmatory RCTs.[43] A complete review of the data surrounding these agents is beyond the scope of this article, but a few additional points are worth considering:

Nitroglycerin is a smooth muscle relaxant that may lower sphincter of Oddi (SO) pressure and increase pancreatic parenchymal blood flow. Seven placebo-controlled RCTs have examined the effect of nitroglycerin on PEP. Three of these studies demonstrated a significant reduction in PEP, whereas the remaining four showed no benefit. Five meta-analyses have demonstrated an approximately 30% to 40% reduction in risk associated with the use of nitroglycerin in the prevention of PEP.[44] Because nitroglycerin is postulated to work by reducing SO pressure, it is unclear whether it would provide incremental benefit over PSP. Nevertheless, sublingual nitroglycerin may have a role in lower-risk cases, in resource-limited environments, or in place of pancreatic stent insertion. A recent small comparative effectiveness RCT demonstrated that the combination of sublingual nitroglycerin plus rectal indomethacin was more effective than indomethacin alone in a study sample that largely did not receive a pancreatic stent.[45] Another methodologically rigorous large-scale multicenter RCT is warranted to confirm the effectiveness of combined sublingual nitroglycerin and rectal indomethacin in the appropriate patient population (high-risk cases in environments where stenting is not widely available). In the interim, sublingual nitroglycerin may be reasonable to consider in patients with NSAID allergy or as an adjunct to rectal NSAIDs in high-risk cases that do not receive a prophylactic pancreatic stent.

Epinephrine sprayed directly on the papilla at the time of ERCP has also been postulated to prevent PEP through direct relaxation of the SO and reduction of papillary edema by decreasing capillary permeability. In addition to a small negative study, a larger trial enrolling 941 subjects undergoing diagnostic ERCP were randomized to 20 mL of 0.02% epinephrine or saline sprayed on the papilla after ERCP.[46] The incidence of pancreatitis was higher in the control group (31 of 480, 6.45%) than in the epinephrine group (9 of 461, 1.95%) ($P = .009$). Limitations of this study include the exclusion of all therapeutic ERCP and the atypical definition of PEP, reducing the external validity of the results in this era of high-quality diagnostic pancreaticobiliary imaging. Because it works primarily by SO relaxation, the impact of topical epinephrine in addition to PSP is unclear, but this agent may be effective as a surrogate stent, or in situations that do not warrant prophylactic stent placement. Even though existing data may not support a definitive RCT, the potential benefit of epinephrine, and its safety, low cost, and widespread availability, may justify a large-scale confirmatory RCT in the appropriate patient population (high-risk therapeutic ERCP, limited availability of pancreatic stents).[47]

Mechanistically, aggressive intravenous fluid (IVF) with lactated Ringer's solution (which attenuates the acidosis that seems to promote zymogen activation and pancreatic inflammation) may be an effective intervention for PEP by favorably affecting physiologic (pH) and microanatomic (pancreatic parenchymal perfusion) parameters. Recently, two observational studies and a pilot RCT[48] have suggested the potential benefit of IVF in reducing the incidence and severity of PEP. This RCT had a very small sample size, defined PEP atypically, and administered IVF over 8 to 10 hours, a schedule that is likely unrealistic in the United States.

Because IVF administration can be dangerous in older persons or in those with sodium-retaining states and the volume of infusion at which the risk-benefit ratio of IVF is optimized remains unknown, additional research is necessary to establish an evidence-based approach. Because data supporting its use in non-ERCP pancreatitis are robust and many practitioners already administer IVF for PEP prevention, large-scale RCTs may be warranted despite the absence of robust preliminary PEP data. Pending these results, it is my personal (non-evidence-based) practice to administer at least 3 L of crystalloid in recovery to young, healthy subjects who have undergone high-risk ERCP and an additional 3 to 5 L within the first 12 hospital hours to those who are admitted with postprocedure pain (depending on the severity of pain, signs of systemic inflammatory response, and assessment of total body volume status).

## REFERENCES

1. Cotton PB, Lehman G, Vennes J, et al. Endoscopic sphincterotomy complications and their management: an attempt at consensus. Gastrointest Endosc 1991;37: 383–93.
2. Kochar B, Akshintala VS, Afghani E, et al. Incidence, severity, and mortality of post-ERCP pancreatitis: a systematic review by using randomized, controlled trials. Gastrointest Endosc 2015;81:143–9.e9.
3. Healthcare cost and utilization project 2012. Available at: http://hcupnet.ahrq.gov. Accessed March 13, 2012.
4. Tse F, Liu L, Barkun AN, et al. EUS: a meta-analysis of test performance in suspected choledocholithiasis. Gastrointest Endosc 2008;67:235–44.
5. Romagnuolo J, Bardou M, Rahme E, et al. Magnetic resonance cholangiopancreatography: a meta-analysis of test performance in suspected biliary disease. Ann Intern Med 2003;139:547–57.
6. Zidi SH, Prat F, Le Guen O, et al. Use of magnetic resonance cholangiography in the diagnosis of choledocholithiasis: prospective comparison with a reference imaging method. Gut 1999;44:118–22.
7. ASGE Standards of Practice Committee, Maple JT, Ben-Menachem T. The role of endoscopy in the evaluation of suspected choledocholithiasis. Gastrointest Endosc 2010;71:1–9.
8. NIH state-of-the-science statement on endoscopic retrograde cholangiopancreatography (ERCP) for diagnosis and therapy. NIH Consens State Sci Statements 2002;19:1–26.
9. Cotton PB, Durkalski V, Romagnuolo J, et al. Effect of endoscopic sphincterotomy for suspected sphincter of Oddi dysfunction on pain-related disability following cholecystectomy: the EPISOD randomized clinical trial. JAMA 2014;311:2101–9.
10. Elmunzer BJ, Debenedet AT, Volk ML, et al. Clinical yield of diagnostic endoscopic retrograde cholangiopancreatography in orthotopic liver transplant recipients with suspected biliary complications. Liver Transpl 2012;18:1479–84.
11. Ding X, Zhang F, Wang Y. Risk factors for post-ERCP pancreatitis: a systematic review and meta-analysis. Surgeon 2014 [pii:S1479-666X(14)00146-2].
12. Chen JJ, Wang XM, Liu XQ, et al. Risk factors for post-ERCP pancreatitis: a systematic review of clinical trials with a large sample size in the past 10 years. Eur J Med Res 2014;19:26.
13. Ghaferi AA, Birkmeyer JD, Dimick JB. Variation in hospital mortality associated with inpatient surgery. N Engl J Med 2009;361:1368–75.
14. Freeman ML, DiSario JA, Nelson DB, et al. Risk factors for post-ERCP pancreatitis: a prospective, multicenter study. Gastrointest Endosc 2001;54:425–34.
15. Cheng CL, Sherman S, Watkins JL, et al. Risk factors for post-ERCP pancreatitis: a prospective multicenter study. Am J Gastroenterol 2006;101:139–47.
16. Freeman ML, Nelson DB, Sherman S, et al. Complications of endoscopic biliary sphincterotomy. N Engl J Med 1996;335:909–18.
17. Tse F, Yuan Y, Moayyedi P, et al. Guidewire-assisted cannulation of the common bile duct for the prevention of post-endoscopic retrograde cholangiopancreatography (ERCP) pancreatitis. Cochrane Database Syst Rev 2012;(12):CD009662.

18. Herreros de Tejada A, Calleja JL, Diaz G, et al. Double-guidewire technique for difficult bile duct cannulation: a multicenter randomized, controlled trial. Gastrointest Endosc 2009;70:700–9.

19. Wang P, Li ZS, Liu F, et al. Risk factors for ERCP-related complications: a prospective multicenter study. Am J Gastroenterol 2009;104:31–40.

20. Nakai Y, Isayama H, Sasahira N, et al. Risk factors for post-ERCP pancreatitis in wire-guided cannulation for therapeutic biliary ERCP. Gastrointest Endosc 2015; 81:119–26.

21. Ito K, Fujita N, Noda Y, et al. Can pancreatic duct stenting prevent post-ERCP pancreatitis in patients who undergo pancreatic duct guidewire placement for achieving selective biliary cannulation? A prospective randomized controlled trial. J Gastroenterol 2010;45:1183–91.

22. Cennamo V, Fuccio L, Zagari RM, et al. Can early precut implementation reduce endoscopic retrograde cholangiopancreatography-related complication risk? Meta-analysis of randomized controlled trials. Endoscopy 2010;42:381–8.

23. Navaneethan U, Konjeti R, Lourdusamy V, et al. Precut sphincterotomy: efficacy for ductal access and the risk of adverse events. Gastrointest Endosc 2014;81: 924–31.

24. Swan MP, Alexander S, Moss A, et al. Needle knife sphincterotomy does not increase the risk of pancreatitis in patients with difficult biliary cannulation. Clin Gastroenterol Hepatol 2013;11:430–6.e1.

25. Liao WC, Tu YK, Wu MS, et al. Balloon dilation with adequate duration is safer than sphincterotomy for extracting bile duct stones: a systematic review and meta-analyses. Clin Gastroenterol Hepatol 2012;10:1101–9.

26. Misra SP, Dwivedi M. Large-diameter balloon dilation after endoscopic sphincterotomy for removal of difficult bile duct stones. Endoscopy 2008;40:209–13.

27. Mazaki T, Mado K, Masuda H, et al. Prophylactic pancreatic stent placement and post-ERCP pancreatitis: an updated meta-analysis. J Gastroenterol 2014;49: 343–55.

28. Choudhary A, Bechtold ML, Arif M, et al. Pancreatic stents for prophylaxis against post-ERCP pancreatitis: a meta-analysis and systematic review. Gastrointest Endosc 2011;73:275–82.

29. Choksi NS, Fogel EL, Cote GA, et al. The risk of post-ERCP pancreatitis and the protective effect of rectal indomethacin in cases of attempted but unsuccessful prophylactic pancreatic stent placement. Gastrointest Endosc 2015;81:150–5.

30. Brackbill S, Young S, Schoenfeld P, Elta G. A survey of physician practices on prophylactic pancreatic stents. Gastrointest Endosc 2006;64:45–52.

31. Dumonceau JM, Andriulli A, Elmunzer BJ, et al. Prophylaxis of post-ERCP pancreatitis: European Society of Gastrointestinal Endoscopy (ESGE) Guideline - updated June 2014. Endoscopy 2014;46:799–815.

32. Das A, Singh P, Sivak MV Jr, et al. Pancreatic-stent placement for prevention of post-ERCP pancreatitis: a cost-effectiveness analysis. Gastrointest Endosc 2007;65:960–8.

33. Freeman ML. Pancreatic stents for prevention of post-endoscopic retrograde cholangiopancreatography pancreatitis. Clin Gastroenterol Hepatol 2007;5:1354–65.

34. Madacsy L, Kurucsai G, Joo I, et al. Rescue ERCP and insertion of a small-caliber pancreatic stent to prevent the evolution of severe post-ERCP pancreatitis: a case-controlled series. Surg Endosc 2009;23:1887–93.

35. Kerdsirichairat T, Attam R, Arain M, et al. Urgent ERCP with pancreatic stent placement or replacement for salvage of post-ERCP pancreatitis. Endoscopy 2014;46:1085–94.

36. Elmunzer BJ, Waljee AK, Elta GH, et al. A meta-analysis of rectal NSAIDs in the prevention of post-ERCP pancreatitis. Gut 2008;57:1262–7.
37. Elmunzer BJ, Scheiman JM, Lehman GA, et al. A randomized trial of rectal indomethacin to prevent post-ERCP pancreatitis. N Engl J Med 2012;366:1414–22.
38. Sun HL, Han B, Zhai HP, et al. Rectal NSAIDs for the prevention of post-ERCP pancreatitis: a meta-analysis of randomized controlled trials. Surgeon 2013;12: 141–7.
39. Sethi S, Sethi N, Wadhwa V, et al. A meta-analysis on the role of rectal diclofenac and indomethacin in the prevention of post-endoscopic retrograde cholangiopancreatography pancreatitis. Pancreas 2014;43:190–7.
40. Dumonceau JM, Andriulli A, Deviere J, et al. European Society of Gastrointestinal Endoscopy (ESGE) Guideline: prophylaxis of post-ERCP pancreatitis. Endoscopy 2010;42:503–15.
41. Elmunzer BJ, Higgins PD, Saini SD, et al. Does rectal indomethacin eliminate the need for prophylactic pancreatic stent placement in patients undergoing high-risk ERCP? Post hoc efficacy and cost-benefit analyses using prospective clinical trial data. Am J Gastroenterol 2013;108:410–5.
42. Akbar A, Abu Dayyeh BK, Baron TH, et al. Rectal nonsteroidal anti-inflammatory drugs are superior to pancreatic duct stents in preventing pancreatitis after endoscopic retrograde cholangiopancreatography: a network meta-analysis. Clin Gastroenterol Hepatol 2013;11:778–83.
43. Kubiliun NM, Adams MA, Akshintala VS, et al. Evaluation of pharmacologic prevention of pancreatitis following endoscopic retrograde cholangiopancreatography: a systematic review. Clin Gastroenterol Hepatol 2015;13:1231–9.
44. Bai Y, Xu C, Yang X, et al. Glyceryl trinitrate for prevention of pancreatitis after endoscopic retrograde cholangiopancreatography: a meta-analysis of randomized, double-blind, placebo-controlled trials. Endoscopy 2009;41:690–5.
45. Sotoudehmanesh R, Eloubeidi MA, Asgari AA, et al. A randomized trial of rectal indomethacin and sublingual nitrates to prevent post-ERCP pancreatitis. Am J Gastroenterol 2014;109:903–9.
46. Hua XL, Bo QJ, Gen GL, et al. Prevention of post-endoscopic retrograde cholangiopancreatography pancreatitis by epinephrine sprayed on the papilla. J Gastroenterol Hepatol 2011;26:1139–44.
47. Singh VK. A randomized trial of rectal indomethacin and papillary spray of epinephrine versus rectal indomethacin to prevent post-ERCP pancreatitis in high risk patients. NCT02116309.
48. Buxbaum J, Yan A, Yeh K, et al. Aggressive hydration with lactated ringer's solution reduces pancreatitis after endoscopic retrograde cholangiopancreatography. Clin Gastroenterol Hepatol 2014;12:303–7.e1.

# Endoscopic Treatment of Recurrent Acute Pancreatitis and Smoldering Acute Pancreatitis

Rohit Das, MD, Dhiraj Yadav, MD, MPH, Georgios I. Papachristou, MD*

## KEYWORDS

- Recurrent acute pancreatitis • Smoldering acute pancreatitis • Endoscopic therapy
- Pancreatic divisum • Idiopathic recurrent acute pancreatitis

## KEY POINTS

- In pancreas divisum–associated recurrent acute pancreatitis (RAP) data from uncontrolled retrospective studies point toward a benefit from minor papillary endoscopic intervention.
- The literature around idiopathic RAP (IRAP), although generally prospective, is heterogeneous, with differing cohort compositions and endoscopic interventions. Randomized data do not support the use of endotherapy in IRAP associated with elevated pancreatic sphincter pressures.
- Smoldering acute pancreatitis (AP) is a poorly defined entity. The role of endotherapy in smoldering AP needs further investigation.

## INTRODUCTION

RAP is a challenging condition, because it leads to significant patient morbidity, has potential for progression to chronic pancreatitis (CP), and has limited management options in many patients. Endoscopic therapy, in the form of papillary sphincterotomy and/or pancreatic duct stenting, is often used as a treatment modality for patients with RAP in the setting of pancreas divisum or idiopathic etiology, aiming to eliminate recurrent attacks and progression to CP.[1–17] The goal of this review is to discuss the role of endoscopic therapy in RAP related to pancreas divisum and IRAP, focusing on the methodology, findings, and limitations of available literature. The endoscopic management of smoldering AP, a poorly defined entity related to AP, also is discussed later.

None of the authors has any relevant financial conflicts to report.
Division of Gastroenterology, Hepatology and Nutrition, University of Pittsburgh Medical Center, PUH, M2, C Wing, 200 Lothrop Street, Pittsburgh, PA 15213, USA
* Corresponding author.
E-mail address: papachri@pitt.edu

Gastrointest Endoscopy Clin N Am 25 (2015) 737–748
http://dx.doi.org/10.1016/j.giec.2015.06.008
1052-5157/15/$ – see front matter Published by Elsevier Inc.

## RECURRENT ACUTE PANCREATITIS

RAP is defined as the occurrence of 2 or more episodes of AP in a given patient, without concurrent clinical or imaging evidence supportive of CP.[18–20] In natural history studies examining the long-term outcomes of patients after an index episode of AP, the incidence of RAP is estimated to be between 3% and 5% per 100 patient-years, with an overall prevalence of 17% to 20%.[19,20] RAP has a variable etiology, with the most common causes alcohol abuse and gallstone disease.[18–20] Pancreatobiliary malformation, specifically pancreas divisum, has also been associated with the development of RAP.[2,20] A significant proportion of patients with RAP, despite thorough work-up, have no etiology identified,[21] and their disease is thus labeled idiopathic.

Irrespective of etiology, RAP is independently associated with the development of CP, although the true incidence and prevalence of this complication, outside of recurrent alcoholic pancreatitis, is unclear.[18–20] Given the socioeconomic impact of CP,[22] alleviation and/or cessation of RAP with etiology-based treatment may have an impact on health care costs and patient morbidity. As discussed previously, endoscopic therapy has been studied as a management option specifically within the context of divisum-associated RAP and IRAP and is the focus of this article.

### Pancreas Divisum–Associated Recurrent Acute Pancreatitis and the Utility of Endoscopic Therapy

During embryologic development of the foregut, the pancreatic parenchyma is formed from the rotation and eventual fusion of the ventral and dorsal anlages. Parenchymal fusion is also associated with ductal fusion in greater than 90% of individuals, and failure of the ventral and dorsal ductal systems to fuse is termed, *pancreas divisum*.[23] Pancreas divisum is the most common congenital anomaly of the pancreas, with a prevalence of 6% to 8% based on prior autopsy and endoscopic retrograde cholangiopancreatography (ERCP) series.[24,25] Pancreas divisum has traditionally been diagnosed via ERCP, although secretin-enhanced magnetic resonance cholangiopancreatography (MRCP) has recently allowed for an accurate, noninvasive mode of diagnosis.

It is controversial as to whether pancreas divisum by itself is a causative factor for the development of RAP. Pathophysiologically, this is thought related to impaired pancreatic ductal drainage through the smaller minor papillary orifice. Retrospective studies have supported this hypothesis and found pancreas divisum significantly more common in patients with RAP compared with normal controls or patients with obscure abdominal pain.[24,26]

In the most recent study investigating this issue, Bertin and colleagues[27] examined the prevalence of pancreas divisum, as diagnosed by MRCP, in patients with RAP and/or CP deemed idiopathic or associated with *CFTR, SPINK1*, and/or *PRSS1* mutations. The frequency of pancreas divisum in the idiopathic group was 5%, not significantly different from the frequency found in both control groups and patients with *SPINK1 or PRSS1* mutations. The frequency of pancreas divisum in patients with concurrent *CFTR* mutation–associated RAP and/or CP was significantly higher at 47%. This finding suggests that pancreas divisum increases the risk of pancreatitis only in combination with another source of pancreatic injury, specifically *CFTR* dysfunction.

### Characteristics of Available Studies for Endoscopic Therapy in Divisum-Associated Recurrent Acute Pancreatitis

The hypothesis of pancreas divisum as an obstructive cause of recurrent pancreatitis and clinical improvement with minor papillary endoscopic intervention were first described by Cotton in 1980[28]. This has subsequently led to numerous studies examining the efficacy of endoscopic therapy in symptomatic pancreas divisum (**Table 1 and 2**).

A majority of studies done thus far have been retrospective in nature and lacking controls— groups of patients who did not receive endotherapy. Prospective studies have been limited, and to date only 1 randomized controlled trial has been performed.[6] In most studies, symptomatic pancreatic divisum has been defined as RAP, with only a minority of studies explicitly mentioning having previous evaluation for alternative etiologies. Other studies have also included patients with divisum-associated CP as well as divisum-associated chronic abdominal pain in the absence of clear biochemical or imaging evidence of pancreatitis.

## Efficacy and Complications

In general, endoscopic therapy for symptomatic pancreas divisum refers to minor papilla sphincterotomy. This may be performed via a pull or needle-knife (NK) technique. Pull sphincterotomy is accomplished by deep cannulation of the papillary orifice with a narrow tip catheter or sphincterotome using contrast or a wire-guided technique. A guide wire is then advanced deep in the accessory duct and a 3- to 4-mm incision is performed with the sphincterotome over the guide wire using pure cut. The NK sphincterotomy technique is accomplished by placing a 3F to 5F pancreatic duct stent into the accessory duct first, followed by performing a free-hand NK sphincterotomy over the pancreatic stent, aiming at the 10- to 12-o'clock position. These 2 techniques have been shown equally effective.[29] Two studies have looked at pancreatic duct stenting without performing sphincterotomy, and 1 report assessed botulinum toxin injection at the minor papilla.[1,6,9]

A recent systematic review was published as an attempt to summarize the currently available data.[8] Overall, 22 studies with a total of 838 patients were included. The review highlighted the variability in study outcomes, with 45% using an objective measure of pancreatitis, 36% using patient-perception based definitions, and the remaining studies having unclear definitions. Technical success of endotherapy was reported in only 4 studies and ranged between 17% and 86%. The overall estimated response rate ranged between 31% and 92% (median 62%), with the highest response rate seen in those presenting with RAP without CP (median 76%). The rate of post-ERCP pancreatitis was 18%, with the majority of cases (90%) mild and self-limited.

## Conclusions Regarding Endoscopic Therapy for Symptomatic Pancreas Divisum

Although the efficacy of endoscopic therapy in divisum-associated RAP is reported at 70% to 80%, this is primarily based on retrospective data, small sample sizes, and a wide variety of outcome definitions. Accordingly, future studies should be prospective, be ideally randomized, and focus on the rate of AP attacks before and after endotherapy so as to garner its true impact on the natural history of divisum-associated RAP.

In the authors' practice, when pancreas divisum is identified on MRCP during a thorough work-up of RAP, endoscopic therapy in the form of minor papillary sphincterotomy and stenting is offered to the patient (**Figs. 1**) after a discussion of the limitations of available evidence. An important consideration in the authors' decision making is the frequency of RAP and its impact on a patient's quality of life. Given the risk for post-ERCP pancreatitis in such cases, the authors routinely administer 1 to 2 L of lactated Ringer solution and 100 mg of indomethacin (rectally) and place pancreatic duct stents perioperatively.[30–32]

**Table 1**
Characteristics of selected studies for endoscopic therapy in symptomatic pancreas divisum

| Author, Year | Type of Study | No. of Patients | Patient Population | Follow-up in Recurrent Acute Pancreatitis Patients | Control Population |
|---|---|---|---|---|---|
| Lans et al,[6] 1992 | Randomized controlled trial | 19 | RAP | 30 mo | Yes—pancreas divisum without RAP |
| Lehman et al,[5] 1993 | Retrospective | 52 | RAP (17), CP (11), chronic pain (24) | 20 mo | No |
| Kozarek et al,[7] 1995 | Retrospective | 39 | RAP (15), CP (19), chronic pain (5) | 26 mo | No |
| Wehrmann et al,[1] 1999 | Prospective | 5 | RAP | 10 mo | No |
| Ertan,[9] 2000 | Prospective | 25 | RAP | 24 mo | No |
| Heyries et al,[17] 2002 | Retrospective | 24 | RAP | 39 mo | No |
| Gerke et al,[16] 2004 | Retrospective | 53 | RAP (30), RAP with chronic pain (14), chronic pain alone (9) | 29 mo | No |
| Chacko et al,[10] 2008 | Retrospective | 57 | RAP (27), CP (20), abdominal pain (8), other (2) | 20 mo | No |
| Kwan et al,[15] 2008 | Retrospective | 21 | RAP | 38 mo | No |
| Borak et al,[11] 2009 | Retrospective | 113 | RAP (62), CP (22), abdominal pain (29) | 47 mo | No |
| Mariani et al,[3] 2014 | Retrospective | 33 | RAP | 54 mo | Yes—pancreas divisum without RAP in past year |

**Table 2**
Reported efficacy of endoscopic therapy for pancreas divisum in selected studies

| Author, Year | Minor Papillary Intervention | Outcome Studied | Results for Recurrent Acute Pancreatitis Group | Complications Overall |
|---|---|---|---|---|
| Lans et al,[6] 1992 | Pancreatic duct stent | No. of subsequent AP episodes | Stent group—1 episode; control group—7 episodes | Stent migration (2) |
| Lehman et al,[5] 1993 | NK minor sphincterotomy | Hospital days for AP, symptom score | 76% Symptom improvement, 92% reduction in hospital days | Post-ERCP pancreatitis (13%), Sphincterotomy bleeding (2%), stent occlusion (47%) |
| Kozarek et al,[7] 1995 | NK minor sphincterotomy and/or pancreatic duct stent | Reduction in frequency of AP episodes | 86% | Post-ERCP pancreatitis (20%), papillary restenosis (12%) |
| Wehrmann et al,[1] 1999 | Minor papillary botulinum toxin injection | Relapse-free period >3 mo | 4/5 Relapse at 1, 7, 9, and 10 mo | None |
| Ertan,[9] 2000 | Pancreatic duct stent | Hospital days for AP, frequency of AP episodes | 83% Reduction in AP episodes, 87% reduction in hospital days | Stent migration (4%), stent occlusion (40%) |
| Heyries et al,[17] 2002 | Pull or NK minor sphincterotomy | Complete resolution in AP episodes | 92% | Post-ERCP pancreatitis (13%), sphincterotomy bleeding (4%), stent migration (4%) |
| Gerke et al,[16] 2004 | Pull or NK minor sphincterotomy | No recurrence of pain symptoms | 43% | Post-ERCP pancreatitis (11%) |
| Chacko et al,[10] 2008 | Pull or NK minor sphincterotomy | >50% Reduction in annual hospitalizations/emergency department visits for AP | 76% | Post-ERCP pancreatitis (11%), perforation (1%) |
| Kwan et al,[15] 2008 | Pull or NK minor sphincterotomy | Complete resolution in AP episodes | 62% | Post-ERCP pancreatitis (10%) |
| Borak et al,[11] 2009 | Pull or NK minor sphincterotomy | Improvement or cure of condition with lack of narcotic use | 71% | Post-ERCP pancreatitis (9%), post-sphincterotomy bleeding (2%) |
| Mariani et al,[3] 2014 | Pull minor sphincterotomy | Complete resolution in AP episodes | 74% | Post-ERCP pancreatitis (12%), post-sphincterotomy bleeding (2%) |

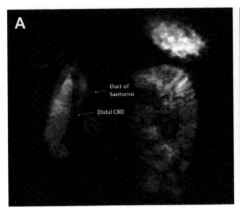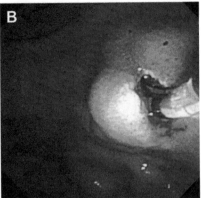

**Fig. 1.** A 55-year-old woman with a history of 3 prior episodes of AP, who was referred to the authors' center for further evaluation and management. Imaging evaluation with secretin-enhanced MRCP (*A*) was diagnostic of complete pancreatic divisum. She subsequently underwent endotherapy, with pull minor sphincterotomy (*B*) and prophylactic pigtail pancreatic duct placement. She has had no further episodes of AP in 1-year follow-up. CBD, common bile duct.

### Idiopathic Recurrent Acute Pancreatitis and the Utility of Endoscopic Therapy

As discussed previously, RAP is most commonly due to alcohol and gallstone disease. When initial evaluation toward these and other causes (hypercalcemia, hypertriglyceridemia, celiac disease, pancreas divisum, and hereditary etiologies) is unrevealing, patients are deemed to have idiopathic disease, which comprises 10% to 30% of those with RAP.[33] In such patients, studies have investigated the utility of ERCP and endoscopic ultrasound to identify causes amenable to endoscopic therapy, such as microlithiasis (biliary sludge) or pancreatic ductal changes related to occult chronic injury.[34–37] Along these lines, several studies have been performed examining the efficacy of empiric endoscopic therapy, mainly biliary and/or pancreatic sphincterotomy, in treating IRAP (**Table 3 and 4**).

### Characteristics of Available Studies for Endoscopic Therapy in Idiopathic Recurrent Acute Pancreatitis

A majority of studies done for endoscopic therapy in IRAP have been prospective in nature, 2 of which were randomized with long-term follow-up). Only 1 study, by Jacob and colleagues,[13] included a truly idiopathic cohort of RAP patients, after exclusion of typical alternative causes, including microlithiasis, sphincter of Odi dysfunction (SOD), and pancreas divisum. Other studies have used advanced endoscopic techniques as both diagnostic and therapeutic tools and have, therefore, included patients who ultimately have a cause identified (ie, microlithiasis) as well as patients with true IRAP. Consequently, interpreting this data in conglomerate is difficult.

### Efficacy and Complications

All studies used a reduction in frequency of attacks or resolution of RAP as their primary outcome (**Table 4**). Endoscopic interventions have varied across studies, ranging from pancreatic duct stenting to biliary sphincterotomy to pancreatic sphincterotomy to dual sphincterotomy. In nonrandomized prospective studies, the nature of the intervention(s) was primarily based on the diagnosis made after manometric and

**Table 3**
Characteristics of selected studies for endoscopic therapy in idiopathic recurrent acute pancreatitis

| Author, Year | Type of Study | No. of Patients | Patient Population | Follow up Duration | Control Population |
|---|---|---|---|---|---|
| Testoni et al,[12] 2000 | Prospective | 40 | IRAP → microlithiasis, SOD, divisum | 41 mo | No |
| Jacob et al,[13] 2001 | Randomized controlled trial | 35 | *True* IRAP | 36 mo | Yes |
| Kaw et al,[42] 2002 | Prospective | 126 | IRAP → microlithiasis, SOD, divisum | 30 mo | No |
| Wehrmann,[40] 2011 | Prospective and retrospective | 37 | IRAP → SOD | 140 mo | No |
| Cote et al,[14] 2012 | Randomized controlled trial | 89 | IRAP → SOD | 78 mo | Yes |

**Table 4**
Reported efficacy of endoscopic therapy in idiopathic recurrent acute pancreatitis in selected studies

| Author, Year | Endoscopic Intervention | Outcome Studied | Efficacy | Complications |
|---|---|---|---|---|
| Testoni et al,[12] 2000 | Biliary sphincterotomy and/or pancreatic sphincterotomy and/or pancreatic duct stent | Complete resolution in AP episodes | 89% | Post-ERCP pancreatitis (9%) |
| Jacob et al,[13] 2001 | Pancreatic duct stent | Frequency of RAP | 11%, vs 53% In the ontrol ($P<.02$) | Post-ERCP pancreatitis (9%), stent occlusion (30%) |
| Kaw et al,[42] 2002 | Biliary and/or pancreatic sphincterotomy | Complete resolution in AP episodes | 67%–100% (Varied based on ultimate diagnosis) | Post-ERCP pancreatitis (16%), post-sphincterotomy bleeding (6%), perforation (0.8%) |
| Wehrmann,[40] 2011 | Biliary and/or pancreatic sphincterotomy with temporary pancreatic duct stent | Complete resolution in AP episodes | 86% After 2 y prospective follow-up, 49% after 8 y additional retrospective follow-up | Not reported |
| Cote et al,[14] 2012 | Pancreatic SOD Biliary vs dual sphincterotomy No pancreatic SOD Biliary vs sham (temporary pancreatic duct stent, both groups) | Complete resolution in AP episodes | No difference in either group | Post-ERCP pancreatitis (15%) |

advanced endoscopic diagnostic studies. Overall, biliary sphincterotomy in these studies has been shown efficacious in 75% to 85% of patients within the context of microlithiasis or biliary sludge (ie, patients without true IRAP).

The utility of pancreatic endotherapy in patients with IRAP is unclear. In general, prior studies have examined this question in patient populations with pancreatic and/or biliary SOD, as documented by manometry. Results of retrospective studies published in abstract form[38–40] reported dual (ie, pancreatic and biliary) sphincterotomy associated with better outcomes compared with biliary sphincterotomy alone. In contrast, Cote and colleagues[14] recently found no efficacy difference after patients with IRAP with elevated pancreatic sphincter pressures were randomized to biliary or dual sphincterotomy, suggesting that pancreatic SOD is more likely an effect, rather than a cause, of RAP.

Only 1 study has addressed the effectiveness of pancreatic endotherapy in IRAP patients with normal sphincter of Oddi pressures and no other alternative etiology.[13] In this small, randomized study, pancreatic duct stenting without pancreatic sphincterotomy led to a significant reduction in the frequency of RAP, although the incidence of persistent pancreatic-type pain was not significantly different.

### Conclusions Regarding the Utility of Endoscopic Therapy in Idiopathic Recurrent Acute Pancreatitis

The efficacy of ablating the pancreatic sphincter in patients with IRAP is unclear (**Fig. 2**). Recent randomized data show no benefit of pancreatic sphincterotomy, even in patients with associated elevation in pancreatic sphincter pressures.[14] There are supportive, randomized data for pancreatic duct stenting as a lone intervention, but they are limited by small sample size and duration of follow-up.[13] Therefore, at this point, pancreatic endotherapy in IRAP cannot be routinely recommended. Future prospective, randomized studies should focus on pancreatic sphincterotomy and/or pancreatic duct stenting in patients with true IRAP.

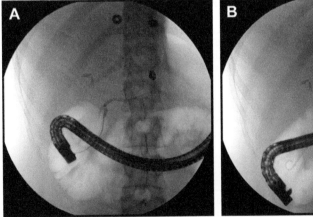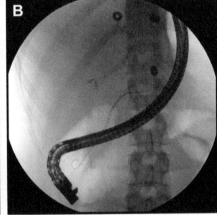

**Fig. 2.** A 19-year-old woman with a history of multiple episodes of RAP without clear etiology despite work-up for metabolic, biliary, autoimmune, anatomic, and genetic causes. Due to her burden of disease, she underwent endoscopic management while an inpatient with an attack of AP. Her pancreatogram was normal (A) and a 5F by 9-cm pigtail pancreatic duct stent was placed (B). Her clinical condition improved dramatically. Two months later, on follow-up ERCP, a pancreatic sphincterotomy was performed. Her next recurrence occurred 2 years after performance of pancreatic endotherapy.

In the authors' practice, after a thorough etiologic evaluation, including genetic studies, pancreatic duct stenting and/or sphincterotomy is considered a last-resort management option in patients with IRAP with a high burden of disease, arbitrarily defined as greater than 3 AP attacks/year. The authors do not perform sphincter of Oddi manometry. Due to a high risk of progression to CP,[41] a strong consideration for total pancreatectomy and auto islet cell transplantation is made in select patients with RAP and associated genetic abnormalities who have a high disease burden.

## SMOLDERING ACUTE PANCREATITIS

Smoldering AP is a poorly defined entity, meant to represent a prolonged course of AP as manifested by persistent pancreatic symptoms, inflammatory changes on CT, and/ or pancreatic enzyme elevations in absence of systemic or local complications (ie, peripancreatic necrosis, parenchymal necrosis, or acute pancreatic fluid collections).

The clinical factors predisposing to smoldering AP are unclear. To date, only 1 study has been published regarding the management of smoldering AP. Varadarajulu and colleagues[43] describe a small case series of 11 patients with smoldering AP treated endoscopically. Patient with smoldering AP, as defined previously, had symptoms lasting for greater than or equal to 10 days. Pancreatograms were normal in 3 patients and otherwise showed ducal irregularities/dilatation in 8. All patients received a pancreatic duct stent, and 10 (91%) had relief of abdominal pain within 9 days and discontinuation of narcotic use in 15 days. No control arm was present in the study. The investigators posit a hypothesis that smoldering AP may be a consequence of functional pancreatic sphincter obstruction from ongoing inflammatory changes, potentially amenable to sphincter ablation with transpapillary stenting.

In retrospective data from an endoscopic database maintained at the authors' center, 16 patients with smoldering AP underwent endoscopic intervention with pancreatic duct stenting. As a first-line therapy, endoscopic management was successful in 10 of 12 (83%) patients and was 100% successful as a second-line therapy in 4

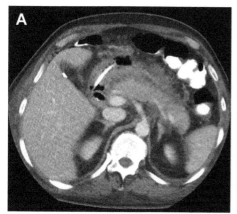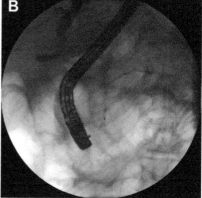

**Fig. 3.** A 56-year-old man with post-ERCP pancreatitis developed smoldering symptoms despite conservative management. There was imaging evidence of ongoing peripancreatic inflammation (*A*) and elevation of pancreatic enzymes, which persisted more than 10 days into his hospitalization, consistent with smoldering acute pancreatitis. He was managed with a nasojejunal feeding tube for pancreatic rest and, ultimately, endotherapy on hospital day 12. His pancreatogram was normal (*B*), and a 5F by 9-cm pancreatic duct stent was placed. He subsequently improved and was discharged on hospital day 17.

patients who first underwent pancreatic rest with a nasojejunal feeding tube. In the authors' practice, patients with smoldering AP receive prolonged pancreatic rest with nasojejunal feeding as a first-line therapy, with endoscopic therapy considered in those with persistent, refractory symptoms despite pancreas rest (**Fig. 3**).

## SUMMARY

In cases of pancreas divisum–associated RAP, data from uncontrolled and primarily retrospective studies point toward a benefit from minor papillary endoscopic intervention. Nevertheless, given the quality of the data, endoscopic management in such patients remains an individualized decision, and randomized controlled studies are needed to ascertain its true long-term benefit.

The literature around IRAP, although generally prospective and in some cases randomized and controlled, is heterogeneous, with differing cohort compositions and endoscopic interventions. Randomized data do not support the use of pancreatic endotherapy in SOD-associated IRAP, and few data exist on the utility of pancreatic endotherapy in IRAP patients with normal sphincter pressures. As such, pancreatic endotherapy in IRAP cannot be routinely recommended and further randomized controlled studies are needed, especially in true IRAP.

Finally, smoldering AP remains a poorly defined manifestation of AP in need of further epidemiologic analysis. Given the paucity of current data, endoscopic management for smoldering AP cannot be routinely recommended, although it remains a management consideration in patients with symptoms refractory to conservative measures.

## REFERENCES

1. Wehrmann T, Schmitt T, Seifert H. Endoscopic botulinum toxin injection into the minor papilla for treatment of idiopathic recurrent pancreatitis in patients with pancreas divisum. Gastrointest Endosc 1999;50(4):545–8.
2. Takuma K, Kamisawa T, Hara S, et al. Etiology of recurrent acute pancreatitis, with special emphasis on pancreaticobiliary malformation. Adv Med Sci 2012;57(2):244–50.
3. Mariani A, Di Leo M, Petrone MC, et al. Outcome of endotherapy for pancreas divisum in patients with acute recurrent pancreatitis. World J Gastroenterol 2014;20(46):17468–75.
4. Liao Z, Gao R, Wang W, et al. A systematic review on endoscopic detection rate, endotherapy, and surgery for pancreas divisum. Endoscopy 2009;41(5):439–44.
5. Lehman GA, Sherman S, Nisi R, et al. Pancreas divisum: results of minor papilla sphincterotomy. Gastrointest Endosc 1993;39(1):1–8.
6. Lans JI, Geenen JE, Johanson JF, et al. Endoscopic therapy in patients with pancreas divisum and acute pancreatitis: a prospective, randomized, controlled clinical trial. Gastrointest Endosc 1992;38(4):430–4.
7. Kozarek RA, Ball TJ, Patterson DJ, et al. Endoscopic approach to pancreas divisum. Dig Dis Sci 1995;40(9):1974–81.
8. Kanth R, Samji NS, Inaganti A, et al. Endotherapy in symptomatic pancreas divisum: a systematic review. Pancreatology 2014;14(4):244–50.
9. Ertan A. Long-term results after endoscopic pancreatic stent placement without pancreatic papillotomy in acute recurrent pancreatitis due to pancreas divisum. Gastrointest Endosc 2000;52(1):9–14.

10. Chacko LN, Chen YK, Shah RJ. Clinical outcomes and nonendoscopic interventions after minor papilla endotherapy in patients with symptomatic pancreas divisum. Gastrointest Endosc 2008;68(4):667–73.

11. Borak GD, Romagnuolo J, Alsolaiman M, et al. Long-term clinical outcomes after endoscopic minor papilla therapy in symptomatic patients with pancreas divisum. Pancreas 2009;38(8):903–6.

12. Testoni PA, Caporuscio S, Bagnolo F, et al. Idiopathic recurrent pancreatitis: long-term results after ERCP, endoscopic sphincterotomy, or ursodeoxycholic acid treatment. Am J Gastroenterol 2000;95(7):1702–7.

13. Jacob L, Geenen JE, Catalano MF, et al. Prevention of pancreatitis in patients with idiopathic recurrent pancreatitis: a prospective nonblinded randomized study using endoscopic stents. Endoscopy 2001;33(7):559–62.

14. Cote GA, Imperiale TF, Schmidt SE, et al. Similar efficacies of biliary, with or without pancreatic, sphincterotomy in treatment of idiopathic recurrent acute pancreatitis. Gastroenterology 2012;143(6):1502–9.e1.

15. Kwan V, Loh SM, Walsh PR, et al. Minor papilla sphincterotomy for pancreatitis due to pancreas divisum. ANZ J Surg 2008;78(4):257–61.

16. Gerke H, Byrne MF, Stiffler HL, et al. Outcome of endoscopic minor papillotomy in patients with symptomatic pancreas divisum. JOP 2004;5(3):122–31.

17. Heyries L, Barthet M, Delvasto C, et al. Long-term results of endoscopic management of pancreas divisum with recurrent acute pancreatitis. Gastrointest Endosc 2002;55(3):376–81.

18. Yadav D, O'Connell M, Papachristou GI. Natural history following the first attack of acute pancreatitis. Am J Gastroenterol 2012;107(7):1096–103.

19. Lankisch PG, Breuer N, Bruns A, et al. Natural history of acute pancreatitis: a long-term population-based study. Am J Gastroenterol 2009;104(11):2797–805.

20. Cavestro GM, Leandro G, Di Leo M, et al. A single-centre prospective, cohort study of the natural history of acute pancreatitis. Dig Liver Dis 2015;47(3):205–10.

21. Sajith KG, Chacko A, Dutta AK. Recurrent acute pancreatitis: clinical profile and an approach to diagnosis. Dig Dis Sci 2010;55(12):3610–6.

22. Hall TC, Garcea G, Webb MA, et al. The socio-economic impact of chronic pancreatitis: a systematic review. J Eval Clin Pract 2014;20(3):203–7.

23. Kozu T, Suda K, Toki F. Pancreatic development and anatomical variation. Gastrointest Endosc Clin N Am 1995;5(1):1–30.

24. Bernard JP, Sahel J, Giovannini M, et al. Pancreas divisum is a probable cause of acute pancreatitis: a report of 137 cases. Pancreas 1990;5(3):248–54.

25. Stimec B, Bulajic M, Korneti V, et al. Ductal morphometry of ventral pancreas in pancreas divisum. Comparison between clinical and anatomical results. Ital J Gastroenterol 1996;28(2):76–80.

26. Dhar A, Goenka MK, Kochhar R, et al. Pancrease divisum: five years' experience in a teaching hospital. Indian J Gastroenterol 1996;15(1):7–9.

27. Bertin C, Pelletier AL, Vullierme MP, et al. Pancreas divisum is not a cause of pancreatitis by itself but acts as a partner of genetic mutations. Am J Gastroenterol 2012;107(2):311–7.

28. Cotton PB. Congenital anomaly of pancreas divisum as cause of obstructive pain and pancreatitis. Gut 1980;21(2):105–14.

29. Attwell A, Borak G, Hawes R, et al. Endoscopic pancreatic sphincterotomy for pancreas divisum by using a needle-knife or standard pull-type technique: safety and reintervention rates. Gastrointest Endosc 2006;64(5):705–11.

30. Buxbaum J, Yan A, Yeh K, et al. Aggressive hydration with lactated Ringer's solution reduces pancreatitis after endoscopic retrograde cholangiopancreatography. Clin Gastroenterol Hepatol 2014;12(2):303–7.e1.
31. Elton E, Howell DA, Parsons WG, et al. Endoscopic pancreatic sphincterotomy: indications, outcome, and a safe stentless technique. Gastrointest Endosc 1998;47(3):240–9.
32. Yaghoobi M, Rolland S, Waschke KA, et al. Meta-analysis: rectal indomethacin for the prevention of post-ERCP pancreatitis. Aliment Pharmacol Ther 2013;38(9): 995–1001.
33. Levy MJ, Geenen JE. Idiopathic acute recurrent pancreatitis. Am J Gastroenterol 2001;96(9):2540–55.
34. Al-Haddad M, Wallace MB. Diagnostic approach to patients with acute idiopathic and recurrent pancreatitis, what should be done? World J Gastroenterol 2008; 14(7):1007–10.
35. Coyle WJ, Pineau BC, Tarnasky PR, et al. Evaluation of unexplained acute and acute recurrent pancreatitis using endoscopic retrograde cholangiopancreatography, sphincter of Oddi manometry and endoscopic ultrasound. Endoscopy 2002;34(8):617–23.
36. Khalid A, Peterson M, Slivka A. Secretin-stimulated magnetic resonance pancreaticogram to assess pancreatic duct outflow obstruction in evaluation of idiopathic acute recurrent pancreatitis: a pilot study. Dig Dis Sci 2003;48(8):1475–81.
37. Wilcox CM, Varadarajulu S, Eloubeidi M. Role of endoscopic evaluation in idiopathic pancreatitis: a systematic review. Gastrointest Endosc 2006;63(7): 1037–45.
38. Jathal A, Sherman S, Fogel EL, et al. Pancreatobiliary sphincterotomy (PBES) versus biliary sphincterotomy (BES) alone in sphincter of oddi dysfunction associated with idiopathic recurrent pancreatitis [abstract]. Gastrointest Endosc 2001; 53:AB93.
39. Guelrud M, Plaz J, Mendoza S, et al. Endoscopic Treatment in Type II Pancreatic Sphincter Dysfunction [abstract]. Gastrointest Endosc 1995;41:389.
40. Wehrmann T. Long-term results (>/= 10 years) of endoscopic therapy for sphincter of Oddi dysfunction in patients with acute recurrent pancreatitis. Endoscopy 2011;43(3):202–7.
41. Howes N, Lerch MM, Greenhalf W, et al. Clinical and genetic characteristics of hereditary pancreatitis in Europe. Clin Gastroenterol Hepatol 2004;2(3):252–61.
42. Kaw M, Brodmerkel GJ Jr. ERCP, biliary crystal analysis, and sphincter of Oddi manometry in idiopathic recurrent pancreatitis. Gastrointest Endosc 2002;55(2): 157–62.
43. Varadarajulu S, Noone T, Hawes RH, et al. Pancreatic duct stent insertion for functional smoldering pancreatitis. Gastrointestinal endoscopy 2003;58(3): 438–41.

# Sphincter of Oddi Dysfunction

Aaron J. Small, MD, MSCE[a], Richard A. Kozarek, MD[b],*

## KEYWORDS

- Sphincter of Oddi dysfunction • Biliary • Pancreatic • Sphincterotomy
- Endoscopic therapy • EPISOD trial • Patient selection

## KEY POINTS

- Sphincter of Oddi dysfunction (SOD) is a benign, acalculous disease that can result in biliary or pancreatic obstructive symptoms.
- Chronic, unrelenting epigastric or right upper quadrant pain is not caused by SOD.
- It is difficult, if not impossible, to diagnose SOD in patients with an intact gallbladder.
- Modified Milwaukee classification is the most relevant classification system in clinical practice.
- The classification and response to sphincterotomy of biliary SOD I to III has been defined by randomized controlled trials, whereas pancreatic SOD classification has not.
- Initial evaluation starts with history taking, biochemistries, and noninvasive imaging before proceeding with endoscopic retrograde cholangiopancreatography (ERCP) and sphincter of Oddi manometry, if necessary.
- Response to sphincterotomy depends largely on the type of disease, with excellent response to type I and variable results with type II.
- Recent level I evidence suggests no role for therapeutic ERCP for type III SOD, which has no better response to treatment than a sham sphincterotomy.

## INTRODUCTION

*Biliary dyskinesia has been known by a number of pseudonyms, including but not limited to ampullary spasm, papillary stenosis, and sphincter of Oddi dysfunction (SOD). The latter name disregards Glisson's 1681 description of the bit of muscle*

---

Disclosure statement: Dr A.J. Small has no conflicts of interest or financial ties to disclose; Dr R.A. Kozarek (Virginia Mason Medical Center) received support from the National Institutes of Health (DK074739-07) as one of the investigators in the EPISOD Study.

[a] Division of Gastroenterology, Digestive Disease Institute, Virginia Mason Medical Center, 1100 Ninth Avenue, Seattle, WA 98101, USA; [b] Division of Gastroenterology, Digestive Disease Institute, Virginia Mason Medical Center, University of Washington, 1100 Ninth Avenue, Seattle, WA 98101, USA
* Corresponding author.
*E-mail address:* Richard.Kozarek@virginiamason.org

*encompassing the distal bile duct and credits Ruggero Oddi, a fourth year medical student at the University of Perugia, Italy, with its description in 1887 and its consequent dysfunction.[1] What neither Glisson nor Oddi envisioned, however, was the controversy surrounding a 6- to 15-mm fragment of smooth muscle that Boyden has divided into three distinct histologic segments to include the sphincter ampullae.[2] Like a theologic trinity, Oddi's sphincter, therefore, has evolved into three. Clinical signs and symptoms accordingly are predicated on which of the subsphincters becomes inflamed, irritated, spastic, patulous, or hormonally belligerent.[3]*

The senior author first wrote this more than 20 years ago.[3] What has happened in the subsequent 2 decades that has made the authors rethink their approach to possible sphincter dysfunction?

The entire paradigm of SOD may currently be unraveling with the questionable utility of effective endoscopic therapies for certain subtypes of SOD. The decision to perform endoscopic retrograde cholangiopancreatography (ERCP) with sphincterotomy for SOD is complex and involves several factors, such as patient characteristics, classification of the disease, local expertise, and potential predictors of response to therapy. When considering therapy for SOD, it is essential to partake in shared decision making with patients and consider each of these variables in order to develop the best approach for each patient having symptoms potentially attributable to the pancreaticobiliary sphincters. This article reviews the current definition of SOD and the various factors to consider before embarking on endoscopic therapy for SOD in light of recent evidence.

## DEFINING SPHINCTER OF ODDI DYSFUNCTION

The sphincter of Oddi (SO) serves as the dynamic gatekeeper for pancreaticobiliary endoscopists as a cylindrical anatomic structure composed of 3 sphincters of smooth muscle fibers that surround the distal common bile duct (CBD), main pancreatic duct, and the ampulla of Vater (**Fig. 1**).[4–6] Given its anatomic position surrounding the intramural portion of the CBD and pancreatic ducts, SO contractility directly regulates the (antegrade) flow of bile and pancreatic juices out into the duodenum and prevents (retrograde) reflux of duodenal fluid into the pancreaticobiliary tree. Dysregulation of SO contractility, involving either of the biliary or pancreatic portions of the sphincter or both, can result in an impedance of flow, alleged to be responsible for biliary colic as well as a source for acute, relapsing pancreatitis. Inflammation and fibrosis at the papillary orifice may also contribute to sphincter spasm or stenosis.[7] The resultant clinical syndrome of this dyskinetic or stenotic sphincter is characterized as SOD. Diagnosis is often made after excluding overt stone disease and other structural causes for pancreatic or biliary pain, including ductal stenosis or stones. A variety of other terms, including *papillary stenosis, sclerosing papillitis, biliary spasms, biliary dyskinesia,* and *postcholecystectomy pain syndrome,* have been linked to SOD, further adding to the confusion of this disease. SOD remains a controversial clinical entity that is multifactorial and may present with complex symptoms.

### Pathogenesis

The cause of SOD is not well understood. It is categorized as a benign, acalculous obstructive disorder at the level of the SO.[8] There are several proposed causes. One is the formation of a stenosis at the ampulla from passage of a gallstone or gravel over an extended time period. A second possibility is attributed to SO hypertension either caused by a congenital hypertrophic sphincter or an overly responsive smooth muscle contraction of the sphincter to neuronal or hormonal stimuli.

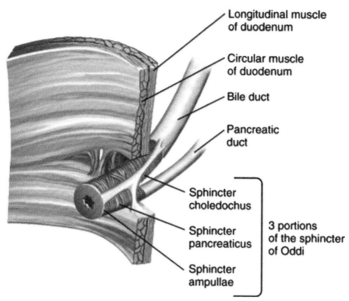

Longitudinal muscle
of duodenum

Circular muscle
of duodenum

Bile duct

Pancreatic
duct

Sphincter
choledochus

Sphincter
pancreaticus

Sphincter
ampullae

3 portions
of the sphincter
of Oddi

**Fig. 1.** SO anatomy. (*From* Elmunzer BJ, Elta GH. Biliary tract motor function and dysfunction. In: Feldman M, Friedman LS, Brandt LJ, editors. Sleisenger and Fordtran's gastrointestinal and liver disease: pathophysiology/diagnosis/management. 9th edition. (PA): Saunders Elsevier; 2010. p. 1068; with permission.)

## Epidemiology

The prevalence of SOD is difficult to ascertain given that the diagnosis is one of exclusion and based on a high level of suspicion, often after response to a biliary and/or pancreatic sphincterotomy. Up to 1.5% of the US population report symptoms consistent with SOD based on survey data, with a 3-fold female predilection.[9] It is estimated that 10% to 20% of patients who undergo cholecystectomy have subsequent recurrent or residual upper abdominal pain; these patients may have SOD.[10–13] Estimates for pancreatic SOD are limited to small cohort studies with 33% to 40% of idiopathic recurrent pancreatitis suspected to be from SOD.[14]

## Classification of Sphincter of Oddi

There have been several reported classification schemes of SOD in an effort to objectify the diagnosis. The most widely adopted is the Milwaukee classification scheme proposed by Hogan and Geenen.[15] In this scheme, SOD is classified into biliary types I, II, and III based on upper abdominal symptoms, biochemical abnormalities, and radiographic results (**Table 1**).[6,15] Subsequently, this classification was broadened to include patients with pancreatic-type pain and relapsing pancreatitis (by single-center expert opinion but never validated in randomized controlled trials [RCTs]). Type I is characterized by (1) dilated CBD or main pancreatic ducts, with some variations in the cutoffs in what is considered a dilated duct (note that the classification fails to consider the degree of bile dilation before and after cholecystectomy); (2) greater than a 1.5- to 2.0-fold elevation in liver-associated enzymes (aminotransferases or alkaline phosphatase levels) or pancreatic enzymes (amylase or lipase) on at least 2 occasions during episodes of pain; and (3) typical, episodic biliary, or pancreatic pain. Type II is suspected when 2 of the 3 aforementioned criteria are present. Finally, type III has been defined by

**Table 1**
**Modified Milwaukee classification scheme**

| Classification | Diagnostic Criteria |
|---|---|
| A. Biliary SOD | |
| Type 1 | 1. Biliary-type pain<br>2. Elevated ALT, AST, AP more than 1.5–2.0 times the upper limit of normal on at least 2 or more occasions<br>3. Bile duct diameter $\geq$10 mm |
| Type 2 | Biliary-type pain with either B or C in the aforementioned criteria |
| Type 3 | Biliary-type pain only with no other abnormalities |
| B. Pancreatic SOD | |
| Type 1 | 1. Pancreatic-type pain<br>2. Elevated serum amylase or lipase more than 1.5–2.0 times the upper limit of normal on at least 2 or more occasions<br>3. Pancreatic duct diameter $\geq$6 mm in the head and $\geq$5 mm in the body |
| Type 2 | Pancreatic-type pain with either B or C in the aforementioned criteria |
| Type 3 | Pancreatic-type pain only with no other abnormalities |

*Abbreviations:* ALT, alanine aminotransferase; AP, alkaline phosphatase; AST, aspartate aminotransferase.

intense biliary or pancreatic-type pain alone with no evidence of laboratory or radiographic abnormalities during episodes of pain or at baseline.

Despite these criteria, some remain skeptical of the diagnosis, contending that type I is rather a consequence of chronic gravel or sludge passage with subsequent papillary stenosis, type II a result of stone passage without stenosis, and type III a functional disorder often associated with gastroparesis, irritable bowel syndrome, nonulcer dyspepsia, and sphincter spasm.[3,16–19] Indeed, recent evidence from a multicenter RCT questions the very validity of the third subtype of SOD. In the Evaluating Predictors and Interventions in Sphincter of Oddi Dysfunction (EPISOD) trial, postcholecystectomy patients with suspected SOD type III had no difference in pain relief following sphincterotomy when compared with those who underwent a sham endoscopic procedure.[20] A similar lack of benefit following sphincterotomy was found in a subset of trial patients who had presumed SOD type II with demonstrated liver test abnormalities. These data point to a lack of therapeutic benefit from sphincter obliteration in this subpopulation, a maneuver that should resolve SO hypertension or spasm and raises many questions about the diagnosis of type III and perhaps even type II disease.[21,22] Such findings are substantial given that half of the patients who have pain following gallbladder removal may have SOD types I or II, and a large number were presumed to have SOD type III.[8,9]

## DIAGNOSTIC EVALUATION

The diagnosis of SOD relies on astute clinical history-taking skills and subsequent laboratory and radiographic tests to rule out other sources of patient discomfort. Rome III criteria can aid in heightening suspicion for functional pancreaticobiliary disease. The diagnostic utility of SO manometry (SOM) and associated high basal pressures has become less reliable, particularly for type III disease.[14]

### Clinical Features

A common presentation for patients suspected to have SOD is disabling, *intermittent, or episodic* pain in the epigastric or right upper quadrant (RUQ) in a middle-aged woman.[8,9] However, the disease is not sex or age definitive. The diagnosis is typically made following cholecystectomy as it is difficult, if not impossible, to diagnose SOD in patients with an intact gallbladder. Biliary SOD can present as episodic, postprandial RUQ pain with or without cholestasis similar to that experienced with choledocholithiasis. Pancreatic SOD generally results in more prolonged pain, radiating to the back, and can be associated with pancreatitis. Conversely, *chronic, unrelenting* epigastric or RUQ pain is not caused by SOD. Physical examination is typically nonspecific for abdominal pain, though an astute practitioner may elicit musculoskeletal pain or a succession splash suggestive of gastroparesis as an alternative diagnosis.

Given the ambiguity in the clinical presentation of patients with SOD, additional screening tools can be helpful to guide one's practice and prompt further testing. The Rome III criteria system is a symptom-based, diagnostic tool developed to aid the classification of functional gastrointestinal disorders when symptoms are not explained by the presence of a structural or tissue abnormality. The most recent criteria, revised in 2006, encompass both biliary and pancreatic SOD with a description of characteristic pain symptoms (**Box 1**).[23] The diagnosis of functional biliary or pancreatic pain, presumably from SOD, is supported with or without evidence of transient enzyme elevations.

### Diagnostic Testing

Patients with SOD are at the highest risk of developing post-ERCP pancreatitis with a prevalence as high as 25%.[10,24,25] Therefore, care must be taken to avoid unnecessary invasive testing to establish a diagnosis. Equally important, if not more so, is to ensure that a diagnosis of occult malignancy is not missed in patients with ductal dilation and abnormal pancreatic or liver function tests. Less invasive imaging to assess ductal dilation, by endoscopic ultrasound, transabdominal ultrasound, helical computed tomography, or magnetic resonance cholangiopancreatography (MRCP), should be used. Provocation with intravenous cholecystokinin or secretin can augment the detection of a dilated bile or pancreatic duct in the setting of sphincter stenosis when coupled with one of the aforementioned noninvasive modalities.[8,9] Other transit studies, the most crude of which is assessment for delayed biliary emptying following a cholangiogram with intraprocedural positional changes, are no longer routinely performed.[26] Recent investigation using serial MRCP following morphine-neostigmine (Prostigmin) stimulation (Nardi provocation test, originally done with transabdominal ultrasound) has been associated with provocative results to include pronounced secretion of pancreatic juice and may someday play a role in the diagnosis of SOD.[27] Hepatobiliary scintigraphy (HIDA) can be used to evaluate underlying gallbladder disease and demonstrate partial biliary obstruction as evident in SOD with prompt hepatic uptake and biliary secretion but poor ductal clearance. However, HIDA can be equivocal if not misleading for biliary dyskinesia depending on patient nutritional and medication intake (ie, narcotic use) preceding the study.[28,29] Variation in radiologist infusion technique can also lead to highly inaccurate HIDA results, although scintigraphic scores have been proposed as an alternative noninvasive test of choice.[30,31]

SOM is considered the gold standard for SOD investigation.[32,33] Expert consensus at a National Institutes of Health conference previously recommended that patients with suspected SOD, particularly types II and III, be referred for manometry rather than diagnostic ERCP alone.[34] High basal sphincter pressures can be confirmatory of a presumptive diagnosis of SOD. However, the performance characteristics have been lackluster. Patients can have fluctuating measurements throughout the day,

**Box 1**
**Rome III diagnostic criteria for functional gallbladder and SODs**

Diagnostic criteria: Episodes of pain located in the epigastrium and/or RUQ and *all* of the following must be included:

1. Episodes last 30 minutes or longer.

2. There are recurrent symptoms occurring at different intervals (not daily).

3. The pain builds up to a steady level.

4. The pain is moderate to severe enough to interrupt patients' daily activities or lead to an emergency department visit.

5. The pain is not relieved by bowel movements.

6. The pain is not relieved by postural change.

7. The pain is not relieved by antacids.

8. Other structural diseases that would explain the symptoms have been excluded.

Supportive criteria: The pain may present with one or more of the following:

1. Associated with nausea and vomiting

2. Radiates to the back and/or right infra-subscapular region

3. Awakens from sleep in the middle of the night

### E1. Functional Gallbladder Disorder

Diagnostic criteria: *All* of the following must be included:

1. Criteria for functional gallbladder and SOD

2. Gallbladder present

3. Normal liver enzymes, conjugated bilirubin, and amylase/lipase

### E2. Functional Biliary SOD

Diagnostic criteria: *Both* of the following must be included:

1. Criteria for functional gallbladder and SOD

2. Normal amylase/lipase

Supportive criterion

1. Elevated serum transaminases, alkaline phosphatase, or conjugated bilirubin are temporally related to at least 2 pain episodes.

### E3. Functional Pancreatic SOD

Diagnostic criteria: *Both* of the following must be included:

1. Criteria for functional gallbladder and SOD

2. Elevated amylase/lipase

and pressure readings can be similar for both symptomatic and normal patients.[8,35–39] Furthermore, SOM has proven to be unreliable as a predictor of response to sphincterotomy, especially for type III disease.[19,40] Even postsphincterotomy patients can have abnormally high manometric readings, questioning its reliability as a diagnostic test for SOD.[39] Patient demographics, pancreaticobiliary enzyme levels, presence of gallbladder disease, pain patterns, use of narcotics, underlying functional disorders, and psychological comorbidities have not been found to correlate with manometric results.[41] Several other limitations of SOM preclude its universal use on all patients with suspected SOD, including (1) need for center expertise and challenging manometry catheter placement; (2) variation in pressure measurements from different types of catheter equipment, variable sphincter lumen size, probe position, and point in time when a spasm is captured; and (3) undue risk involved in catheter insertion during diagnostic ERCP. Measurement of liver enzymes and biliary dilation may be sufficient, if not superior, to manometry for diagnosis and predicting response to therapy.[14,42,43] The latter strategy seems cost-effective when factoring in the patients and endoscopists' time, center resources, and potential hospitalization risks incurred with diagnostic SOM; yet, to date, there are no cost analysis studies that validate this claim.

## TREATMENT AND PREDICTORS OF RESPONSE

The goal of therapy is to relieve pain and prevent recurrence induced by high, fixed or spastic, SO pressures causing backflow of bile or pancreatic secretions. Several pharmacologic agents have been tried. Surgical options have been supplanted by endoscopic interventions, although recent data have refuted decades of practice by revealing that endoscopic treatment is no better than placebo in select patients.[19] The classification of disease based on the Milwaukee classification remains the biggest predictor of response to endoscopic therapy.

### Medical Treatment

The application of pharmacologic therapies for SOD has been limited to proof of concept and small placebo-controlled trials. Several smooth muscle relaxation agents have been tested. Intrasphincteric injection of botulinum toxin and topical application of a nitric oxide carrier showed initial promise in animal models, but efficacy was not as reliable in humans.[44,45] Nifedipine had initial short-acting benefit, particularly for type II disease, but the long-acting effects were no different from placebo.[46,47] Nitrate therapy (ie, glyceryl trinitrate), phosphodiesterase inhibitors (ie, vardenafil), and receptor modulators affecting gastrointestinal motility (ie, trimebutine) have all been tried in a small number of patients with promising results.[6] Future application of these agents will depend on their reproducibility in efficacy in larger trials. Antidepressants, amitriptyline, and antispasmodics (ie, hyoscyamine sulfate) can ameliorate symptoms and should be offered to mitigate pain and potential concomitant psychosomatic stress. Alternative therapies, such as self-administered electroacupuncture, may also have a role in achieving symptomatic relief.[48]

### Endoscopic Treatment

Endoscopic measures to eradicate sphincter dyskinesia or stenosis have been a mainstay therapy. The first available evidence on the therapeutic benefit of ERCP sphincterotomy for biliary SOD was reported in 1989.[49] Since then, several other clinical trials have demonstrated similar efficacy of endoscopic sphincter ablation in patients with manometrically reported hypertension.[29,50] Various other observational studies have replicated this benefit albeit at a lower rate and with discordance between manometric pressures and symptomatic response.[17] The inclusion of a mixed study population of SOD types I, II, and III has created substantial heterogeneity in the literature and, thus, varying response rates. Patients with biliary type I generally respond well to endoscopic intervention even in patients with normal basal sphincter pressures. In one small study exclusive to only patients with type I, all had symptomatic relief up to 2 years with biliary sphincterotomy, including the one-third of patients who had normal sphincter pressures.[51]

The data are less convincing for type II disease with varying response rates depending on manometric findings. In the initial landmark trial demonstrating efficacy of biliary sphincterotomy, patients with type II disease had a marked difference in response rate when they had abnormal basal sphincter pressures.[41] A second trial confirmed similar clinical success in patients with type II disease with elevated baseline manometric results or abnormal pressures following cholecystokinin provocation.[34] Thus, the concept of manometric-directed endoscopic therapy was conceived. Although directed therapy is applicable principally for type II SOD, manometric results can be an inadequate predictor of response to therapy and comparable clinical results can be achieved without manometry.[50,52] In addition, many patients have their sphincters ablated before referral into a center with manometry capabilities.[17]

Therapy for SOD type III has long been problematic. Traditionally described as the group of patients most likely to be injured by a procedure that benefits them the least, these patients had a reported 50% chance, at best, of symptomatic relief whether one or both sphincters were ablated.[53,54] The EPISOD trial has affirmed long-held suspicions and generated a paradigm shift away from practices in favor of sphincterotomy for patients with SOD type III. These results may also be true for some patients with type II disease. In the EPISOD trial, 214 patients with presumed type III SOD were randomized to sham biliary sphincterotomy, biliary, or dual sphincterotomy regardless of the biliary and pancreatic manometry results.[19] At the 1-year follow-up, patients who did not undergo sphincterotomy had a statistically significant better outcome (37%) than those who received either biliary or dual sphincterotomy (23%). The evidence is clear: sphincterotomy for patients with postcholecystectomy pain who met the Rome III criteria and the definition for SOD type III is not only ineffective but even less effective than a diagnostic cholangiogram. A caveat to these results is that many patients with SOD III have underlying duodenal visceral hyperalgesia, psychosomatic disorders, and central sensitization, disorders that will not improve despite sphincter obliteration.[17,55–61]

Endoscopic therapy may also have a role for suspected pancreatic SOD type I and II. Sphincterotomy has been reported as efficacious at preventing future recurrent attacks for patients with idiopathic relapsing pancreatitis attributed to pancreatic SOD type I or II.[62–64] Several cohort studies have demonstrated this risk reduction with biliary or dual sphincterotomy, with a prolonged interval between episodes of pancreatitis.[26,62,63,65] In a landmark trial by the Indiana group, patients with SOD with idiopathic acute relapsing pancreatitis had a similar benefit whether they underwent a biliary (51.5%) or a combined biliary and pancreatic sphincterotomy (52.8%), suggesting that a pancreatic sphincterotomy should not be performed for these patients, especially given the high rate of iatrogenic late restenosis and other adverse events.[64,66,67] The same investigators demonstrated that patients with abnormal pancreatic manometry had a 4-fold higher risk of having another episode of pancreatitis than those who had normal manometric results.[56] These findings are particularly important when considering that up to 40% of patients with idiopathic pancreatitis may have abnormal manometric pressures.[68] Nevertheless, although endoscopic sphincterotomy can reduce the risk of relapse in patients with acute relapsing pancreatitis and suspected SOD, this risk is not nil, with up to 50% of patients developing another flare on long-term follow-up.[63]

Endoscopic intervention for either biliary or pancreatic SOD is risky and can have limited value, even for types I and II. Given that SOD, particularly type III, has long been reported to be associated with concomitant psychosocial and somatic disorders, some experts advocate for a formal psychological evaluation before proceeding with ERCP.[69,70] Others have advocated for sphincter botulinum injection or transpapillary stenting as a therapeutic trial before committing patients to a sphincterotomy.[71,72] If the decision is made to offer endoscopic treatment after exhausting optimal medical therapy, a candid discussion about the risks and benefits of ERCP for this indication is mandatory. The endoscopist should emphasize that although the risk of post-ERCP pancreatitis can be reduced with the use of rectal indomethacin and prophylactic pancreatic duct stenting (both of which are highly recommended in this population), this risk remains substantial, especially when compared with potentially ineffective therapy.[73,74] Management of these patients should occur at experienced centers where routine placement of prophylactic pancreatic duct stenting is performed.

## Predictors of Response

In the ideal situation, the endoscopist would be able to recognize which patients best respond to endoscopic therapy before an attempt is made. Manometric pressures offer some guidance but can be inconsistent. Patients with high basal pressures (>40 mm Hg) tend to respond more commonly than those with marginal pressures for biliary SOD. This response is especially apparent in biliary SOD type II in which the response rate to sphincterotomy has been reported to be 80% to 90% for high pressures and only 30% to 35% for pressures less than 40 mm Hg.[75] The authors' group as well as others have demonstrated that manometry is a dynamic test; sphincter pressures can differ dramatically depending on the day, further confounding whether patients should undergo endoscopic intervention.[14] Several studies have explored patient factors associated with the higher likelihood of response to sphincterotomy. Aside from manometry, the best predictor of response remains the Milwaukee classification, with type I being the most likely to respond (up to 70%–100%) and type III the least (equivalent to placebo) (**Box 2**).[57] However, note that this response is for biliary classification only and that pancreatic SOD, in the authors' opinion, has not undergone a comparable level of scrutiny. Chronic narcotic use, older age, gastroparesis, pain patterns, and pancreatic manometric pressures have been implicated as

---

**Box 2**
**Selection for endoscopic sphincterotomy based on classification type**

After exhausting all other potential causes and medical therapies and assuming documented evidence of abnormal biochemistries and/or imaging above thresholds

*Patients who should be treated*

- SOD type I

*Patients who should not be treated*

- SOD type III

*Patients who should possibly be treated*

- SOD type II (with high manometric pressures)

predictors of positive or negative response to treatment. However, others have not reproduced these associations.[19,33,76]

### Surgical Treatment

Surgical options have been largely reserved for patients in whom endoscopic sphincterotomy is not technically feasible or in cases of restenosis following endoscopic measures. Transduodenal sphincteroplasty with transpapillary septoplasty is the traditional open operative approach. Clinical success rates are similar to endoscopic sphincterotomy, ranging from 43% to 75%, and depend highly on SOD type.[4,6,77–79]

## CHALLENGES AND FUTURE CONSIDERATIONS

SOD remains one of the most enigmatic entities in the spectrum of pancreaticobiliary diseases. Using a classification scheme predicated on laboratory and radiographic

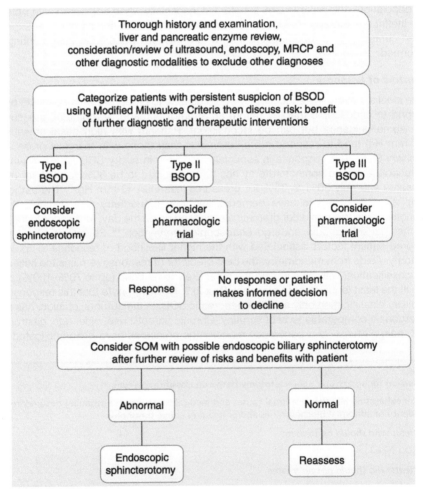

**Fig. 2.** Proposed algorithm for approach of a patient with suspected biliary SOD (BSOD). (*Adapted from* Rehman A, Affronti J, Rao S. Sphincter of Oddi dysfunction: an evidence-based review. Expert Rev Gastroenterol Hepatol 2013;7:719; with permission; and *Courtesy of* Informa Healthcare, London, UK; with permission.)

cutoffs conceived by expert opinion, how does one categorize patients who fall just less than these threshold levels? How does one categorize patients with atypical biliary colic and normal pancreaticobiliary enzymes but found to have a dilated bile duct to 15 mm? Similarly, how does one diagnose a patient with profound nausea and acute on chronic epigastric pain and an intact gallbladder with no evidence of choledocholithiasis but found to have a 1.5-fold aminotransferase elevation? Is this microlithiasis, acalculous cholecystitis, or SOD? The diagnosis changes if this patient's bile duct measures 10 mm in diameter rather than 4 mm, so should the management as well? How does one classify a patient with aminotransferase elevations 1.4 times the normal level, a bile duct measuring 8 to 9 mm on cross-sectional imaging, and who presents to the office with debilitating, recurrent RUQ pain after cholecystectomy? Is this SOD type I, II, or neither? Should an ERCP with sphincterotomy be performed knowing this patient has a high risk (up to 25%) of developing post-ERCP complications, such as bleeding, pancreatitis, and its sequelae, that can result in prolonged hospitalization and even mortality? Recent evidence has unraveled the very existence of certain subtypes of SOD.[19,43] Further investigation to evaluate the application of manometry-directed biliary or dual sphincterotomy for SOD II in a trial setting is underway. Finally, can we identify which patients respond to therapy, beyond the imperfections of sphincter manometry and the classification scheme? Likewise, which patients will have durable relief? These questions have yet to be validated in large cohort studies or randomized trials with meaningful results. Predictive biomarkers to stratify patients are still lacking. Until further data emerge, the authors propose a treatment algorithm (**Fig. 2**) following referral to a center with pancreaticobiliary expertise.

## SUMMARY

Patient selection for endoscopic sphincterotomy starts with patient education regarding risks of ERCP and an unpredictable response to treatment. Moreover, both practitioner and patients need to be aware that clinical response in initial responders may be short and result in recurrent reliance on the biliary endoscopist. The endoscopist must consider repeat high-risk ERCP at the beckoning of a patient who received brief relief of pain that may be unrelated to sphincter dysfunction. It is the authors' opinion that endoscopic therapy should be reserved for referral centers meeting quality metrics in pancreaticobiliary endoscopy given the relatively high complication rate in this population. There are evolving data on the utility of endoscopic therapy for SOD type I and type II, but overall endoscopic therapy remains a reasonable option for this patient group. However, unless further studies suggest otherwise, endoscopic therapy is problematic for SOD type III and currently not advisable. Currently, endoscopic sphincterotomy remains the preferred strategy for SOD type I. However, endoscopic therapy of any kind requires a commitment to patient counseling and a high threshold to reserve this invasive and potentially high-risk procedure for the subset of postcholecystectomy patients who have clearly shown benefit from sphincterotomy. Lastly, predictors of response and failure to achieve sustained pain relief are areas in which additional data are sorely needed.

## REFERENCES

1. Okazaki K, Yamamoto Y, Kagigama S, et al. Pressure of papillary sphincter zone and pancreatic main duct in patients with chronic pancreatitis in the early stage. Scand J Gastroenterol 1988;23:501–7.
2. Boyden EA. The anatomy of the choledochoduodenal junction in man. Surgery 1957;104:641–52.

3. Kozarek RA. Biliary dyskinesia: are we any closer to defining an entity? Gastrointest Endosc Clin N Am 1993;3:167–78.
4. Oddi R. D'une disposition a sphincter speciale de l'ouverture du canal choledoque. Arch Ital Biol 1887;8:317.
5. Eichhorn EP Jr, Boyden EA. The choledochoduodenal junction in the dog; a restudy of Oddi's sphincter. Am J Anat 1955;97:431–59.
6. Leung WD, Sherman S. Endoscopic approach to the patient with motility disorders of the bile duct and sphincter of Oddi. Gastrointest Endosc Clin N Am 2013;23:405–34.
7. Elmunzer BJ, Elta GH. Biliary tract motor function and dysfunction. In: Feldman M, Friedman LS, Brandt LJ, editors. Sleisenger and Fordtran's gastrointestinal and liver disease: pathophysiology/diagnosis/management. 9th edition. (PA): Saunders Elsevier; 2010. p. 1067–73.
8. Rehman A, Affronti J, Rao S. Sphincter of Oddi dysfunction: an evidence-based review. Expert Rev Gastroenterol Hepatol 2013;7:713–22.
9. Drossman DA, Li Z, Andruzzi E, et al. US householder survey of functional gastrointestinal disorders: prevalence, sociodemography, and health impact. Dig Dis Sci 1993;38:1569–80.
10. Petersen BT. An evidence-based review of sphincter of Oddi dysfunction, I: presentations with "objective" biliary findings (types I and II). Gastrointest Endosc 2004;59:525–34.
11. Petersen BT. Sphincter of Oddi dysfunction, II: evidence-based review of the presentations with "objective" pancreatic findings (types I and II) and presumptive type III. Gastrointest Endosc 2004;59:670–87.
12. Tarnasky PR, Palesch YY, Cunningham JT, et al. Pancreatic stenting prevents pancreatitis after biliary sphincterotomy in patients with sphincter of Oddi dysfunction. Gastroenterology 1998;115:1518–24.
13. Kakuyama S, Nobutani K, Masuda A, et al. Sphincter of Oddi manometry using guide-wire type manometer is feasible for examination of sphincter of Oddi motility. J Gastroenterol 2013;48:1144–50.
14. Kaw M, Brodmerkel GJ. ERCP, biliary crystal analysis, and sphincter of Oddi manometry in idiopathic recurrent pancreatitis. Gastrointest Endosc 2002;55:157–62.
15. Hogan WJ, Geenen JE. Biliary dyskinesia. Endoscopy 1988;20:179–83.
16. Kozarek RA. Sphincter of Oddi dysfunction: stones, spasm, or stenosis? Gastroenterol Hepatol 2007;3:708–9.
17. Menees S, Elta GH. Sphincter of Oddi dysfunction. Curr Treat Options Gastroenterol 2005;8:109–15.
18. Baillie J. Sphincter of Oddi dysfunction: overdue for an overhaul. Am J Gastroenterol 2005;100:1217–20.
19. Rastogi A, Slivka A, Moser AJ, et al. Controversies concerning pathophysiology and management of acalculous biliary-type abdominal pain. Dig Dis Sci 2005; 50:1391–401.
20. Cotton PB, Durkalski V, Romangnuolo J, et al. Effect of endoscopic sphincterotomy for suspected sphincter of Oddi dysfunction on pain-related disability following cholecystectomy: the EPISOD randomized clinical trial. JAMA 2014; 311:2101–9.
21. Mosko JD, Chuttani R. EPISOD puts an end to sphincter of Oddi dysfunction type III. Ann Gastroenterol 2014;27:427–8.
22. Dawwas MF, Bruno MJ, Lee JG. Endoscopic sphincterotomy for sphincter of Oddi dysfunction: inefficacious therapy for a fictitious disease. Gastroenterology 2015;148(2):440–3.

23. Longstreth GF, Thompson WG, Chey WD, et al. Functional bowel disorders. Gastroenterology 2006;130:1480–91.

24. Freeman ML, Nelson DB, Sherman S, et al. Complications of endoscopic biliary sphincterotomy. N Engl J Med 1996;335:909–18.

25. Imler TD, Sherman S, McHenry L, et al. Low yield of significant findings on endoscopic retrograde cholangiopancreatography in patients with pancreaticobiliary pain and no objective findings. Dig Dis Sci 2012;57:3252–7.

26. Baillie J. Sphincter of Oddi dysfunction. Curr Gastroenterol Rep 2010;12:130–4.

27. Chowdhury AH, Humes DJ, Pritchard SE, et al. The effects of morphine-neostigmine and secretin provocation on pancreaticobiliary morphology in healthy subjects: a randomized, double-blind crossover study using serial MRCP. World J Surg 2011;35:2102–9.

28. Morris-Stiff G, Falk G, Kraynak L, et al. Cholecystokinin provocation HIDA test. J Gastrointest Surg 2011;15:1658–9.

29. Bertalan V, Szepes A, Lonovics J, et al. Assessment of the reproducibility of quantitative hepatobiliary scintigraphy (QHBS) in patients with sphincter of Oddi dysfunction (SOD)- inappropriate method or intermittent disease? Hepatogastroenterology 2006;53:160–5.

30. Ziessman HA. Hepatobiliary scintigraphy in 2014. J Nucl Med 2014;55:967–75.

31. Sostre S, Kalloo AN, Spiegler EJ, et al. A noninvasive test of sphincter of Oddi dysfunction in postcholecystectomy patients: the scintigraphic score. J Nucl Med 1992;33:1216–22.

32. Lehman GA. Endoscopic sphincter of Oddi manometry: a clinical practice and research tool. Gastrointest Endosc 1991;37:490–2.

33. Lans JL, Parikh NP, Geenen JE. Application of sphincter of Oddi manometry in routine clinical investigations. Endoscopy 1991;23:139–43.

34. Cohen S, Bacon BR, Berlin JA, et al. National Institutes of Health State-of-the-Science Conference Statement: ERCP for diagnosis and therapy. Gastrointest Endosc 2002;56:803–9.

35. Seetharam P, Rodrigues G. Sphincter of Oddi and its dysfunction. Saudi J Gastroenterol 2008;14:1–6.

36. Varadarajulu S, Hawes RH, Cotton PB. Determination of sphincter of Oddi dysfunction in patients with prior normal manometry. Gastrointest Endosc 2003;58:341–4.

37. Thune A, Scicchitano J, Roberts-Thomson I, et al. Reproducibility of endoscopic sphincter of Oddi manometry. Dig Dis Sci 1991;36:1401–5.

38. Khashab MA, Watkins JL, McHenry L Jr, et al. Frequency of sphincter of Oddi dysfunction in patients with previously normal sphincter of Oddi manometry studies. Endoscopy 2010;42:369–74.

39. Eversman D, Fogel EL, Rusche M, et al. Frequency of abnormal pancreatic and biliary sphincter manometry compared with clinical suspicion of sphincter of Oddi dysfunction. Gastrointest Endosc 1999;50:637–41.

40. Sgouros SN, Pereira SP. Systematic review: sphincter of Oddi dysfunction- noninvasive diagnostic methods and long-term outcome after endoscopic sphincterotomy. Aliment Pharmacol Ther 2006;24:237–46.

41. Romagnuolo J, Cotton PB, Durkalski V, et al. Can patient and pain characteristics predict manometric sphincter of Oddi dysfunction in patients with clinically suspected sphincter of Oddi dysfunction? Gastrointest Endosc 2014;79:765–72.

42. Toouli J, Roberts-Thomson IC, Kellow J, et al. Manometry based randomised trial of endoscopic sphincterotomy for sphincter of Oddi dysfunction. Gut 2000;46:98–102.

43. Sherman S, Lehman GA. Sphincter of Oddi dysfunction: diagnosis and treatment. JOP 2001;2:382–400.
44. Pasricha PJ, Miskovsky EP, Kalloo AN. Intrasphincteric injection of botulinum toxin for suspected sphincter of Oddi dysfunction. Gut 1994;35:1319–21.
45. Slivka A, Chuttani R, Carr-Locke DL, et al. Inhibition of sphincter of Oddi function by the nitric oxide carrier S-nitroso-N-acetylcysteine in rabbits and humans. J Clin Invest 1994;94:1792–8.
46. Sand J, Nordback I, Koskinen M, et al. Nifedipine for suspected type II sphincter of Oddi dyskinesia. Am J Gastroenterol 1993;88:530–5.
47. Craig AG, Toouli J. Slow release nifedipine for patients with sphincter of Oddi dyskinesia: results of a pilot study. Intern Med J 2002;32:119–20.
48. Walter WA, Curtis HC. Self-administered electroacupuncture provides symptomatic relief in a patient with sphincter of Oddi dysfunction: a patient's report. Acupunct Med 2013;31:430–4.
49. Geenen JE, Hogan WJ, Dodds WJ, et al. The efficacy of endoscopic sphincterotomy after cholecystectomy in patients with sphincter-of-Oddi dysfunction. N Engl J Med 1989;320:82–7.
50. Botoman VA, Kozarek RA, Novell LA, et al. Long-term outcome after endoscopic sphincterotomy in patients with biliary colic and suspected sphincter of Oddi dysfunction. Gastrointest Endosc 1994;40:165–70.
51. Rolny P, Geenen JE, Hogan WJ. Post-cholecystectomy patients with "objective signs" of partial bile outflow obstruction: clinical characteristics, sphincter of Oddi manometry findings, and results of therapy. Gastrointest Endosc 1993;39:778–81.
52. Kalaitzakis E, Ambrose T, Phillips-Hughes J, et al. Management of patients with biliary sphincter of Oddi disorder without sphincter of Oddi manometry. BMC Gastroenterol 2010;10:124.
53. Cotton PB. ERCP is most dangerous for people who need it the least. Gastrointest Endosc 2001;54:535–6.
54. Beltz S, Sarkar A, Loren DE, et al. Risk stratification for the development of post-ERCP pancreatitis by sphincter of Oddi dysfunction classification. South Med J 2013;106:298–302.
55. Cote GA, Tarnasky PR, Wilcox CM. Sphincter of Oddi: ERCP plus sphincterotomy- yes or no? ASGE Leading Edge 2014;4:1–10.
56. Desautels SG, Slivka A, Hutson WR, et al. Postcholecystectomy pain syndrome: pathophysiology of abdominal pain in sphincter of Oddi type III. Gastroenterology 1999;116:900–5.
57. Kurucsai G, Joo I, Fejes R, et al. Somatosensory hypersensitivity in the referred pain area in patients with chronic biliary pain and a sphincter of Oddi dysfunction: new aspects of an almost forgotten pathogenetic mechanism. Am J Gastroenterol 2008;103:2717–25.
58. Abraham HD, Anderson C, Lee D. Somatization disorder in sphincter of Oddi dysfunction. Psychosom Med 1997;59:553–7.
59. Bennett E, Evans P, Dowsett J, et al. Sphincter of Oddi dysfunction: psychosocial distress correlates with manometric dyskinesia but not stenosis. World J Gastroenterol 2009;15:6080–5.
60. Winstead NS, Wilcox CM. Health-related quality of life, somatization, and abuse in sphincter of Oddi dysfunction. J Clin Gastroenterol 2007;41:773–6.
61. Seminowicz DA, Labus JS, Bueller JA, et al. Regional gray matter density changes in brains of patients with irritable bowel syndrome. Gastroenterology 2010;139:48–57.

62. Wehrmann T. Long-term results (> 10 years) of endoscopic therapy for sphincter of Oddi dysfunction in patients with acute recurrent pancreatitis. Endoscopy 2011;43:202–7.

63. Okolo PI, Pasricha PJ, Kalloo AN. What are the long-term results of endoscopic pancreatic sphincterotomy. Gastrointest Endosc 2000;52:15–9.

64. Cote GA, Imperiale TF, Schmidt SE, et al. Similar efficacies of biliary, with or without pancreatic, sphincterotomy in treatment of idiopathic recurrent acute pancreatitis. Gastroenterology 2012;143:1502–9.

65. Guelrud M, Plaz J, Mendoza S, et al. Endoscopic treatment in type II pancreatic sphincter dysfunction. Gastrointest Endosc 1995;41:A398.

66. Kozarek RA, Ball TJ, Patterson DJ, et al. Endoscopic pancreatic duct sphincterotomy: indications, technique, and analysis of results. Gastrointest Endosc 1994; 40:592–8.

67. Elton E, Howell DA, Parsons WG, et al. Endoscopic pancreatic sphincterotomy: indications, outcome, and a safe stentless technique. Gastrointest Endosc 1998;47:240–9.

68. Fischer M, Hassan A, Sipe BW, et al. Endoscopic retrograde cholangiopancreatography and manometry findings in 1,241 idiopathic pancreatitis patients. Pancreatology 2010;10:444–52.

69. Brawman-Mintzer O, Durkalski V, Romagnuolo J, et al. Psychosocial characteristics and pain burden of patients with suspected sphincter of Oddi dysfunction in the EPISOD multicenter trial. Am J Gastroenterol 2014;109:436–42.

70. Moffatt DC, Barkay O, Cote GA, et al. Abnormal psychometric profiles in patients with suspected sphincter of Oddi dysfunction. Gastrointest Endosc 2011;73: AB341.

71. Hall TC, Dennison AR, Garcea G. The diagnosis and management of sphincter of Oddi dysfunction: a systematic review. Langenbecks Arch Surg 2012;397: 889–98.

72. Murray WR. Botulinum toxin-induced relaxation of the sphincter of Oddi may select patients with acalculous biliary pain who will benefit from cholecystectomy. Surg Endosc 2011;25:813–6.

73. Cotton PB, Garrow DA, Gallagher J, et al. Risk factors for complications after ERCP: a multivariate analysis of 11,497 procedures over 12 years. Gastrointest Endosc 2009;70:80–8.

74. Pahk A, Rigaux J, Poreddy V, et al. Prophylactic pancreatic stents: does size matter? A comparison of 4-Fr and 5-Fr stents in reference to post-ERCP pancreatitis and migration rate. Dig Dis Sci 2011;56:3058–64.

75. Tarnasky PR, Hawes RH. Pancreaticobiliary pain and suspected sphincter of Oddi dysfunction. In: Baron TH, Kozarek RA, Carr-Locke DL, editors. ERCP. 2nd edition. (PA): Saunders Elsevier; 2013. p. 419–29.

76. Freeman ML, Gill M, Overby C, et al. Predictors of outcomes after biliary and pancreatic sphincterotomy for sphincter of Oddi dysfunction. J Clin Gastroenterol 2007;41:94–102.

77. Moody FG, Vecchio R, Calabuig R, et al. Transduodenal sphincteroplasty with transampullary septectomy for stenosing papillitis. Am J Surg 1991;161:213–8.

78. Hastbacka J, Jarvinen H, Kivilaakso E, et al. Results of sphincteroplasty in patients with spastic sphincter of Oddi. Predictive value of operative biliary manometry and provocation tests. Scand J Gastroenterol 1986;21:516–20.

79. Stephens RV, Burdick GE. Microscopic transduodenal sphincteroplasty and transampullary septoplasty for papillary stenosis. Am J Surg 1986;152:621–7.

# Pancreatic Endotherapy for Chronic Pancreatitis

Rupjyoti Talukdar, MD[a], Duvvur Nageshwar Reddy, MD, DM[b],*

## KEYWORDS

- Painful chronic pancreatitis • Pancreatic calculi • Stricture • Pseudocyst
- Endoscopic retrograde cholangiopancreatography
- Extracorporeal shock wave lithotripsy • Multiple plastic stent • Metal stents

## KEY POINTS

- Extracorporeal shock wave lithotripsy (ESWL) is recommended as the first-line therapy for large (>5-mm) obstructive pancreatic ductal stones.
- Dominant pancreatic duct strictures should be initially managed with a wide-bore single plastic stent with 3 monthly exchanges for a year, even in asymptomatic patients.
- Recent studies have evaluated multiple plastic and self-expanding covered metal stents for refractory pancreatic ductal stricture.
- Pancreatic pseudocysts (PPs) should be treated endoscopically with or without endoscopic ultrasound (EUS) guidance.

## INTRODUCTION

Intractable abdominal pain and associated morphologic abnormalities in the pancreatobiliary system are the major determinants of interventional therapy in chronic pancreatitis (CP). Pain mechanisms in CP are multipronged, and recent experimental evidence suggests that pancreatic ductal hypertension can activate pancreatic stellate cells, which in turn can generate oxidative stress and subsequent inflammation.[1] The penultimate phenotype of pain in CP emanates from a composite of chronic inflammation and oxidative stress–induced nociception, mechanical allodynia and inflammatory hyperalgesia, pancreatic neuropathy, and peripheral and central neuroplasticity.[2] Complications, such as PPs, gastric outlet obstruction, biliary obstruction, and pancreatic cancer, are important contributors to pain in CP. The evidence that pancreatic ductal

Commercial and Financial Conflicts of Interest: None.
Funding Source: None.
[a] Wellcome-DBT India Alliance Laboratory, Asian Healthcare Foundation, Department of Medical Gastroenterology, Asian Institute of Gastroenterology, 6-3-661, Somajiguda, Hyderabad 500082, India; [b] Department of Medical Gastroenterology, Asian Institute of Gastroenterology, 6-3-661, Somajiguda, Hyderabad 500082, India
* Corresponding author.
*E-mail address:* aigindia@yahoo.co.in

Gastrointest Endoscopy Clin N Am 25 (2015) 765–777
http://dx.doi.org/10.1016/j.giec.2015.06.010
giendo.theclinics.com

hypertension can result in inflammation and pain justifies ductal decompression for amelioration of pain. Decompression can be performed using endoscopic and surgical approaches, with endoscopic approach currently recommended as the first-line modality by the European Society of Gastrointestinal Endoscopy (ESGE).[3]

It is mandatory to perform a meticulous morphologic evaluation for assessment of the disease magnitude and confounding local anatomic alterations prior to endotherapy. It is also mandatory to rule out pancreatic cancer, especially in patients over age 50 years, of female gender, of white race, with presence of jaundice and overt exocrine insufficiency, and with absence of pancreatic calcifications.[4,5] Size and distribution of pancreatic ductal calculi can be best evaluated by CT, even though transabdominal ultrasonography also provides a fairly good assessment. Presence of pancreatic ductal strictures, biliary strictures, and anatomic variants, such as pancreas divisum, can be best identified with magnetic resonance cholangiopancreatography (MRCP). MRCP is also advantageous over EUS and CT in differentiating a PP from a walled-off necrosis (in patients with CP with recent acute exacerbation).[6,7]

## INDICATIONS AND CONTRAINDICATIONS OF PANCREATIC ENDOTHERAPY

Intractable pain is the single most common and compelling indication for pancreatic endotherapy in patients with CP, and the modality of choice depends on the morphology.

- Presence of small stones can be extracted by endoscopic retrograde cholangiopancreatography (ERCP) with pancreatic sphincterotomy using Dormia baskets and balloons. Stones larger than 5 mm can be best fragmented by lithotripsy with or without pancreatic ductal stenting. Currently, ESWL has been recommended as the first choice by the ESGE.[3] **Box 1** depicts the contraindications of ESWL.
- Pancreatic ductal strictures can be managed by pancreatic sphincterotomy and stenting with or without dilatation.
- PPs should be treated in the presence of pseudocyst infection, symptomatic intracystic bleeding, biliary obstruction, gastric outlet obstruction, early satiety, abdominal pain, weight loss, and enlarging pseudocyst size.[3] It has been suggested that prophylactic treatment of asymptomatic pseudocyst may be considered in the presence of compression of major vessels, pancreaticopleural fistula, pseudocyst size greater than 5 cm that does not regress after 6 weeks, and pseudocyst wall thickness of greater than 5 mm.[8,9]
- EUS finds a place in the drainage of the dilated pancreatic duct using rendezvous techniques when transpapillary access is not possible.
- Treatment of pain refractory to standard intervention can be attempted with EUS-guided celiac plexus block.

---

**Box 1**
**Contraindications for extracorporeal shock wave lithotripsy**

- Stones all along the MPD
- Isolated calculi in tail region
- Multiple MPD strictures
- Presence of moderate to massive ascites
- PP
- Pancreatic head mass

---

## TECHNIQUE/PROCEDURE
### Endotherapy for Pancreatic Ductal Calculi

Over the years, several techniques to fragment and remove pancreatic ductal calculi have evolved. These include techniques requiring intraductal access, such as mechanical lithotripsy, electrohydraulic lithotripsy, and laser-guided lithotripsy, or extracorporeal intervention, such as ESWL.

- Intraductal mechanical lithotripsy, which is performed using a through-the-scope mechanical lithotripter, is technically challenging with a high complication rate[10] and currently is seldom used.
- Electrohydraulic lithotripsy is performed under direct pancreatoscopic visualization using a mother-daughter scope system and has the advantage of delivering energy to a focused area on the calculi.[11] Even though technical modifications, such as use of a single-operator SpyGlass systems[12] and laser lithotripsy using holmium laser, have evolved over time, evidence in the literature is limited, thereby mandating further safety and outcome studies.[13] Furthermore, availability of these techniques precludes widespread utility.
- ESWL is currently the first-line modality to manage large (>5-mm) painful obstructive pancreatic ductal calculi, particularly for those located in the head and body regions.[3] The goal is to reduce the stones to fragments lower than 3 mm. The technique of ESWL consists of 4 components, namely a shock wave generator, a focusing system, a coupling mechanism, and a localizing unit, all of which are packed in the same machine.[14] Best results are obtained by the third-generation lithotripters, which are equipped with bidimensional fluoroscopic and ultrasonic targeting system. ESWL should be performed on a slightly lateral decubitus, and a maximum of 5000 shocks per session with an intensity of 15,000 to 16,000, KV and 90 shocks per minute is usually delivered for optimal stone fragmentation.[15] The fragmented stones are usually removed with an ERCP and pancreatic sphincterotomy after ESWL. Concomitant pancreatic ductal stenting may be performed in the presence of a pancreatic ductal stricture. For radiolucent stones, a pre-ESWL pancreatic sphincterotomy with a nasopancreatic tube placement can aid in accurate focusing for ESWL.[16] In the presence of multiple ductal stones, the one located nearest to the pancreatic duct orifice should be targeted first. Isolated intraductal stones located in the tail need not be treated with ESWL because these stones are unlikely to result in sufficient upstream ductal pressure to cause pain. Furthermore, attempts to fragment ductal stones in the tail could result in collateral splenic injury. Recent evidence suggests that use of secretin for pancreatic ESWL results in a fluid-stone interface from the ductal secretions, akin to that in ureteral stones, that can translate in a more effective stone fragmentation.[17]

Even though ESWL has traditionally been performed under general anesthesia, the authors prefer to use thoracic epidural anesthesia with 0.25% bupivacaine (with or without clonidine) to cause D6 to D12 segmental block. Epidural anesthesia also offers the advantage of a reduced procedural time compared with use of total IV anesthesia.[18]

### Endotherapy for Main Pancreatic Duct Stricture

Strictures in the main pancreatic duct (MPD) are seen in up to 18% patients with CP.

- Currently, placement of a single 10F polyethylene stent with planned stent exchanges within 1 year even in the absence of symptoms is the first-line treatment of dominant pancreatic duct stricture.[3] Dominant strictures might require prior dilatation with bougies, balloons, or a Soehendra stent retriever.[19]

- Even though straight or pigtailed plastic stents have been widely used for treating MPD strictures, there still does not exist an ideal stent. Several modifications have so far been made in pancreatic stent technology, namely development of the S-shaped,[20] winged type,[21] and the bumpy[20,22] stents. These stents, however, have been tested on either animal models or in short-term clinical trials with small sample sizes. Data on validation of these results and long-term data on efficacy and safety need to be generated before these stents can be used routinely.
- An evolving technique to treat MPD strictures that persist beyond 12 months of single plastic stenting is to deploy multiple plastic stents placed side by side simultaneously.[23]
- Another approach that has been advocated in the recent years for refractory strictures is the temporary placement of fully covered self-expandable metallic stents (FCSEMSs).[24]

### Endotherapy for Pancreatic Pseudocysts

PPs are seen in 20% to 40% of patients with CP.[25] Endoscopic drainage of pseudo-cysts can be performed by transmural and transpapillary approaches.[14]

- It is important to evaluate for abnormal ductal anatomy, including pancreatic ductal leak and communication with the pseudocyst, with a pretreatment MRCP or ERCP. An increase in pseudocyst size on serial imaging could be a clue to ductal communication with the pseudocyst. Presence of ductal obstruction should be managed prior to endotherapy for pseudocysts to achieve better success and prevent recurrence. Similarly, arterial pseudoaneurysms, if detected, should be embolized prior to endotherapy because mortality associated with bleeding from pseudoaneurysms close to pseudocysts is high.[26]
- Transpapillary drainage during ERCP is useful for small, solitary, and communicating pseudocysts situated in relation to the head and body of the pancreas. This type of drainage has also been shown feasible and useful in large and multiple pseudocysts.[27]
- Transmural drainage can be performed by creating a communication between the pseudocyst and the stomach (cystogastrostomy) or duodenum (cystoduodenostomy). After puncture, at least 2 double pigtailed plastic stents should be placed across the puncture to keep the opening between the pseudocyst and the stomach/duodenum patent.[28] The stent should not be removed prior to at least 2 months of insertion and a cross-sectional imaging should be mandatorily performed to evaluate cyst resolution prior to stent removal.[29] If there is imaging evidence of a disconnected pancreatic duct, the stent needs to be kept in situ indefinitely to achieve the best results.[30] An attempt to bridge the ductal rupture, if possible, is also associated with good long-term success. Prior to the use of EUS in pseudocyst drainage, presence of a visible bulge on the gastric or duodenal wall was essential, through which the puncture was made. Under linear-array echoendoscopic guidance, drainage can be performed for even non-bulging pseudocysts that are located even beyond far away from the gastric or duodenal lumen with superior results.[31] EUS can also help in mapping out an avascular area for puncture, which is of added help in patients with extensive collaterals secondary to portal hypertension. EUS offers an additional aid in distinguishing pseudocysts from cystic neoplasms.[32]

### Endoscopic Ultrasound–Guided Access and Drainage After Failed Endoscopic Retrograde Cholangiopancreatography

The development of linear-array echoendoscope has enabled newer approaches for drainage of the pancreatobiliary system when conventional ERCP fails.

After the initial demonstration by Harada and colleagues in 1995,[33] several studies evaluated the feasibility and efficacy of EUS-guided pancreatobiliary drainage. The fundamental principle is to puncture the MPD under EUS guidance through the gastric or duodenal wall with a large-bore needle. Once successful access to the MPD is achieved, ductal drainage can be performed by either rendezvous techniques or the transmural route. In view of the technical challenge posed by EUS-guided rendezvous procedures and the high frequency of complications, it is currently recommended for only selected patients in tertiary care centers with appropriate infrastructure and expertise.

### Endoscopic Ultrasound–Guided Celiac Plexus Block

Celiac plexus block with a local anesthetic (bupivacaine) with or without a combination of steroid (triamcinolone) is another modality for treatment of pain in CP.[34]

Celiac plexus block can be performed percutaneously; however, EUS-guided procedure has better results and lesser risk of complications, such as paraplegia, which is associated with percutaneous technique.[35] In view of doubtful efficacy (short-lived pain relief, if any at all) and frequent complications, celiac plexus block should be kept as rescue or bridge therapy for patients who do not respond to conventional medical and endoscopic therapy and are not ideal surgical candidates. Even though EUS-guided celiac ganglion neurolysis with absolute alcohol is justified in pancreatic cancer, it should be avoided in CP, because fibrosis resulting from alcohol injection could make subsequent surgery technically difficult.

## COMPLICATIONS

- Even though intraductal mechanical and electrohydraulic lithotripsy procedures are associated with higher complication risk, ESWL is a relatively safe procedure. Usual complications of ESWL include acute pancreatitis (AP), splenic injury, skin petechiae, bleeding, Steinstrasse, and perforation, with AP being the most important. A recent study involving 1470 ESWL procedures reported an overall complication rate of 6.7%. The study documented an odds ratio of 1.28 each for developing post-ESWL complications in the presence of pancreas divisum and the interval between diagnosis of CP, respectively. On the other hand, male gender emerged as a potential independent protective factor against moderate to severe complications, with an odds ratio 0.19.[36]
- Common problems encountered with pancreatic stents include stent migration and clogging. Patency duration of pancreatic stents usually range from 6 to 12 months.[37]
- Complications of endoscopic pseudocyst drainage include bleeding, infection, and retroperitoneal leak, respectively, seen in approximately 4% patients. Mortality, however, is usually low (0.5%).[38] Complications, such as bleeding and rupture, are lower in the transpapillary method, but risk of infection is higher.
- Complications of celiac plexus block commonly include transient diarrhea, pain exacerbation, hypotension, occasionally infections, and rarely death.[39,40]

## OUTCOMES
### Extracorporeal Shock Wave Lithotripsy

Efficacy of ESWL is usually measured in terms of complete stone fragmentation, stone clearance, and pain relief.

- It has been recently shown that solitary and lower-density stone are independent predictors of complete stone clearance with ESWL.[41] **Table 1** lists the important studies that have reported complete duct clearance and pain relief in response to ESWL with or without ERCP.[14,37]
- The authors' group has recently demonstrated complete pain relief in 68.7% and 60.3% patients on intermediate (2–5 y) and long-term (>5-y) follow-up, respectively, after ESWL in a follow-up cohort of 636.[42] Complete ductal clearance was observed in 77.5% and 76% of patients in the intermediate and long-term follow-up groups, respectively. Even though 14.1% in the intermediate follow-up group and 22.8% in the long-term group had stone recurrence, merely 3.8% patients on intermediate follow-up whereas none in the long-term follow-up required repeat ESWL. This study suggested that if ESWL is initiated early on, then pain relief is likely to persist for a longer duration.
- Seven and colleagues,[43] in a study involving of 120 patients, showed pain relief in 85% patients after a mean follow-up of 4.3 years. Complete pain relief was seen in 50% patients, and there was a significant improvement in quality-of-life scores (Visual analog scale VAS) (7.3 [2.7] versus 3.7 [2.4]; $P<.001$). The proportion of pain-free patients followed over 4 years was significantly higher than those who underwent surgery (61% versus 21%; $P = .009$). The longest follow-up period in this study was more than 7 years.

**Table 1**
**Studies showing results of extracorporeal shock wave lithotripsy with and without endoscopic retrograde cholangiopancreatography on pain relief and duct clearance in patients with chronic pancreatitis**

| Author, Year | N | Follow-up Period (mo) | Treatment | Overall (Complete) Pain Relief (%) | Complete Duct Clearance (%) |
|---|---|---|---|---|---|
| Delahaye et al,[64] 1992 | 123 | 14 | ESWL + ERCP | 85 (45) | 59 |
| Schneider et al,[65] 1994 | 50 | 20 | ESWL + ERCP | 90 (62) | 60 |
| Dumonceau et al,[66] 1996 | 41 | 24 | ESWL + ERCP | 54 | 50 |
| Johanns et al,[67] 1996 | 35 | 23 | ESWL + ERCP | 83 | 46 |
| Ohara et al,[68] 1996 | 32 | 44 | ESWL | 86 | 75 |
| Costamagna et al,[69] 1997 | 35 | 27 | ESWL + ERCP | 72 | 74 |
| Adamek et al,[70] 1999 | 83 | 40 | ESWL + ERCP | 76 | NA |
| Brand et al,[71] 2000 | 48 | 7 | ESWL + ERCP | 82 | 44 |
| Kozarek et al,[72] 2002 | 40 | 30 | ESWL + ERCP | 80 | NA |
| Farnbacher et al,[73] 2004 | 125 | 29 | ESWL + ERCP | (48) | 64 |
| Delahaye et al,[74] 2004 | 56 | 173 | ESWL + ERCP | 85 (45) | 48 |
| Iniu et al,[75] 2005 | 237 | 44 | ESWL + ERCP | 91 | 73 |
| | 318 | | ESWL | | 70 |
| Dumonceau,[76] & Vonlaufen,[38] 2007 | 29 | 52 | ESWL + ERCP | 55 | NA |
| | 26 | | ESWL | 58 | NA |
| Tandan et al,[16] 2010 | 1006 | 6 | ESWL + ERCP | 84 | 76 |
| Seven et al,[43] 2012 | 120 | 51 | ESWL + ERCP | 50 | NA |
| Tandan et al,[42] 2013 | 636 | 96 | ESWL + ERCP | 60.3 | 77.2 |

*Data from* Nguyen-Tang T, Dumonceau J-M. Endoscopic treatment in chronic pancreatitis, timing, duration and type of intervention. Best Pract Res Clin Gastroenterol 2010;24:281–98; and Tringali A, Boskoski I, Costamagna G, et al. The role of endsccopy in the therapy of chronic pancreatitis. Best Pract Res Clin Gastroenterol 2008;22:145–65; with permission.

- Use of secretin prior to ESWL was shown to result in more stone clearance in a recent study by Choi and colleagues.[17] In this study, intravenous administration of 16 μg secretin prior to ESWL was shown to result in 63% stone clearance compared with 46% when secretin was not used. Multiple logistic regression suggested use of secretin and pre-ESWL pancreatic stenting as independent predictors of complete or near-complete stone clearance.
- ESWL is safe and effective in stone clearance and amelioration of pain even in children.[44] The authors have shown, in a recent study, that 34.9% of children who had pancreatic ductal calculi greater than 5 mm in size were effectively treated with a total of 57 ESWL sessions (range 1–3 session per patient). There were no intraprocedural adverse events, and only 8 (4.8%) patients overall (which also included children undergoing only ERCP) developed postprocedure adverse events in the form of mild AP in 2 and abdominal pain in 6.

### *Pancreatic Duct Stenting for Strictures*

**Table 2**[14,37] lists important studies that have evaluated the role of pancreatic ductal stenting for MPD strictures.

- Long-term clinical success for MPD stenting for strictures is usually considered as absence of pain at 1 year after stent retrieval.[3] Cessation of further stenting is marked by adequate pancreaticoduodenal outflow of contrast medium for 1 to 2 minutes after ductal filling upstream of a stricture and easy passage of a 6F catheter through the stricture.
- Pancreatic stenting is technically successful in 85% to 98% cases[45,46] and is associated with immediate pain relief in 65% to 95% patients that is sustained in 32% to 68% on follow-up of up to 14 to 58 months.[47–49] In a recent study of 17 patients who underwent pancreatic stenting, 57% remained completely pain-free (no relapse) at the end of 5 years.[50]

**Table 2**
Studies showing results of main pancreatic duct stenting for pancreatic ductal strictures and clinical outcomes in patients with chronic pancreatitis

| Author, Year | N | Follow-up Period (mo) | Stent Diameter (F) | Stricture Resolution (%) | Early/ Sustained Pain Relief (%) | Need for Surgery (%) |
|---|---|---|---|---|---|---|
| Cremer et al,[45] 1991 | 75 | 37 | 10 | 9 | 94/NA | 15 |
| Binmoeller et al,[49] 1995 | 93 | 58 | 5, 7, and 10 | NA | 74/65 | 26 |
| Ponchon et al,[46] 1995 | 23 | 14 | 10 | 48 | 74/52 | 15 |
| Smits et al,[77] 1995 | 49 | 34 | 10 | NA | 82/82 | 6 |
| Morgan et al,[78] 2003 | 25 | NA | 5–7–8.5 | NA | 65/NA | NA |
| Vitale et al,[79] 2004 | 89 | 43 | 5–7–10 | NA | 83/68 | 12 |
| Eliftheriadis et al,[80] 2005 | 100 | 69 | 8.5–10 | 62 | 70/62 | 4 |
| Ishihara et al,[20] 2006 | 20 | 21 | 10 | NA | 95/90 | NA |
| Weber et al,[47] 2007 | 17 | 24 | 7–11.5 | NA | 89/83 | NA |

*Data from* Nguyen-Tang T, Dumonceau J-M. Endoscopic treatment in chronic pancreatitis, timing, duration and type of intervention. Best Pract Res Clin Gastroenterol 2010;24:281–98; and Tringali A, Boskoski I, Costamagna G, et al. The role of endsccopy in the therapy of chronic pancreatitis. Best Pract Res Clin Gastroenterol 2008;22:145–65; with permission.

- Multiple plastic stenting has been shown to have technical and functional success rates of 100% and 94.7%, respectively, along with pain relief in 84.2%. Stent migration and reintervention were seen in 10.5% and 15.8%, respectively.[23]
- Use of FCSEMSs was associated with 100% technical and functional success. Although 85.2% patients were pain-free at short-term follow-up, complications were observed in 26.8%, with stent migration in 8.2% and reintervention in 9.8% patients.[24] Currently, use of FCSEMSs is recommended only under clinical trial settings with planned exchanges within 1 year because the patency of these stents in the pancreatic duct is limited to that duration.

### Drainage of Pancreatic Pseudocysts

- Even though procedure-related morbidity and pseudocyst recurrence is similar with endoscopic and surgical drainage in the long term, procedure-related mortality is significantly lower with endoscopic drainage (0.2% vs 2.5%).[51] Other variables that have been found significantly better with endotherapy compared with surgery include cost, length of hospital stay, and quality of life up to 3 months after drainage.[52]
- Both transpapillary and transmural drainage of pseudocysts have been found to yield similar long-term success whereas the former was found to have lower morbidity (1.8% vs 15.4%; $P = .008$). Even though transmural pseudocyst drainage can be performed by both conventional and EUS-guided drainage, success rate is higher with EUS-guided drainage because it does not require presence of an intraluminal bulge.[53,54] Results are most favorable for pseudocyst located in the head of pancreas
- Between the 2 routes of transmural drainage, namely transgastric and transduodenal, the latter was found to have greater long-term success (83.1% vs 64.0%; $P = .019$),[55,56] whereas mortality was same as that with transgastric drainage.
- Treatment failure for endoscopic drainage of PPs was found independently associated with placement of single (straight) stent and stenting duration of less than 6 weeks in a retrospective study.[28] A recent randomized controlled trial has shown that recurrence of pseudocyst was associated with early stent removal.[29]
- A majority of studies have evaluated the role of endotherapy in pseudocyst drainage resulting from both AP and CP. It is now increasingly recognized, after the revision of the Atlanta classification,[57] that PPs are uncommon in AP.[58,59] It is likely that many of so-called pseudocysts in patients with AP in those studies were actually walled-off necrosis. Therefore, it is likely that the results obtained from studies on pseudocyst drainage would be even better if only patients with CP with true pseudocyst were considered.

### Endoscopic Ultrasound–Guided Access and Drainage After Failed Endoscopic Retrograde Cholangiopancreatography

A recent study by Shah and colleagues[60] reported a success rate of up to 75% for EUS-guided rendezvous pancreatic procedure. Another Spanish multicenter study[61] of 125 patients showed an overall technical and clinical success rates of 67.2% and 63.2%, respectively, for EUS-guided biliopancreatic access. In another study by Ergun and colleagues,[62] significant reductions in pain score and MPD diameter (mean [SD]), from 7 (1.1) cm and 8.1 (4.1) mm to 1.6 (0.6) cm and 3.9 (1.0) mm, respectively, were observed on long-term follow-up (median [range] of 38 [3–120] months) of patients who underwent successful EUS-guided drainage.

### Endoscopic Ultrasound–Guided Celiac Plexus Block

The role of EUS-guided celiac plexus block for pain relief in CP has been controversial.

- Even if it is beneficial, the effect is short-lived, with 55% patients showing improvement after 4 to 8 weeks that reduces to 26% and 10% after 12 and 24 weeks, respectively.[63]
- Results are even poorer for patients under 45 years of age who had undergone previous pancreatic surgery.

## REFERENCES

1. Asaumi H, Watanabe S, Taguchi M, et al. Externally applied pressure activates pancreatic stellate cells through the generation of intracellular reactive oxygen species. Am J Physiol Gastrointest Liver Physiol 2007;293:G972–8.
2. Talukdar R, Reddy DN. Pain in chronic pancreatitis: managing beyond the pancreatic duct. World J Gastroenterol 2013;19:6319–28.
3. Dumonceau JM, Delhaye M, Tringali A, et al. Endoscopic treatment of chronic pancreatitis: European Society of Gastrointestinal Endoscopy (ESGE) Clinical Guideline. Endoscopy 2012;44:784–800.
4. Varadarajulu S, Tamhane A, Eloubeidi MA, et al. Yield of EUS guided pancreatic masses in the presence or the absence of chronic pancreatitis. Gastrointest Endosc 2005;62:728–36.
5. Arvanitakis M, Van Laethem JL, Parma J, et al. Predictive factors for pancreatic cancer in patients with chronic pancreatitis in association with k-Ras gene mutation. Endoscopy 2004;36:535–42.
6. Morgan DE, Baron TH, Smith JK, et al. Pancreatic fluid collections prior to intervention: evaluation with MR imaging compared with CT and US. Radiology 1997; 203:773–8.
7. Pamuklar E, Semelka RC. MR imaging of the pancreas. Magn Reson Imaging Clin N Am 2005;13:313–30.
8. Vitas GJ, Sarr MG. Selected management of pancreatic pseudocysts: operative versus expectant management. Surgery 1992;111:123–30.
9. Yeo CJ, Bastidas JA, Lynch-Nyhan A, et al. The natural history of pancreatic pseudocysts documented by computed tomography. Surg Gynecol Obstet 1990;170:411–7.
10. Freeman ML. Mechanical lithotripsy forpancreatic duct stones. Gastrointest Endosc 1996;44:333–6.
11. Howell DA, Dy RM, Hanson BL, et al. Endoscopic treatment of pancreatic duct stones using a10F pancreatoscope and electrohydraulic lithotripsy. Gastrointest Endosc 1999;50:829–33.
12. Chen YK, Taransky PR, Raijman I, et al. Peroral pancreatic stone therapy and investigation of suspected pancreatic lesions- first human experience using the spyglass direc visualization system (SDVS). Gastrointest Endosc 2008;67: AB108.
13. Maydeo A, Kwek BE, Bhandari S, et al. Single-operator cholangioscopy-guided laser lithotripsy in patients with difficult biliary and pancreatic ductal stones (with videos). Gastrointest Endosc 2011;74(6):1308–14.
14. Nguyen-Tang T, Dumonceau J-M. Endoscopic treatment in chronic pancreatitis, timing, duration and type of intervention. Best Pract Res Clin Gastroenterol 2010;24:281–98.

15. Ong WC, Tandan M, Reddy V, et al. Multiple pancreatic duct stones in tropical chronic pancreatitis: safe clearance with extracorporeal shock wave lithotripsy. J Gastroenterol Hepatol 2006;21:1514–8.

16. Tandan M, Reddy DN, Santosh D, et al. Extracorporeal shock wave lithotripsy and endotherapy for pancreatic calculi- a large single center experience. Indian J Gastroenterol 2010;29:143–8.

17. Choi EK, McHenry L, Watkins JL, et al. Use of intravenous secretin during extracorporeal shock wave lithotripsy to facilitate endoscopic clearance of pancreatic duct stones. Pancreatology 2012;12:272–5.

18. Darisetty S, Tandan M, Reddy DN, et al. Epidural anesthesia is effective for extracorporeal shock wave lithotripsy of pancreatic and biliary calculi. World J Gastrointest Surg 2010;2:165–8.

19. Binmoeller KF, Ratod VD, Soehendra N. Endoscopic therapy of pancreatic strictures. Gastrointest Endosc Clin N Am 1998;8:125–42.

20. Ishihara T, Yamaguchi T, Seza K, et al. Efficacy of s-type stents for the treatment of main pancreatic duct stricture in patients with chronic pancreatitis. Scand J Gastroenterol 2006;41:744–50.

21. Raju GS, Gomez G, Xiao SY, et al. Effect of a novel pancreatic stent design on short-term pancreatic injury in a canine model. Endoscopy 2006;38:260–5.

22. Park do H, Kim MH, Moon SH, et al. Feasibility and safety of placement of a newly designed, fully covered self-expandable metal stent for refractory benign pancreatic ductal stricture: a pilot study. Gastrointest Endosc 2008;68:1182–9.

23. Costamagna G, Bulajic M, Tringali A, et al. Multiple stenting of refractory pancreatic duct strictures in severe chronic pancreatitis: long term results. Endoscopy 2006;38:254–9.

24. Shen Y, Liu M, Chen M, et al. Covered metal stent or multiple plastic stents for refractory pancreatic ductal strictures in chronic pancreatitis: a systematic review. Pancreatology 2014;14:87–90.

25. Andren-Sandberg A, Dervenis C. Pancreatic pseudocysts in the 21st century. Part 1: classification, pathophysiology, anatomic consideration and treatment. JOP 2004;5:8–24.

26. Balachandra S, Siriwerdena AK. Systematic appraisal of management of the major vascular complications of pancreatitis. Am J Surg 2005;109:489–95.

27. Bhasin DK, Rana SS, Nanda M, et al. Endoscopic management of pancreatic pseudocysts at atypical locations. Surg Endosc 2010;24(5):1085–91.

28. Cahen D, Rauws E, Fockens P, et al. Endoscopic drainage of pancreatic pseudocysts: long-term outcome and procedural factors associated with safe and successful treatment. Endoscopy 2005;37:977–83.

29. Arvanitakis M, Delahaye M, Bali MA, et al. Pancreatic fluid collections: a randomized controlled trial regarding stent removal after endoscopic transmural drainage. Gastrointest Endosc 2007;65:609–19.

30. Deviere J, Antaki F. Disconnected pancreatic tail syndrome: a plea for multidisciplinarity. Gastrointest Endosc 2008;67:680–2.

31. Sanchez Cortes E, Maalak A, Le Moine O, et al. Endoscopic cystenterostomy of non-bulging pancreatic fluid collections. Gastrointest Endosc 2002;56:380–6.

32. Bruggie WR. Approaches to drainage of pancreatic pseudocysts. Curr Opin Gastroenterol 2004;20:488–92.

33. Harada N, Kouzu T, Arima M, et al. Endoscopic ultrasound-guided pancreatography: a case report. Endoscopy 1995;27:612–5.

34. Talukdar R, Nageshwar Reddy D. Endoscopic therapy for chronic pancreatitis. Curr Opin Gastroenterol 2014;30:484–9.

35. Gress F, Schmitt C, Sherman S, et al. A prospective randomized comparison of endoscopic ultrasound and computed tomography-guided celiac plexus block for managing chronic pancreatitis. Am J Gastroenterol 1999;94:900–5.

36. Li BR, Liao Z, Du TT, et al. Risk factors for complications of pancreatic extracorporeal shock wave lithotripsy. Endoscopy 2014;46:1092–100.

37. Tringali A, Boskoski I, Costamagna G, et al. The role of endsccopy in the therapy of chronic pancreatitis. Best Pract Res Clin Gastroenterol 2008;22:145–65.

38. Dumonceau JM, Vonlaufen A. Pancreatic endoscopic retrograde cholangiopancreatography (ERCP). Endoscopy 2007;39:124–30.

39. Kaufman M, Singh G, Das S, et al. Efficacy of endoscopic ultrasound-guided celiac plexus block and celiac plexus neurolysis for managing abdominal pain associated with chronic pancreatitis and pancreatic cancer. J Clin Gastroenterol 2010;44:127–34.

40. Gimeno-Garcia AZ, Elwassief A, Paquin SC, et al. Fatal complication after endoscopic ultrasound-guided celiac plexus neurolysis. Endoscopy 2012;44(Suppl 2 UCTN):E267.

41. Ohyama H, Mikata R, Ishihara T, et al. Efficacy of stone density on noncontrast computed tomography in predicting the outcome of extracorporeal shock wave lithotripsy for patients with pancreatic stones. Pancreas 2015;44(3):422–8.

42. Tandan M, Reddy DN, Talukdar R, et al. Long-term clinical outcomes of extracorporeal shockwave lithotripsy in painful chronic calcific pancreatitis. Gastrointest Endosc 2013;78:726–33.

43. Seven G, Schreiner MA, Ross AS, et al. Long-term outcomes associated with pancreatic extracorporeal shock wave lithotripsy for chronic calcific pancreatitis. Gastrointest Endosc 2012;75:997–1004.

44. Agarwal J, Nageshwar Reddy D, Talukdar R, et al. ERCP in the management of pancreatic diseases in children. Gastrointest Endosc 2014;79:271–8.

45. Cremer M, Deviere J, Delahaye M, et al. Stenting in severe chronic pancreatitis: results in medium-term follow up in seventy six patients. Endoscopy 1991;23:171–6.

46. Ponchon T, Bory RM, Hedelius F, et al. Endoscopic stenting for pain relief in chronic pancreatitis: results of a standardized protocol. Gastrointest Endosc 1995;42:452–6.

47. Weber A, Schneider J, Neu B, et al. Endoscopic stents for patients with chronic pancreatitis: results from a prospective follow-up study. Pancreas 2007;34:287–94.

48. Farnbacher MJ, Muhldorfer S, Wehler M, et al. Interventional endoscopic therapy in chronic pancreatitis in chronic pancreatitis including temporary stenting: a definitive treatment? Scand J Gastroenterol 2006;41:111–7.

49. Binmoeller KF, Jue P, Seifert H, et al. Endoscopic stent drainage in chronic pancreatitis and a dominant stricture: long-term results. Endoscopy 1995;27:638–44.

50. Weber A, Schneider J, Neu B, et al. Endoscopic stent therapy in chronic pancreatitis: a 5-year follow-up study. World J Gastroenterol 2013;19:715–20.

51. Rosso E, Alexakis N, Ghaneh P, et al. Pancreatic pseudocysts in chronic pancreatitis: endoscopic and surgical treatment. Dig Surg 2003;20:397–406.

52. Varadarajulu S, Band JY, Sutton BS, et al. Equal efficacy of endoscopic and surgical cystogastrostomy for pancreatic pseudocyst drainage in a randomized trial. Gastroenterology 2013;145:583–90.

53. Park DH, Lee SS, Moon S-H, et al. Endoscopic ultrasound guided versus conventional transmural drainage for panceatic pseudocysts: a prospective randomized trial. Endoscopy 2009;41:842–8.

54. Binmoeller FK, Seifert H, Walter A, et al. Transpapillary and tansmural drainage of pancreatic pseudocysts. Gastrointest Endosc 1995;42:219–24.
55. Beckinghem IJ, Krige JE, Bornman PC, et al. Endoscopic management of pancreatic pseudocysts. Br J Surg 1997;84:1638–45.
56. Cremer M, Deviere J, Engelholm L. Endoscopic management of cysts and pseudocysts in chronic pancreatitis: long-term follow up after 7 years of experience. Gastrointest Endosc 1989;35:1–9.
57. Banks PA, Bollen TL, Dervenis C, et al. Classification of acute pancreatitis-2012: revision of the Atlanta classification and definitions by international consensus. Gut 2013;62:102–11.
58. Acevedo-Piedra NG, Moya-Hoyo N, Rey-Riveiro M, et al. Validation of the determinant-based classification and revision of the Atlanta classification systems for acute pancreatitis. Clin Gastroenterol Hepatol 2014;12:311–6.
59. Talukdar R, Bhattacharyya A, Rao B, et al. Validation of the revised Atlanta definitions of severity of acute pancreatitis: have all loose ends being tied? Pancreatology 2013;13:S6–7.
60. Shah JN, Marson F, Weilert F, et al. Single-operator, single-session EUS-guided anterograde cholangiopancreatography in failed ERCP or inaccessible papilla. Gastrointest Endosc 2012;75:56–64.
61. Vila JJ, Perez-Miranda M, Vazquez-Sequiros E, et al. Initial experience with EUS-guided cholangiopancreatography for biliary and pancreatic duct drainage: a Spanish national survey. Gastrointest Endosc 2012;75:1133–41.
62. Ergun M, Aouattah T, Gigot J-F, et al. Endoscopic ultrasound-guided transluminal drainage of pancreatic duct obstruction: long-term outcome. Endoscopy 2011; 43:518–25.
63. Gress F, Schmitt C, Sherman S, et al. Endoscopic ultrasound-guided celiac plexus block for managing abdominal pain associated with chronic pancreatitis: a prospective single center experience. Am J Gastroenterol 2001;96:409–16.
64. Delhaye M, Vandermeeren A, Baize M, et al. Extracorporeal shock-wave lithotripsy of pancreatic calculi. Gastroenterology 1992;102:610–20.
65. Schneider HT, May A, Benninger J, et al. Piezoelectric shock wave lithotripsy of pancreatic duct stones. Am J Gastroenterology 1994;89:2042–8.
66. Dumonceau JM, Deviere J, Le Moine O, et al. Endoscopic pancreatic drainage in chronic pancreatitis associated with ductal stones: long term results. Gastrointest Endosc 1996;43:547–55.
67. Johanns W, Jakobeit C, Greiner L, et al. Ultrasound-guided extracorporeal shock wave lithotripsy of pancreatic ductal stones: six years' experience. Can J Gastroenterol 1996;10(7):471–5.
68. Ohara H, Hoshino M, Hayakawa T, et al. Single application extracorporeal shock wave lithotripsy is the first choice for patients with pancreatic duct stones. Am J Gastroenterol 1996;91:1388–94.
69. Costamagna G, Gabbrielli A, Mutignani M, et al. Extracorporeal shock wave lithotripsy of pancreatic stones in chronic pancreatitis: immediate and medium-term results. Gastrointest Endosc 1997;46(3):231–6.
70. Adamek HE, Jakobs R, Buttmann A, et al. Long term follow up of patients with chronic pancreatitis and pancreatic stones treated with extracorporeal shock wave lithotripsy. Gut 1999;45:402–5.
71. Brand B, Kahl M, Sindhu S, et al. Prospective evaluation of morphology, function and quality of life after the extracorporeal shockwave lithotripsy and endoscopic treatment of chronic calcific pancreatitis. Am J Gastroenterol 2000;95: 3428–38.

72. Kozarek RA, Brandabur JJ, Ball TJ, et al. Clinical outcomes in patients who undergo extracorporeal shock wave lithotripsy for chronic calcific pancreatitis. Gastrointest Endosc 2002;56:496–500.
73. Farnbacher MJ, Schoen C, Rabenstein T, et al. Pancreatic duct stones in chronic pancreatitis: criteria for treatment intensity and success. Gatrointest Endosc 2002;56:501–6.
74. Delhaye M, Arvanitakis M, Verset G, et al. Long term clinical outcome after endoscopic pancreatic ductal drainage for patients with painful chronic pancreatitis. Clin Gastroenterol Hepatol 2004;2:1096–106.
75. Inui K, Tazuma S, Yamaguchi T, et al. Treatment of pancreatic stones with extracorporeal shock wave lithotripsy: results of a multi center survey. Pnacreas 2005; 30:26–30.
76. Dumonceau M, Costamagna G, Tringali A, et al. Treatment of painful calcified chronic pancreatitis: extracorporeal shock wave lithotripsy versus endoscopic treatment: a randomised controlled trial. Gut 2007;56:545–52.
77. Smits ME, Badiga SM, Rauws EA, et al. Long term results of pancreatic stents in chronic pancreatitis. Gastrointest Endosc 1995;42:461–7.
78. Morgan DE, Smith JK, Hawkins K, et al. Endoscopic stent therapy in advanced chronic pancreatitis: relationships between ductal changes, clinical response and stent patency. Am J Gastroenterol 2003;98:821–6.
79. Vitale GC, Cothron K, Vitale EA, et al. Role of pancreatic duct stenting in the treatment of chronic pancreatitis. Surg Endosc 2004;18:1431–4.
80. Eleftherlandis N, Dinu F, Delhaya M, et al. Long term outcome of pancreatitic stenting in severe chronic pancreatitis. Endoscopy 2005;37:223–30.

# Innovations in Intraductal Endoscopy

## Cholangioscopy and Pancreatoscopy

Raj J. Shah, MD

### KEYWORDS

- ERCP • Cholangioscopy • Pancreatoscopy • Cholangiocarcinoma • Bile duct stone
- Pancreatic duct stone • Biliary stricture • IPMN

### KEY POINTS

- Cholangiopancreatoscopy (CP) is an adjunct to endoscopic retrograde cholangiopancreatography (ERCP) and can be used for the clarification of indeterminate lesions and for guiding therapy of malignancy.
- CP is an established modality in successfully treating difficult pancreaticobiliary stones.
- CP imaging has both fiberoptic and digital technologies and is available in endoscope and catheter-based systems.
- CP is currently widely available, although its use should be limited to those endoscopists who are proficient in performing complex ERCP.

## INTRODUCTION: NATURE OF THE PROBLEM

Miniature endoscopes and optical catheters permit direct visualization of the bile and pancreatic ducts. These are usually passed through the working channel of a standard therapeutic duodenoscope during endoscopic retrograde cholangiopancreatography (ERCP).

The first cholangioscope was described in 1941,[1] and the per-oral approach was subsequently introduced in the early 1970s.[2,3] Per-oral pancreatoscopy (POP) was first described in Japan in 1975.[4] Presently, the 10F platforms provide a working channel, tip deflection, and either fiberoptic or digital/video chips; slim gastroscopes are used without a duodenoscope for direct cholangioscopy.[5–9]

## INDICATIONS/CONTRAINDICATIONS

For indications and contraindications to cholangiopancreatoscopy, see **Table 1**.

Pancreaticobiliary Endoscopy, University of Colorado Anschutz Medical Campus, 1635 Aurora Ct, Mail Stop F735, AIP 2.031, Aurora, CO 80045, USA
*E-mail address:* Raj.Shah@UCdenver.edu

Gastrointest Endoscopy Clin N Am 25 (2015) 779–792
http://dx.doi.org/10.1016/j.giec.2015.06.012          giendo.theclinics.com

**Table 1**
**Indications and contraindications to cholangiopancreatoscopy**

| Indications | Contraindications |
|---|---|
| Established<br>• Therapy of difficult pancreatic and biliary stones<br>• Indeterminate biliary and pancreatic strictures<br>• Evaluation of equivocal findings during cholangiopancreatography<br>• Assessment of the extent of cholangiocarcinoma or main duct IPMN before surgery<br>• Guiding selective wire access across strictures and the cystic duct/gallbladder<br>Equivocal Evidence<br>• Assess for residual stones in dilated bile or pancreatic ducts not seen on cholangiopancreatography<br>• Evaluate dominant stenoses in primary sclerosing cholangitis<br>• Delivery of biliary photodynamic therapy<br>• Guiding treatment margins for biliary radiofrequency ablation | • Active cholangitis<br>• Small duct (<5 mm) in diameter |

## TECHNIQUE/PROCEDURE PREPARATION
### Sedation

General anesthesia is recommended. Intraductal irrigation can lead to reflux of fluids and pooling within the stomach, increasing the risk of aspiration.[10] For "mother-daughter" systems, trained secondary personnel (ie, a registered nurse, technician, or assisting endoscopist) handle the "daughter" scope.

### Antibiotic Prophylaxis

Preprocedural broad-spectrum intravenous antibiotic prophylaxis is recommended due to a potentially higher rate of cholangitis when compared with those patients undergoing ERCP without cholangioscopy.[11,12]

### Patient Positioning

We prefer the semiprone position.

### Equipment

Systems available in the United States for cholangioscopy include endoscope-based dual-operator systems, commonly referred to as "mother-daughter" (Olympus America, Center Valley, PA, and Pentax, Montvale, NJ) and a catheter-based system, commonly referred to as "single-operator" cholangioscopy (SpyGlass DS Direct Visualization System, Boston Scientific Endoscopy, Marlboro, MA). In addition, cholangioscopy can be performed using a slim (4.9–5.9 mm outer diameter) gastroscope or even standard gastroscope in patients with a dilated common bile duct.[9]

Fiberoptic cholangioscopes range in diameter from 3.1 to 3.4 mm, with a working channel of 1.2 mm that permits passage of forceps and lithotripsy fibers, and have up/down tip deflection.[7,8] Video cholangioscopes are prototypes. The fully disposable single-operator catheter-based system is approved by the Food and Drug Administration for pancreatic duct inspection, has 4-way tip deflection, a 1.2-mm working channel diameter, and two 0.6-mm irrigation ports.[7,8,13] Pancreatoscopy is primarily performed with scopes and catheters designed for inspection of the bile duct. A detailed review of the available cholangiopancreatoscopes has been summarized in a technical status evaluation report by the American Society of Gastrointestinal Endoscopy's Technology committee and other technical reviews.[7,13,14]

Slim gastroscopes (5–6-mm diameters) can be used in patients with dilated common bile ducts generally larger than 10 mm in diameter.[9,15–18] The larger working channel accommodates argon plasma coagulation probes, larger biopsy forceps, and lithotripsy fibers. Insufflation with sterile saline, water, or $CO_2$ is preferable, as air insufflation has been associated with air embolism.[18]

## Technique

### Scope insertion

CP is carried out during ERCP, and generally following cholangiopancreatography to map the target areas. A long (450-cm) 0.035-inch guidewire is advanced to the intrahepatics or pancreatic tail and the cholangiopancreatoscope is advanced over the guidewire through a therapeutic duodenoscope. For endoscope-based systems, a "transfer tube" is placed into the biopsy port to allow wire exit from the working channel to permit counter-traction to help minimize duodenoscope elevator use. Sphincterotomy and/or stricture dilation are performed, unless the orifice is patulous, to facilitate scope passage.[13] If a slim gastroscope is being used, it may be inserted into the duct over a guidewire placed during ERCP or by way of a free-hand technique.[9] Pediatric forceps may be used to gently grasp intraductal mucosa or prototype anchoring balloons to permit advancement of the slim gastroscope toward the intrahepatics.[9,16,17] For the single-operator catheter-based system, the endoscopist has control of the 4-way steering dials and may periodically lock the dials for fine movements of the catheter to stabilize visualization of a target during biopsy.

Once the cholangioscope is advanced to the desired location within the duct, the guidewire is removed to enhance visualization and to permit use of the working channel.

Narrow duct diameters or tight strictures complicate or prohibit scope passage. Circumferential visualization also may be compromised in the evaluation of a markedly dilated duct.

The angle to the pancreatic orifice from the duodenoscope is more oblique than compared with the bile duct, and initial transpapillary advancement is often simpler than traversing the biliary orifice, which is often at a right angle. However, traversing the minor papilla is more difficult due to acute angulation.[19,20] To negotiate downstream narrowed caliber ducts, dilation with a 4-mm or 6-mm balloon before attempting device introduction may be required. The inherent angulation at the relatively fixed genu may limit circumferential inspection of the area.

## TECHNIQUES TO IMPROVE VISUALIZATION

Irrigation rates should be kept as low as possible to permit sufficient view. Periodic duodenoscope suctioning and aspiration using the CP is encouraged. For the digital catheter-based system, a separate port for suction via the working channel can be attached to wall suction. This is effective even when devices such as biopsy forceps or electrohydraulic lithotripsy (EHL) are present in the working channel (Shah, personal observation, 2015). The endoscope-based fiberoptic systems also have suction capability. A "closed circuit" technique of irrigation and suctioning in the catheter-based system may be used to reduce debris obscuring visualization.

### Intraductal Lithotripsy

EHL or laser lithotripsy can be used to treat large bile and pancreatic duct stones under direct visualization. EHL has 2 coaxially insulated electrodes ending at an open tip.

During water immersion, sparks are generated that produce high-amplitude hydraulic pressure waves for stone fragmentation.[21] A generator produces a series of high-voltage electrical impulses at a frequency of 1 to 20 per second, with power settings ranging from 50% to 100%. The tip of the EHL fiber should protrude no more than 2 to 3 mm from the scope and be positioned en face with the stone.[13] Pulsed laser is transmitted via a flexible quartz fiber through the working channel of the cholangioscope. The application of repetitive pulses of laser energy to the stone leads to the formation of a gaseous collection of ions and free electrons of high kinetic energy (eg, plasma). Absorption of the laser energy rapidly expands and collapses the plasma, inducing a spherical mechanical shockwave between the laser fiber and stone, leading to stone fragmentation.[22]

### Intraductal Biopsy

Two methods can be used to obtain targeted biopsies from the bile or pancreatic duct: CP-directed biopsy and CP-assisted biopsy. CP-directed biopsy is performed by passing a miniature biopsy forceps under direct visualization. For CP-assisted biopsy, the target site is localized using CP visualization and a fluoroscopic spot film of the CP tip positioned at the lesion. After CP removal, a biliary or conventional biopsy forceps is passed through the working channel of the duodenoscope alongside the guidewire to obtain tissue samples under fluoroscopic guidance.[23]

## DEVICE INSERTION SUGGESTIONS

If there is failure to pass accessories through the CP channel, withdrawing the CP to the distal duct, advancing the device, followed by advancement of the CP may be helpful to traverse the angulation between the elevator and the orifice. Alternatively, advancement of the CP toward the bifurcation may also facilitate device passage. For the disposable catheter-based system and forceps passage, rapid open and closure of the forceps when resistance is encountered can be helpful. This is not recommended for endoscope-based systems because of the potential for damage to the working channel. If the target lesion is distal, passage of the miniature forceps or lithotripsy fiber may be difficult and CP-assisted biopsies can be obtained or preloading of fibers followed by free-hand cannulation, respectively.[13]

## COMPLICATIONS AND MANAGEMENT

Complications specific to the performance of cholangiopancreatoscopy include cholangitis, which is related to intraductal fluid irrigation, and, uncommonly, hemobilia and bile leaks attributable to intraductal lithotripsy.[7,11,24] Our center retrospectively assessed patients undergoing ERCP with or without cholangiopancreatoscopy and found that CP had higher consensus complications (pancreatitis, perforation, cholangitis, or bleeding; 4.2% vs 2.2%), and specifically postprocedural cholangitis (1.0% vs 0.2%).[11] For pancreatoscopy, it is likely that higher rates of pancreatitis may be seen that are inherent to pancreatic endotherapy.[19]

## POSTOPERATIVE CARE

When cholangioscopy is performed in the setting of hilar or intrahepatic strictures or leaks, we recommend the use of postprocedural antibiotics for 5 to 7 days as prophylaxis of cholangitis and infection, respectively.[12] Further, for index pancreatic endotherapy to include sphincterotomy, therapeutic stenting, and intraductal lithotripsy, we generally recommend postprocedure 23-hour observation and judicious periprocedural intravenous fluids.

## REPORTING, FOLLOW-UP, AND CLINICAL IMPLICATIONS

Cholangioscopy findings are included in a separate paragraph in the ERCP report. In the highly suspicious clinical setting, if malignant findings are suggested based on cholangioscopy visualization, surgical resection may be recommended.[25] If the examination is equivocal for malignancy and tissue sampling is nondiagnostic, a close interval for repeat tissue sampling is planned. For pancreatoscopy, we recommend prophylactic stenting.

## OUTCOMES
### Cholangioscopy Outcomes

#### Bile duct stones
Preliminary data from our center categorized complex biliary stones that required endoscopic papillary large balloon dilation, mechanical lithotripsy, or intraductal lithotripsy. There were 211 patients with primarily extrahepatic stones who required these advanced techniques, and complete clearance was achieved in 99%; 79% at index ERCP and 20% at subsequent ERCP. Patients in the intraductal lithotripsy group had significantly larger stones.[26] CP is less successful with associated strictures or intrahepatic stones[24,27,28] (**Fig. 1, Table 2**).

The use of direct cholangioscopy using 5-mm to 6-mm slim gastroscopes has gained momentum in recent years. Lee and colleagues[35] reported on 48 patients with duct diameter greater than 10 mm who were felt to have complete clearance of stones by balloon occlusion cholangiography. Subsequent direct cholangioscopy was successful in 46, 13 of whom (28%) had residual stones.

#### Suspected biliary malignancies
In patients with indeterminate strictures or filling defects at cholangiography, cholangioscopy permits direct inspection (**Fig. 2**). However, stent-associated changes and trauma related to stricture dilation may alter the mucosal appearance.

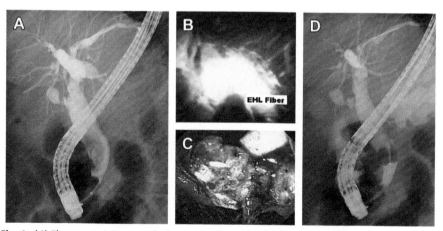

**Fig. 1.** (*A*) Fluoroscopic image of a large extrahepatic bile duct stone. (*B*) Digital single operator cholangioscopy (SOC) image of the stone and EHL fiber. (*C*) Endoscopic image of extracted bile duct stone fragments. (*D*) Fluoroscopic image of a cleared bile duct.

**Table 2**
**Results of cholangioscopy-guided intraductal lithotripsy for biliary stones**

| Author (n = Number of Patients) | Location of Stones and Method (EHL or LL) | Clearance, % | Morbidity, % |
|---|---|---|---|
| Chen et al,[29,30] 2011 (66) ~15 Centers | Mostly extrahepatic (EHL and LL) | 92 | Variable |
| Patel[30] (69) 4 Centers | Extrahepatic/Intrahepatic (LL) | 97 | 4 |
| Arya et al,[24] 2004 (94) | Extrahepatic/Intrahepatic (EHL) | 90 | 17 |
| Farrell et al,[32] 2005 (26) | Extrahepatic (EHL) | 100 | 0 |
| Maydeo et al,[33] 2011 (60) | Extrahepatic (LL) | 100 | 14 |
| Piraka et al,[27] 2007 (32) | Extrahepatic/Intrahepatic (EHL) | 81 | 6 |
| Sepe et al,[31] 2012 (13) | Cystic duct (EHL) | 77 | 0 |
| Okugawa et al,[28] 2002 (36) | Intrahepatic (EHL); 1/3 had ESWL | 64 | 3 |
| Neuhaus et al,[34] 1998 (60) | Extrahepatic: ESWL vs LL | 73 vs 97 ($P<.05$) | 7 |

*Abbreviations:* EHL, electrohydraulic lithotripsy; ESWL, extracorporeal shock wave lithotripsy; LL, laser lithotripsy.

Cholangioscopic visualization of "tumor vessels" (irregularly dilated and tortuous blood vessels), intraductal nodules, masses, infiltrative (eg, irregular margins with partial occlusion of the lumen) or ulcerated strictures, and papillary or villous mucosal projections may indicate malignancy and should prompt biopsies.[36,37] Prospective case series using either endoscope-based or catheter-based systems have shown that cholangioscopic visualization with or without biopsy has a sensitivity of 78% to 100% and a specificity of 79% to 98% for detecting biliary malignancies[23,29,37–41] (**Table 3**).

### Primary sclerosing cholangitis
In a prospective ERCP study of 53 patients with primary sclerosing cholangitis (PSC), cholangioscopy compared with cholangiography had higher sensitivity (92% vs 66%)

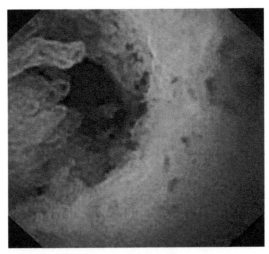

**Fig. 2.** Video NBI cholangioscopy view of a biliary villous mass.

**Table 3**
**Select larger series of cholangioscopy for evaluation of biliary strictures**

| Author (Number of Patients) | Cholangioscope | Sensitivity/Specificity | Comments |
|---|---|---|---|
| Shah et al,[23] 2006 (62) | Endoscope-based | 89%/96% (biliary and pancreatic combined) | First consecutive series of per-oral cholangiopancreatoscopy–directed sampling |
| Manta et al,[42] 2013 (52) | Fiberoptic catheter-based | 88%/94% (cholangioscopy-directed biopsies) | 43/45 had successful cholangioscopy-directed biopsies |
| Chen et al,[29] 2011 (95) | Fiberoptic catheter-based | 78%/82% (visual) 49%/98% (cholangioscopy-directed biopsies) | International, multicenter Cholangiogram impression had 51% sensitivity |
| Itoi et al,[43] 2007 (87) | Video NBI cholangioscope | 92% (visual)/N/A | Prospective, multicenter Asian series |
| Mounzer et al,[37] 2015 (89) | Video NBI cholangioscope | 93%/85% (visual) | Single-center US series |

*Abbreviations:* N/A, not available; NBI, narrow band imaging.

and specificity (93% vs 51%).[44] However, this yield has not been duplicated by other centers.[45] Features traditionally classified as malignant on cholangioscopy, such as nodular and infiltrative strictures, may be present in benign PSC.[46] The use of video narrow band imaging (NBI) in one small series did not translate to an improvement of detection of dysplasia and there was overlap in benign and malignant cholangioscopic findings.[46]

*Pancreatic stones*
The potential advantage of ERCP with POP over extracorporeal shock wave lithotripsy is that it may address stones and concurrent pancreatic duct (PD) strictures that likely contribute to stone formation, all at the index ERCP[47–51] (**Table 4**). The published experience of POP for the treatment of pancreatic duct stones remains limited but will continue to emerge and become a primary modality at select referral centers (**Fig. 3**).

**Table 4**
**Pancreatoscopy and intraductal lithotripsy for pancreatic duct stones**

| Author (Patients) | EHL, LL | Complete or Partial Clearance | Complications | Median Follow-up |
|---|---|---|---|---|
| Howell[27] (6) | EHL | 83% (combined) | None | n/a |
| Attwell et al,[52] 2014 (46) Single center | 39 patients with lithotripsy (33 EHL, 6 LL) | 70% Complete 21% Partial | 10% (mild) | 18 mo 74% Clinical success |
| US multicenter[53] (28) | LL (1–4 sessions and one-third had incomplete ESWL) | 79% Complete 11% Partial | 29% (mild) | 13 mo 89% Clinical success |

*Abbreviations:* EHL, electrohydraulic lithotripsy; ESWL, extracorporeal shock wave lithotripsy; LL, laser lithotripsy.

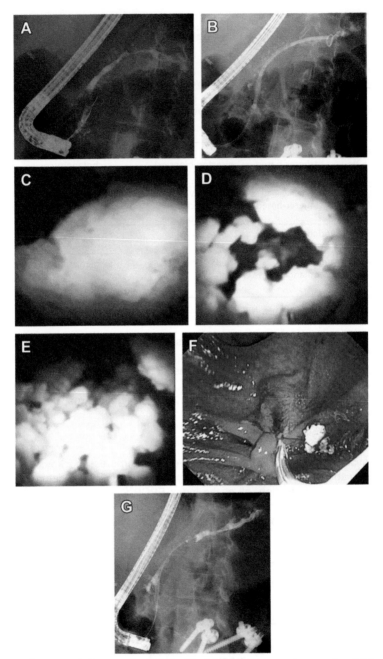

**Fig. 3.** (*A*) Fluoroscopic image of a pancreatic duct tail stone upstream of a stricture; the filling defect in the genu is an "air bubble." (*B*) Fluoroscopic image of the digital SOC in the tail of the pancreas. (*C*) Digital SOC image of the pancreatic duct stone in the tail. (*D* and *E*) Digital SOC images of fragmented pancreatic duct stone following EHL. (*F*) Endoscopic image of extracted pancreatic duct stone fragments. (*G*) Fluoroscopic image of the pancreatic duct tail stone cleared after EHL fragmentation and balloon extraction.

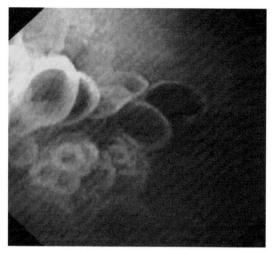

**Fig. 4.** Video NBI pancreatoscopy view of an IPMN "fish-egg" lesion.

### Intraductal papillary mucinous neoplasia

For a video NBI pancreatoscopy view of an intraductal papillary mucinous neoplasia (IPMN) "fish-egg" lesion and a video NBI pancreatoscopy view of an IPMN villous mass lesion, see **Figs. 4** and **5**. For pancreatoscopy outcomes from select series of IPMNs, see **Table 5**.

Pancreatoscopy outcomes from select series of indeterminate pancreatic pathology:

- A series of 44 patients with indeterminate pancreatic pathology used single-operator pancreatoscopy and 41 reached the target region. Of the 17 patients with main duct-IPMN, 76% were correctly identified by pancreatoscopy. The incidence of post-ERCP pancreatitis was higher than previous series (17%).[57]

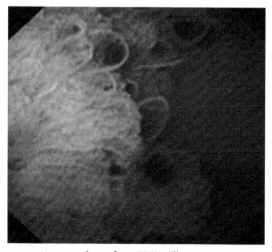

**Fig. 5.** Video NBI pancreatoscopy view of an IPMN villous mass lesion.

**Table 5**
**Pancreatoscopy outcomes from select series of IPMN**

| Author (Patients) | IPMN Types | Malignancy Predictors | Complications | Median Follow-up |
|---|---|---|---|---|
| Hara et al,[54] 2002 (60) | I: granular; II: fish-egg without vascular images; III: fish-egg with vascular images; IV: villous; V: vegetative mass | Types III, IV, V Sensitivity:68% Specificity: 87% | None | n/a |
| Yamaguchi et al,[55] 2005 (103) | n/a | POP aspiration had a higher sensitivity (62% vs 38%) compared with catheter aspiration | 10% (mild) | 18 mo 74% Clinical success |
| Miura et al,[56] 2010 (21) video POP | 7 type IV, 2 type V, 9 adenocarcinoma | Sessile or semipedunculated predictive of adenoma or hyperplasia | n/a | n/a |

Abbreviations: IPMN, intraductal papillary mucinous neoplasia; POP, per-oral pancreatoscopy.

- Our group has preliminary data on 78 patients with suspected pancreatic duct neoplasia evaluated over 13 years. Main duct-IPMN was noted in 21 patients, 6 of whom had dysplasia (Type IV = 5 and Type V = 1). POP was useful in localizing main duct-IPMN to guide resection, excluding lesions in the head for anticipated extended pancreatic tail resection, and evaluating for mixed IPMN in patients with established side branch-IPMN. The POP visual impression had a sensitivity of 91% and specificity of 96%.[58]

## CURRENT CONTROVERSIES/FUTURE CONSIDERATIONS

The introduction of the catheter-based (eg, single-operator) cholangioscopy system has led to wider availability and utilization and the digital version is fully disposable. The endoscope-based system has limited availability. The target provider to perform cholangioscopy should be adept in the performance of complex ERCP. Proficiency in performing cholangioscopy should be achieved before attempting pancreatoscopy, which tends to be more technically demanding and of higher risk.

For difficult biliary stones (eg, cuboidal, impacted, or larger than the downstream duct), whether proceeding immediately to cholangioscopy and intraductal lithotripsy would lead to shorter procedure times, fewer repeat procedures, and be more cost-effective compared with attempts at large papillary balloon dilation and/or mechanical lithotripsy remains to be determined.

For indeterminate biliary strictures, early use of cholangioscopy and directed sampling may be preferred to multiple, repeated attempts at ERCP with conventional sampling to reduce the time to diagnosis.

## SUMMARY

- Cholangiopancreatoscopy is performed using endoscope or catheter-based systems.

- Cholangioscopy with intraductal lithotripsy is an established modality in the treatment of difficult biliary stones, obviating the need for open bile duct exploration. For the evaluation of suspected biliary malignancies, it has an improved sensitivity and specificity over cholangiography alone, with or without biopsy.
- Pancreatoscopy has a high success rate in patients with dilated pancreatic ducts and carries an acceptable risk profile. It is a useful adjunct to ERCP, endoscopic ultrasonography, and noninvasive imaging to improve the detection of pancreatic duct neoplasia with specific attention to IPMN. POP has an emerging role in pancreatic stone therapy.
- Complications specific to the performance of cholangiopancreatoscopy include cholangitis, which is related to intraductal fluid irrigation and pancreatitis in the setting of pancreatoscopy.

## REFERENCES

1. McIver MA. An instrument for visualizing the interior of the common duct at operation. Surgery 1941;9:112.
2. Kawai K, Nakajima M, Akasaka Y, et al. A new endoscopic method: the peroral choledocho-pancreatoscopy (author's transl). Leber Magen Darm 1976;6:121 [in German].
3. Vennes JA, Silvis SE. Endoscopic visualization of bile and pancreatic ducts. Gastrointest Endosc 1972;18:149–52.
4. Takekoshi T, Maruyama M, Sugiyama N, et al. Retrograde pancreatocholangioscopy. Gastrointest Endosc 1975;17:678–83.
5. Urakami Y, Seifert E, Butke H. Peroral direct cholangioscopy (PDCS) using routine straight-view endoscope: first report. Endoscopy 1977;9:27–30.
6. Soda K, Shitou K, Yoshida Y, et al. Peroral cholangioscopy using new fine-caliber flexible scope for detailed examination without papillotomy. Gastrointest Endosc 1996;43:233–8.
7. ASGE Technology Committee, Shah RJ, Adler DG, et al. Cholangiopancreatoscopy. Gastrointest Endosc 2008;68:411–21.
8. Chen YK, Pleskow DK. SpyGlass single-operator peroral cholangiopancreatoscopy system for the diagnosis and therapy of bile-duct disorders: a clinical feasibility study (with video). Gastrointest Endosc 2007;65:832–41.
9. Brauer BC, Chen YK, Shah RJ. Single-step direct cholangioscopy by freehand intubation using standard endoscopes for diagnosis and therapy of biliary diseases. Am J Gastroenterol 2012;107:1030–5.
10. American Society of Anesthesiologists Committee. Practice guidelines for preoperative fasting and the use of pharmacologic agents to reduce the risk of pulmonary aspiration: application to healthy patients undergoing elective procedures: an updated report by the American Society of Anesthesiologists Committee on Standards and Practice Parameters. Anesthesiology 2011;114:495.
11. Sethi A, Chen YK, Austin GL, et al. ERCP with cholangiopancreatoscopy may be associated with higher rates of complications than ERCP alone: a single-center experience. Gastrointest Endosc 2011;73:251–6.
12. Banerjee S, Shen B, Baron TH, et al. Antibiotic prophylaxis in GI endoscopy. Gastrointest Endosc 2008;67:791–8.
13. Shah RJ, Chen YK. Transpapillary and percutaneous choledochoscopy in the evaluation and management of biliary strictures and stones. Tech Gastrointest Endosc 2007;9:161–8.

14. Nguyen NQ, Binmoeller KF, Shah JN. Cholangioscopy and pancreatoscopy (with videos). Gastrointest Endosc 2009;70:1200–10.

15. Larghi A, Waxman I. Endoscopic direct cholangioscopy by using an ultra-slim upper endoscope: a feasibility study. Gastrointest Endosc 2006;63:853–7.

16. Choi HJ, Moon JH, Ko BM. Overtube-balloon–assisted direct peroral cholangioscopy by using an ultra-slim upper endoscope (with videos). Gastrointest Endosc 2009;69:935–40.

17. Moon JH, Ko BM, Choi HJ, et al. Intraductal balloon-guided direct peroral cholangioscopy with an ultraslim upper endoscope (with videos). Gastrointest Endosc 2009;70:297–302.

18. Albert JG, Friedrich-Rust M, Elhendawy M, et al. Peroral cholangioscopy for diagnosis and therapy of biliary tract disease using an ultra-slim gastroscope. Endoscopy 2011;43:1004–9.

19. Brauer BC, Chen YK, Ringold DA, et al. Peroral pancreatoscopy via the minor papilla for diagnosis and therapy of pancreatic diseases. Gastrointest Endosc 2013;78(3):545–9.

20. Ringold DA, Shah RJ. Peroral pancreatoscopy in the diagnosis and management of intraductal papillary mucinous neoplasia and indeterminate pancreatic duct pathology. Gastrointest Endosc Clin N Am 2009;19(4):601–13.

21. Sievert CE Jr, Silvis SE. Evaluation of electrohydraulic lithotripsy as a means of gallstone fragmentation in a canine model. Gastrointest Endosc 1987;33:233–5.

22. Hochberger J, Gruber E, Wirtz P, et al. Lithotripsy of gallstones by means of a quality-switched giant-pulse neodymium:yttrium-aluminum-garnet laser. Basic in vitro studies using a highly flexible fiber system. Gastroenterology 1991;101: 1391–8.

23. Shah RJ, Langer DA, Antillon MR, et al. Cholangioscopy and cholangioscopic forceps biopsy in patients with indeterminate pancreaticobiliary pathology. Clin Gastroenterol Hepatol 2006;4:219–25.

24. Arya N, Nelles SE, Haber GB, et al. Electrohydraulic lithotripsy in 111 patients: a safe and effective therapy for difficult bile duct stones. Am J Gastroenterol 2004; 99:2330–4.

25. Asbun HJ, Conlon K, Fernandez-Cruz L, et al. When to perform a pancreatoduodenectomy in the absence of positive histology? A consensus statement by the International Study Group of Pancreatic Surgery. Surgery 2014;155(5): 887–92.

26. Camilo J, Nordstrom E, Brown NG, et al. Per oral cholangioscopy (POC) with intraductal lithotripsy, mechanical lithotripsy (ML), and large balloon papillary dilation (LBPD) for extraction of complex biliary stones: a 12-year single academic center experience in 222 patients. Gastrointest Endosc 2013;77:AB313.

27. Howell DA, Dy RM, Hanson BL, et al. Gastrointest Endosc 1999;50(6):829–33.

28. Okugawa T, Tsuyuguchi T, K C S, et al. Peroral cholangioscopic treatment of hepatolithiasis: long-term results. Gastrointest Endosc 2002;56:366–71.

29. Chen YK, Parsi MA, Binmoeller KF, et al. Single-operator cholangioscopy in patients requiring evaluation of bile duct disease or therapy of biliary stones (with videos). Gastrointest Endosc 2011;74:805.

30. Patel SN, Rosenkranz L, Hooks B, et al. Holmium-yttrium aluminum garnet laser lithotripsy in the treatment of biliary calculi using single-operator cholangioscopy: a multicenter experience (with video). Gastrointest Endosc 2014;79(2):344–8.

31. Sepe PS, Berzin TM, Sanaka S, et al. Single-operator cholangioscopy for the extraction of cystic duct stones (with video). Gastrointest Endosc 2012;75(1): 206–10.

32. Farrell JJ, Bounds BC, Al-Shalabi S, et al. Single-operator duodenoscope-assisted cholangioscopy is an effective alternative in the management of choledocholithiasis not removed by conventional methods, including mechanical lithotripsy. Endoscopy 2005;37:542–7.

33. Maydeo A, Kwek BE, Bhandari S, et al. Single-operator cholangioscopy-guided laser lithotripsy in patients with difficult biliary and pancreatic ductal stones (with videos). Gastrointest Endosc 2011;74(6):1308–14.

34. Neuhaus H, Zillinger C, Born P, et al. Randomized study of intracorporeal laser lithotripsy versus extracorporeal shock-wave lithotripsy for difficult bile duct stones. Gastrointest Endosc 1998;47:327–34.

35. Lee YN, Moon JH, Choi HJ, et al. Direct peroral cholangioscopy using an ultraslim upper endoscope for management of residual stones after mechanical lithotripsy for retained common bile duct stones. Endoscopy 2012;44:819–24.

36. Seo DW, Lee SK, Yoo KS, et al. Cholangioscopic findings in bile duct tumors. Gastrointest Endosc 2000;52:630–4.

37. Mounzer R, Austin G, Fukami N, et al. PerOral video cholangiopancreatoscopy with narrow-band imaging for the evaluation if indeterminate pancreaticobiliary disease: a single-center US experience. Gastrointest Endosc 2015;81(5): AB143.

38. Fukuda Y, Tsuyuguchi T, Sakai Y, et al. Diagnostic utility of peroral cholangioscopy for various bile-duct lesions. Gastrointest Endosc 2005;62:374–82.

39. Ramchandani M, Reddy DN, Gupta R, et al. Role of single-operator peroral cholangioscopy in the diagnosis of indeterminate biliary lesions: a single-center, prospective study. Gastrointest Endosc 2011;74:511–9.

40. Siddiqui AA, Mehendiratta V, Jackson W, et al. Identification of cholangiocarcinoma by using the Spyglass Spyscope system for peroral cholangioscopy and biopsy collection. Clin Gastroenterol Hepatol 2012;10:466–71.

41. Osanai M, Itoi T, Igarashi Y, et al. Peroral video cholangioscopy to evaluate indeterminate bile duct lesions and preoperative mucosal cancerous extension: a prospective multicenter study. Endoscopy 2013;45:635–42.

42. Manta R, Frazzoni M, Conigliaro R, et al. SpyGlass single-operator peroral cholangioscopy in the evaluation of indeterminate biliary lesions: a single-center, prospective, cohort study. Surg Endosc 2013;27(5):1569–72.

43. Itoi T, Sofuni A, Itokawa F, et al. Peroral cholangioscopic diagnosis of biliary-tract diseases by using narrow-band imaging (with videos). Gastrointest Endosc 2007; 66:730–6.

44. Tischendorf JJ, Krüger M, Trautwein C, et al. Cholangioscopic characterization of dominant bile duct stenoses in patients with primary sclerosing cholangitis. Endoscopy 2006;38:665–9.

45. Awadallah NS, Chen YK, Piraka C, et al. Is there a role for cholangioscopy in patients with primary sclerosing cholangitis? Am J Gastroenterol 2006;101: 284–91.

46. Azeem N, Gostout CJ, Knipschield M, et al. Cholangioscopy with narrow-band imaging in patients with primary sclerosing cholangitis undergoing ERCP. Gastrointest Endosc 2014;79(5):773–9.

47. Costamagna G, Gabbrielli A, Mutignani M, et al. Extracorporeal shock wave lithotripsy of pancreatic stones in chronic pancreatitis: immediate and medium-term results. Gastrointest Endosc 1997;46:231–6.

48. Adamek HE, Jakobs R, Buttmann A, et al. Long term follow up of patients with chronic pancreatitis and pancreatic stones treated with extracorporeal shock wave lithotripsy. Gut 1999;45:402–5.

49. Kozarek RA, Brandabur JJ, Ball TJ, et al. Clinical outcomes in patients who undergo extracorporeal shock wave lithotripsy for chronic calcific pancreatitis. Gastrointest Endosc 2002;56:496–500.

50. Brand B, Kahl M, Sidhu S, et al. Prospective evaluation of morphology, function, and quality of life after extracorporeal shock wave lithotripsy and endoscopic treatment of chronic calcific pancreatitis. Am J Gastroenterol 2000;95:3428–38.

51. Seven G, Schreiner MA, Ross AS, et al. Long-term outcomes associated with pancreatic extracorporeal shock wave lithotriopsy for chronic calcific pancreatitis. Gastrointest Endosc 2012;75:997–1004.

52. Attwell AR, Brauer BC, Chen YK, et al. Endoscopic retrograde cholangiopancreatography with per oral pancreatoscopy for calcific chronic pancreatitis using endoscope and catheter-based pancreatoscopes: a 10-year single-center experience. Pancreas 2014;43(2):268–74.

53. Attwell AR, Patel S, Kahaleh M, et al. ERCP with per-oral pancreatoscopy-guided laser lithotripsy for calcific chronic pancreatitis: a multicenter U.S. experience. Gastrointest Endosc 2015;82(2):311–8.

54. Hara T, Yamaguchi T, Ishihara T, et al. Diagnosis and patient management of intraductal papillary-mucinous tumor of the pancreas by using peroral pancreatoscopy and intraductal ultrasonography. Gastroenterology 2002;122(1):34–43.

55. Yamaguchi T, Shirai Y, Ishihara T, et al. Pancreatic juice cytology in the diagnosis of intraductal papillary mucinous neoplasm of the pancreas: significance of sampling by peroral pancreatoscopy. Cancer 2005;104(12):2830–6.

56. Miura T, Igarashi Y, Okano N, et al. Endoscopic diagnosis of intraductal papillary-mucinous neoplasm of the pancreas by means of peroral pancreatoscopy using a small-diameter videoscope and narrow-band imaging. Dig Endosc 2010;22(2): 119–23.

57. Arnelo U, Siiki A, Swahn F, et al. Single-operator pancreatoscopy is helpful in the evaluation of suspected intraductal papillary mucinous neoplasms (IPMN). Pancreatology 2014;14(6):510–4.

58. El Hajj I, Brauer B, Fukami N, et al. Role of peroral pancreatoscopy (POP) in the evaluation of suspected main pancreatic duct neoplasia: a 13-year U.S. single center experience. Gastrointest Endosc 2014;79(5):AB130 [abstract].

# Biliary Tumor Ablation with Photodynamic Therapy and Radiofrequency Ablation

 CrossMark

Ioana Smith, MD[a], Michel Kahaleh, MD[b],*

## KEYWORDS

- Biliary disease • Cholangiocarcinoma • Bile duct • PDT • RFA
- Radiofrequency ablation • Photodynamic therapy

## KEY POINTS

- Most patients with hilar cholangiocarcinoma have unresectable disease and require palliation with biliary stenting.
- Photodynamic therapy (PDT) is a local ablative method that uses a systemic photosensitizing agent that preferentially accumulates in malignant cells and is activated by a nonthermal light causing destruction of the malignant cells through a process mediated by oxygen-free radicals.
- Potential treatment options for PDT include palliation in combination with chemotherapy, palliation in combination with stenting, postoperatively for recurrent tumor, or downstaging a patient for curative surgery.
- Radiofrequency ablation (RFA) using thermal energy is emerging as a potentially effective treatment of malignant biliary occlusion and has been used before insertion of biliary stents and as a treatment of metal stent occlusion.
- In the limited existing studies, RFA was effective in achieving local tumor control and may offer a therapeutic option for patients with recurrent or primary cholangiocarcinoma.

Funding sources: None.
Conflicts of Interest: M. Kahaleh has received grant support from Boston Scientific, Fujinon, EMcison, Xlumena, Inc, W.L. Gore, MaunaKea, Apollo Endosurgery, Cook Endoscopy, ASPIRE Bariatrics, GI Dynamics, and MI Tech, and is a consultant for Boston Scientific and Xlumena, Inc.
[a] Division of Gastroenterology and Hepatology, University of Alabama at Birmingham, 1720 2nd Avenue South BDB 380, Birmingham, AL 35294, USA; [b] Division of Gastroenterology and Hepatology, Weill Cornell Medical College, 1305 York Avenue 4th floor, New York, NY 10021, USA
* Corresponding author.
*E-mail address:* mkahaleh@gmail.com

Gastrointest Endoscopy Clin N Am 25 (2015) 793–804
http://dx.doi.org/10.1016/j.giec.2015.06.013
1052-5157/15/$ – see front matter © 2015 Elsevier Inc. All rights reserved.

## INTRODUCTION

The incidence of cholangiocarcinoma accounts for 2% of all gastrointestinal malignancies, and fewer than 20% of patients are considered to have resectable tumors at the time of diagnosis.[1] Given that most cholangiocarcinomas are unresectable, the goal of intervention is biliary decompression.[2] Jaundice, pruritis, secondary biliary cirrhosis, cholangitis, coagulopathy, and weight loss are consequences of obstruction.[1] Recent data have suggested that it is useful to drain more than 50% of the liver volume for favorable long-term results.[3] Metal stents (bare metal mesh) are usually preferred and carry the advantage of longer duration of patency compared with plastic stents.[4] There is controversy over unilateral versus bilateral stents in unresectable hilar biliary obstruction, as only a portion of the liver will be drained with a single stent.[2] Tumor ablation combined with stenting can reduce cholestasis and improve median survival time in patients with cholangiocarcinoma.[5] Photodynamic therapy (PDT) and, more recently, radiofrequency ablation (RFA), have been used as adjuvant therapies to improve results of biliary stenting.[3] Ultimately, endoscopic biliary drainage may enable patients to receive additional chemotherapy.[2]

## PHOTODYNAMIC THERAPY
### Photodynamic Therapy Technique

#### Preparation
Antibiotic prophylaxis should be given to patients with anticipated incomplete biliary drainage. There are multiple photosensitizing agents available for cholangiocarcinoma, with hematoporphyrin derivatives (eg, Photofrin II, Photosan-3) being the most commonly used.[1] This intravenous agent preferentially accumulates in cancer cells.[6] For instance, Porfimer sodium (Photofrin; Axcan Pharma Inc, Birmingham, AL), which is the only photosensitizer approved by the Food and Drug Administration (FDA), is injected intravenously at a dosage of 2 mg/kg body weight 48 hours before laser activation.[7] All the procedures are done under general anesthesia. Considerations before ablation therapy include assessing resectability or not, determination of atrophic segments, antibiotic prophylaxis, and patient education (**Box 1**).

#### Patient position/approach
Patients are placed in the prone or supine position. Endoscopic retrograde cholangiopancreatography (ERCP) is performed as a standard of care at the time of PDT.

---

**Box 1**
**Considerations before ablation**

- Resectable versus unresectable disease
  - Surgery is indicated for resectable disease
- Determine what area of the liver is atrophic and not draining
- Liver metastasis versus cholangiocarcinoma
  - Patients with liver metastasis are not candidates for photodynamic therapy (PDT)
- Antibiotic therapy is required for prevention of cholangitis
- Patients need to be educated about PDT side effects: photosensitivity

*Data from* Kahaleh M. Photodynamic therapy in cholangiocarcinoma. J Natl Compr Canc Netw 2012;10(Suppl 2):S44–7; with permission.

*Technique/procedure*

Forty-eight hours after systemic administration of the photosensitizing agent, light activation is performed using a quartz fiber mounted with a cylindrical diffuser tip coupled to a diode laser emitting a particular wavelength.[1]

Endoscopic retrograde cholangiography is performed using a large-channel duodenoscope.[7] After cannulation into the biliary tract, a cholangiogram is performed to help define the anatomic distribution of malignant tissue.[7] Then, selective bougie and balloon dilation of the stricture(s) to be treated is performed.[7]

PDT is delivered through a 3.0-m-length fiber with a 2.5-cm-long cylindrical diffuser at its distal end (Pioneer Optics, Windsor Locks, CT).[7] The diffuser can be inserted into a 10-F sheath of a plastic stent delivery system and placed at the level of the stricture being treated (**Figs. 1–3**).[7] Alternatively, cholangioscopy can be used as a platform to administer PDT.[1,2,7]

A diode laser system (InGaAlP Laser Diode; Diomed Inc, Andover, MA) with a maximum power output of 2000 mW and a wavelength of 633 $\pm$ 3 nm is used as a light source.[7] Photoactivation is performed at 630 nm with a light dose of 180 J/cm$^2$, fluence of 0.250 W/cm$^2$, and irradiation time of 750 seconds (3).[7]

At the completion of the laser application, plastic endoprostheses or external drainage tubes are inserted given that the PDT site induces swelling and coagulation necrotic changes for up to a 1 week after PDT (4).[6] The depth of tumor necrosis with hematoporphyrin derivates is 4 to 6 mm (**Fig. 4**), thus primary tumors with deeper invasion cannot be eradicated with this method alone.[1,6]

## Photodynamic Therapy Complications/Management

- Most of the complications with PDT are from the ERCP and the biliary stenting themselves
- A relevant side effect of PDT includes phototoxicity, which can last 4 to 6 weeks after drug administration[6]
- Cutaneous complications include[8] the following:
  - Serious phototoxicity requiring oral corticosteroid treatment

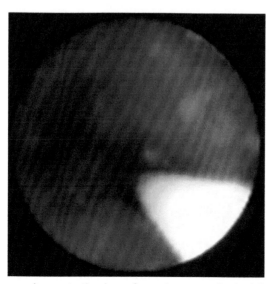

**Fig. 1.** Cholangioscopy demonstrating large fungating cancer in the bile duct (patient A).

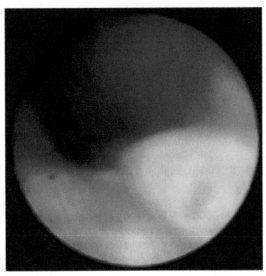

**Fig. 2.** Position of the PDT probe into the malignant stricture (patient A).

- o Herpes zoster requiring hospitalization and intravenous antiviral treatment
- o Erythema multiforme drug reaction requiring symptomatic treatment with antihistamines, analgesics, and local skin care

### Postoperative Care

Antibiotics should be continued in cases of incomplete biliary drainage. Postoperatively, patients treated with PDT are advised to remain out of direct sunlight because

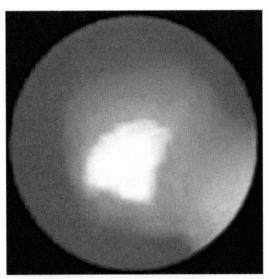

**Fig. 3.** Administration of red light (photodynamic therapy) into the malignant stricture (patient A).

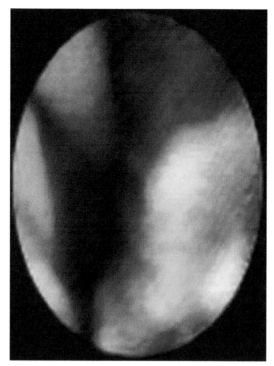

**Fig. 4.** Demonstration of necrosis induced by PDT after 3 months (patient A).

porfimer sodium may cause prolonged photosensitivity lasting 30 to 90 days.[7] The photosensitivity effects of the drug last 4 to 6 weeks in decreasing intensity[1]; therefore, repeated PDT sessions are often necessary.[2] PDT is typically repeated at 3-month intervals, at which time all stents should be replaced.[7]

## Outcomes

Potential treatment options for PDT include palliation in combination with chemotherapy, palliation in combination with stenting, postoperatively for recurrent tumor, or downstaging option for a patient before curative surgery (**Table 1**). PDT with chemotherapy and more than 2 sessions of PDT were significant independent predictors of longer survival in advanced cholangiocarcinoma in the study by Hong and colleagues[9] ($P$ = .013). In a prospective randomized trial, patients receiving PDT with chemotherapy showed higher 1-year survival rate compared with those with PDT alone (76.2% vs 32%, $P$ = .003) and prolonged overall survival (median 17 vs 8 months, $P$ = .005).[10] Combination of stenting and subsequent PDT prolonged survival over stenting alone (493 vs 98 days, $P<.0001$).[11] In Lee and colleagues'[5] review article, it was concluded that PDT improves survival and quality of life, and reduces tumor growth while treating cholestasis. In Leggett and colleagues'[12] review article, compared with biliary stenting, PDT was associated with a statistically significant increase in the length of survival (weighted mean difference [WMD] 265 days), improvement in Karnofsky scores (WMD 7.74), and a trend for decline in serum bilirubin (WMD −2.92 mg/dL).

**Table 1**
**Studies of PDT in patients with malignant biliary lesions**

| Study, Year of Study | No. of Patients in Each Treatment Arm | Findings |
|---|---|---|
| Hong et al,[9] 2014 | 16 treated with PDT and chemotherapy; 58 treated with PDT | Patients receiving PDT and chemotherapy had a median survival of 538 vs 334 d in those receiving PDT alone ($P = .05$) |
| Ortner et al,[11] 2003 | 20 treated with PDT and stenting; 19 treated with stenting | Combination of stenting and subsequent PDT prolonged survival over stenting alone (493 vs 98 d, $P < .0001$) |
| Cheon et al,[26] 2012 | 72 treated with PDT and stenting; 71 treated with stenting | Patients receiving PDT with stenting survived longer than those not treated with PDT (9.8 vs 7.3 mo, $P = .029$) |
| Park et al,[10] 2014 | 21 treated with PDT and chemotherapy; 22 treated with PDT | Patients receiving PDT with chemotherapy showed higher 1-y survival rate compared with those receiving PDT alone (76.2% vs 32%, $P = .003$) and prolonged overall survival (median 17 vs 8 mo, $P = .005$) |
| Talreja et al,[27] 2013 | 20 received chemotherapy and radiation therapy; 5 received chemotherapy only; and 1 received radiation therapy only | Survival means of patients who received PDT and chemotherapy/radiation therapy (median survival 257 d) vs those who received PDT only (median survival 183 d) showed no significant difference (log-rank $P = .20$) |
| Lee et al,[28] 2012 | 18 treated with stenting and PDT; 15 treated with stenting | PDT and stenting was associated with significantly prolonged stent patency (median 244 vs 177 d, $P = .002$) and longer patient survival (median 356 vs 230 d, $P = .006$) |

*Abbreviation:* PDT, photodynamic therapy.

Neoadjuvant PDT was evaluated in 7 patients with advanced hilar cholangiocarcinomas (advanced Bismuth type III and IV carcinoma) thought to be unresectable.[13] After PDT at the area of tumor infiltration and 2 cm beyond, a curative resection could be performed in all patients after a mean period of 6 weeks. Eighty-three percent were recurrence free after 1 year.[13] In a small study of 8 patients who underwent PDT postoperatively for recurrent tumor, adjuvant PDT was a safe and useful option for a better survival benefit in these patients.[14]

In a study, 11 patients with hilar cholangiocarcinoma (Bismuth III-IV) were treated with temoporfin PDT and stenting and 10 could be analyzed for local tumor response.[15] Tumoricidal efficacy was 90%; 4 patients showed tumoricidal depth of greater than or equal to 7.5; and cholestasis and palliation improved in 8 patients with an overall median survival of 18 months after the first PDT.[15] In another study, combined stenting and PDT performed with a low Foscan dose resulted in equal and potentially longer survival times compared with standard Photofrin PDT and lowered the risk of side effects strongly.[16] Unfortunately, those drugs are not FDA approved in the United States.

### Current Controversy/Future Considerations

PDT for palliation of unresectable cholangiocarcinoma is accepted, although more data are needed on PDT for recurrent tumors after surgery and neoadjuvant PDT. Newer photosensitizers with greater penetration depth and shorter photosensitivity are needed. Recently, a polymeric photosensitizer-embedded self-expanding nonvascular metal stent (PDT-stent) was designed and allowed repeatable photodynamic treatment of cholangiocarcinoma without systemic injection of photosensitizer in animals.[17] The PDT-stent sustained its photodynamic activities for at least 2 months.[17] Further randomized trials are necessary to strengthen the use of PDT in recurrent tumors after surgery and the use of PDT as a neoadjuvant treatment.[5]

There is a need for novel techniques in direct visualization of the bile duct to permit PDT. In a study, the median survival of patients treated with PDT only was 200 days compared with 386 days in those treated with cholangioscopy with direct PDT ($P = .45$).[18] Cholangioscopy permitted targeted therapy during PDT while simultaneously reducing exposure to radiation (21.1 vs 11.1 minutes, $P<.0001$).[18] In a small prospective study, PDT under direct peroral cholangioscopy with an ultraslim upper endoscope was successfully performed in 7 of 9 patients and in 15 of 17 sessions.[19] Biliary drainage under direct peroral cholangioscopy was possible in 7 of 7 patients who needed it after PDT.[19]

## RADIOFREQUENCY ABLATION
### Radiofrequency Ablation Technique

#### Preparation
Antibiotic prophylaxis should be given to patients with anticipated incomplete biliary drainage. All the procedures are done under general anesthesia.

#### Patient position/approach
Patients are placed in the prone or supine position. ERCP is performed as a standard of care.

#### Technique/procedure
After cannulation into the biliary tract, a cholangiogram is performed to define stricture length and diameter.[20] RFA achieves localized tumor necrosis via thermal energy and can be performed through an endobiliary and percutaneous intraductal technique. The RFA catheter (Habib Endo HPB; EMcision Ltd, London, UK) is a single-use, bipolar device used for endoluminal delivery of RFA into the biliary tree over a 0.035-inch guide wire.[21] It has an 8-F catheter with a 180-cm working length and can be deployed through endoscope working channels of at least 3.2 mm in diameter.[21,22] The distal end of the RFA catheter has a 5-mm leading tip, proximal to which there are 2 circumferential, 8-mm-wide stainless steel electrodes separated by a distance of 8 mm providing a cylindrical ablation over a 25-mm length.[21] The proximal end of the catheter permits connection to a power source.[21,22] Ablation using a RITA 1500X RF generator (Angiodynamics, Latham, NY) or ERBE generator (Marietta, Georgia)[20] set at 7 to 10 W for a time period of 2 minutes can be conducted (**Fig. 5**). A 1-minute resting period after energy delivery should be allowed before moving the catheter and biliary stents are placed after RFA (**Fig. 6**) (5–6).[20]

### Radiofrequency Ablation Complications/Management

- Most of the complications with RFA are from the ERCP and the biliary stenting themselves
- Complications reported include the following: hematobilia, gallbladder empyema, cholangitis, cholangiosepsis, cholecystitis, gallbladder empyema, hepatic coma, 1 partial liver infarction, biliary bleeding, and clinical and asymptomatic pancreatitis[21,23,24]
- Bile duct perforation, bile leak, and thermal injury to the duodenum or pancreas have not been reported[21]

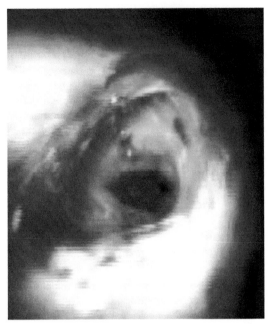

**Fig. 5.** Digital cholangioscopy showing malignant biliary stricture before RFA (patient B).

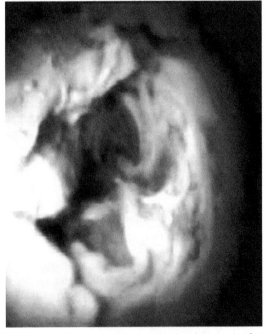

**Fig. 6.** Digital cholangioscopy demonstrating intense local necrosis after RFA (patient B).

**Table 2**
**Studies of RFA in patients with malignant biliary lesions**

| Study, Year of Study | No. of Patients in Each Treatment Arm | Findings |
|---|---|---|
| Butros et al,[29] 2014 | 7 patients and 9 tumors treated with RFA | RFA achieved technique effectiveness and local tumor control in 89% (8/9 tumors) of the patients, respectively, with a mean overall survival of 38.5 mo |
| Mizandari et al,[30] 2013 | 39 patients treated with RFA after external biliary decompression and before metal stent insertion | 28 are alive and 10 died with a median survival of 89.5 d and median stent patency of 84.5 d |
| Dolak et al,[23] 2014 | 58 patients underwent 84 RFA procedures | Median stent patency after last electively performed RFA: 170 d. Median survival was 10.6 mo from the time of the first RFA |
| Pai et al,[31] 2014 | 9 patients with malignant biliary obstruction and blocked metal stents underwent RFA following external biliary decompression | All 9 patients had their stent patency restored successfully without the use of secondary stents; 6 patients are alive and 3 patients are dead with a median stent patency of 102.5 d; 3 patients with stent blockage at 321, 290, and 65 d postprocedure underwent percutaneous transhepatic drain insertion and repeat ablation |
| Sharaiha et al,[20] 2014 | 26 patients underwent RFA with stenting and 40 patients underwent stenting alone | RFA was an independent predictor of survival as well as age and receipt of chemotherapy. Overall stent patency rates were the same across both groups |
| Steel et al,[32] 2011 | 22 patients underwent RFA | Deployment of an RFA catheter was successful in 21 patients. One patient failed to have successful biliary decompression after SEMS placement and died within 90 d. At 90-d follow-up, 1 additional patient had died with a patent stent and 3 patients had occluded biliary stents |
| Tal et al,[24] 2014 | 12 patients underwent 19 RFA procedures | Deployment of RFA was successful in all patients. Systemic chemotherapy was administered in 4 patients. Seven patients died during follow-up and median survival was 6.4 mo from the time of the first RFA |
| Figueroa-Barojas et al,[33] 2013 | 20 patients underwent RFA with stenting | 25 strictures were treated. Mean stricture length treated was 15.2 mm. Mean stricture diameter before RFA was 1.7 mm, and the mean diameter after RFA was 5.2 mm. There was a significant increase of 3.5 mm in the bile duct diameter after RFA |
| Alis et al,[34] 2013 | 10 patients underwent RFA with stenting | Morbidity and mortality rate within the first 30 d after the procedure was 20% and 0%, respectively. Endobiliary decompression was not achieved in 1 patient. Median duration of stent patency was 9 mo |

*Abbreviations:* RFA, radiofrequency ablation; SEMS, self-expandable metallic stent.

## Outcomes

In the review article of malignant biliary obstruction by Rustagi and Jamidar,[21] there was significant improvement in mean stricture diameter. The calculated overall mean stricture length was 25 mm with range from 3.5 to 60 mm, suggesting endobiliary RFA is feasible for short and long biliary strictures.[23] In one of the largest experiences with biliary RFA in malignant biliary obstruction, except for one severe interventional complication (hepatic infarct), RFA was a technically feasible and safe therapeutic option for the palliative treatment of malignant biliary obstruction[23] **(Table 2)**. A recent retrospective study published by Strand and colleagues[25] compared RFA with PDT in cholangiocarcinoma, but failed to provide matched patients in terms of staging and number of sessions, therefore ending up comparing apples and oranges.

## Current Controversy/Future Considerations

Endoscopically applicable RFA is emerging as a potentially effective treatment of malignant biliary occlusion and has been used before insertion of biliary stents and as a treatment of metal stent occlusion. Given the potential risk of thermal injury to adjacent structures, accurate pre-interventional imaging assessment of the tumor surroundings is necessary, especially for proximal strictures.[23] Prospective trials are warranted to further assess the efficacy and safety of this technique in biliary tumors as well as its cost-effectiveness. Further head-to-head comparisons between RFA and PDT in cholangiocarcinoma are also warranted.

## SUMMARY

PDT improves survival and quality of life, and reduces tumor growth while treating cholestasis. RFA is emerging as a potentially effective treatment of malignant biliary occlusion and has been used before insertion of biliary stents and as a treatment of self-expandable metallic stent occlusion. In the few existing studies, RFA was effective in achieving local tumor control; in the future, it may offer a therapeutic option for patients with recurrent or primary cholangiocarcinoma. Further randomized trials with RFA in malignant biliary obstruction with longer follow-up are needed.

## REFERENCES

1. Webb K, Saunders M. Endoscopic management of malignant bile duct strictures. Gastrointest Endosc Clin N Am 2013;23(2):313–31.
2. Kahaleh M. Photodynamic therapy in cholangiocarcinoma. J Natl Compr Canc Netw 2012;10(Suppl 2):S44–7.
3. Goenka MK, Goenka U. Palliation: Hilar cholangiocarcinoma. World J Hepatol 2014;6(8):559–69.
4. Marsh Rde W, Alonzo M, Bajaj S, et al. Comprehensive review of the diagnosis and treatment of biliary tract cancer 2012. Part II: multidisciplinary management. J Surg Oncol 2012;106:339–45.
5. Lee TY, Cheon YK, Shim CS. Current status of photodynamic therapy for bile duct cancer. Clin Endosc 2013;46:38–44.
6. Cheon YK. The role of photodynamic therapy for hilar cholangiocarcinoma. Korean J Intern Med 2010;25(4):345–52.
7. Talreja JP, Kahaleh M. Photodynamic therapy for cholangiocarcinoma. Gut Liver 2010;4(Suppl 1):S62–6.

8. Wolfsen HC, Ng CS. Cutaneous consequences of photodynamic therapy. Cutis 2002;69:140–2.

9. Hong MJ, Cheon YK, Lee EJ. Long-term outcome of photodynamic therapy with systemic chemotherapy compared to photodynamic therapy alone in patients with advanced Hilar cholangiocarcinoma. Gut Liver 2014;8(3):318–23.

10. Park do H, Lee SS, Park SE, et al. Randomised phase II trial of photodynamic therapy plus oral fluoropyrimidine, S-1, versus photodynamic therapy alone for unresectable hilar cholangiocarcinoma. Eur J Cancer 2014;50(7):1259–68.

11. Ortner ME, Caca K, Berr F, et al. Successful photodynamic therapy for nonresectable cholangiocarcinoma: a randomized prospective study. Gastroenterology 2003;125(5):1355–63.

12. Leggett CL, Gorospe EC, Murad MH, et al. Photodynamic therapy for unresectable cholangiocarcinoma: a comparative effectiveness systematic review and meta-analyses. Photodiagnosis Photodyn Ther 2012;9:189–95.

13. Wiedmann M, Caca K, Berr F, et al. Neoadjuvant photodynamic therapy as a new approach to treating hilar cholangiocarcinoma: a phase II pilot study. Cancer 2003;97:2783–90.

14. Nanashima A, Yamaguchi H, Shibasaki S, et al. Adjuvant photodynamic therapy for bile duct carcinoma after surgery: a preliminary study. J Gastroenterol 2004; 39(11):1095–101.

15. Wagner A, Kiesslich T, Neureiter D, et al. Photodynamic therapy for hilar bile duct cancer: clinical evidence for improved tumoricidal tissue penetration by temoporfin. Photochem Photobiol Sci 2013;12(6):1065–73.

16. Kniebühler G, Pongratz T, Betz CS, et al. Photodynamic therapy for cholangiocarcinoma using low dose mTHPC (Foscan(®)). Photodiagnosis Photodyn Ther 2013;10(3):220–8.

17. Bae BC, Yang SG, Jeong S, et al. Polymeric photosensitizer-embedded self-expanding metal stent for repeatable endoscopic photodynamic therapy of cholangiocarcinoma. Biomaterials 2014;35(30):8487–95.

18. Talreja JP, DeGaetani M, Sauer BG, et al. Photodynamic therapy for unresectable cholangiocarcinoma: contribution of single operator cholangioscopy for targeted treatment. Photochem Photobiol Sci 2011;10(7):1233–8.

19. Choi HJ, Moon JH, Ko BM, et al. Clinical feasibility of direct peroral cholangioscopy-guided photodynamic therapy for inoperable cholangiocarcinoma performed by using an ultra-slim upper endoscope (with videos). Gastrointest Endosc 2011;73(4):808–13.

20. Sharaiha RZ, Natov N, Glockenberg KS, et al. Comparison of metal stenting with radiofrequency ablation versus stenting alone for treating malignant biliary strictures: is there an added benefit? Dig Dis Sci 2014;59(12):3099–102.

21. Rustagi T, Jamidar PA. Intraductal radiofrequency ablation for management of malignant biliary obstruction. Dig Dis Sci 2014;59(11):2635–41.

22. Wadsworth CA, Westaby D, Khan SA. Endoscopic radiofrequency ablation for cholangiocarcinoma. Curr Opin Gastroenterol 2013;29(3):305–11.

23. Dolak W, Schreiber F, Schwaighofer H, et al. Endoscopic radiofrequency ablation for malignant biliary obstruction: a nationwide retrospective study of 84 consecutive applications. Surg Endosc 2014;28(3):854–60.

24. Tal AO, Vermehren J, Friedrich-Rust M, et al. Intraductal endoscopic radiofrequency ablation for the treatment of hilar non-resectable malignant bile duct obstruction. World J Gastrointest Endosc 2014;6(1):13–9.

25. Strand DS, Cosgrove ND, Patrie JT, et al. ERCP-directed radiofrequency ablation and photodynamic therapy are associated with comparable survival in the

treatment of unresectable cholangiocarcinoma. Gastrointest Endosc 2014;80(5): 794–804.

26. Cheon YK, Lee TY, Lee SM, et al. Longterm outcome of photodynamic therapy compared with biliary stenting alone in patients with advanced hilar cholangiocarcinoma. HPB (Oxford) 2012;14(3):185–93.

27. Talreja JP, Degaetani M, Ellen K, et al. Photodynamic therapy in unresectable cholangiocarcinoma: not for the uncommitted. Clin Endosc 2013;46(4):390–4.

28. Lee TY, Cheon YK, Shim CS, et al. Photodynamic therapy prolongs metal stent patency in patients with unresectable hilar cholangiocarcinoma. World J Gastroenterol 2012;18(39):5589–94.

29. Butros SR, Shenoy-Bhangle A, Mueller PR, et al. Radiofrequency ablation of intrahepatic cholangiocarcinoma: feasibility, local tumor control, and long-term outcome. Clin Imaging 2014;38(4):490–4.

30. Mizandari M, Pai M, Xi F, et al. Percutaneous intraductal radiofrequency ablation is a safe treatment for malignant biliary obstruction: feasibility and early results. Cardiovasc Intervent Radiol 2013;36(3):814–9.

31. Pai M, Valek V, Tomas A, et al. Percutaneous intraductal radiofrequency ablation for clearance of occluded metal stent in malignant biliary obstruction: feasibility and early results. Cardiovasc Intervent Radiol 2014;37(1):235–40.

32. Steel AW, Postgate AJ, Khorsandi S, et al. Endoscopically applied radiofrequency ablation appears to be safe in the treatment of malignant biliary obstruction. Gastrointest Endosc 2011;73(1):149–53.

33. Figueroa-Barojas P, Bakhru MR, Habib NA, et al. Safety and efficacy of radiofrequency ablation in the management of unresectable bile duct and pancreatic cancer: a novel palliation technique. J Oncol 2013;2013:910897.

34. Alis H, Sengoz C, Gonenc M, et al. Endobiliary radiofrequency ablation for malignant biliary obstruction. Hepatobiliary Pancreat Dis Int 2013;12(4):423–7.

# Endoscopic Ultrasound–Assisted Pancreaticobiliary Access

Frank Weilert, MD[a], Kenneth F. Binmoeller, MD[b],*

## KEYWORDS

- Endoscopic ultrasound • Pancreaticobiliary access
- Endoscopic retrograde cholangiopancreatography
- Endoscopic ultrasound–guided anterograde cholangiopancreatography

## KEY POINTS

- Endoscopic ultrasound (EUS)–guided pancreaticobiliary access allows a variety of drainage options when endoscopic retrograde cholangiopancreatography fails.
- EUS-guided drainage has high clinical success when performed by interventional endoscopists with an acceptable adverse event profile.
- Standardized algorithms should be used for EUS-guided access and drainage to allow comparative data collection and reporting.
- Specialized tools for transluminal drainage allow extended indications for access and intervention in reach of the therapeutic endoscopist.

 **Video of single-step endoscopic ultrasound–guided gallbladder stenting with a cautery-equipped stent delivery system for the lumen-apposing stent accompanies this article at http://www.giendo.theclinics.com/**

## INTRODUCTION

Endoscopic retrograde cholangiopancreatography (ERCP) is the primary approach to drain an obstructed pancreatic or biliary duct.[1] In approximately 10% to 15% of cases, endoscopic biliary access may fail (**Box 1**). Failed biliary drainage is traditionally referred for percutaneous transhepatic biliary drainage (PTBD) or surgical bypass, which carry significantly higher morbidity and mortality rates compared with ERCP

Disclosures: K.F. Binmoeller is the inventor of the AXIOS stent and the founder and chief medical officer for Xlumena Inc.
[a] Waikato Hospital, Waikato District Health Board, Hamilton, New Zealand; [b] Interventional Endoscopy Services, California Pacific Medical Center, San Francisco, CA, USA
* Corresponding author.
*E-mail address:* BinmoeK@sutterhealth.org

Gastrointest Endoscopy Clin N Am 25 (2015) 805–826
http://dx.doi.org/10.1016/j.giec.2015.06.003
1052-5157/15/$ – see front matter © 2015 Elsevier Inc. All rights reserved.

---

**Box 1**
**Causes of failed retrograde access to the bile and pancreatic ducts**

*Failed ductal cannulation*

Unidentifiable papilla

Tumor infiltration of the papilla

Juxtapapillary diverticulum

High-grade ductal stricture

Difficult anatomy

*Inability to reach the papilla (or ductal anastomosis)*

Gastric outlet obstruction

High-grade duodenal stenosis

   Postpeptic structuring

   Malignant infiltration

Postsurgical anatomy

Gastrectomy

Gastric bypass

Whipple procedure

Hepaticojejunostomy

Billroth II gastrectomy

---

and transpapillary drainage.[2,3] Endoscopic ultrasound (EUS) provides a real-time imaging platform to access and deliver therapy to organs and tissues outside of the bowel lumen. The bile and pancreatic ducts can be directly accessed from the stomach and duodenum, offering an alternative to ERCP when this fails or is not feasible.[4]

### Background

EUS-guided cholangiopancreatography was first described in 1996.[4] Using a curved linear array (CLA) echoendoscope, a standard fine-needle aspiration (FNA) needle is guided under real-time visualization into the bile or pancreatic duct and contrast injected for cholangiopancreatography or pancreatography. The route of access is anterograde, in contrast to the retrograde approach of ERCP. The authors prefer the term EUS-guided anterograde cholangiopancreatography (EACP) to cover the spectrum of EUS-guided techniques for accessing and draining the bile and pancreatic ducts (**Box 2**). Patients with known difficult anatomy (eg, altered anatomy or gastric outlet obstruction) or prior failed ductal access are more likely to require EACP. All patients referred for therapeutic ERCP should be consented for both ERCP and EACP to allow same-session EUS-guided drainage when ERCP fails.

There are theoretic advantages of EACP over ERCP. By avoiding the ampulla and accidental cannulation or injection of the pancreatic duct, EACP eliminates the risk of pancreatitis. EACP is reserved for failed ERCP but could eliminate the problem of difficult cannulation altogether if used as a primary access strategy. Anterograde transenteric drainage can obviate all instrumentation (wire passage, dilation, and stenting) of the downstream stricture. Additionally, creating a natural fistula at a distance from the obstructing tumor resolves the problem of tumor ingrowth and overgrowth, which can cause stent obstruction.

| Box 2 |
| --- |
| **Classification of EUS-guided pancreatobiliary interventions** |
| *Anterograde-retrograde access and downstream drainage* |
| EUS-guided rendezvous procedure |
| *Anterograde access and upstream drainage* |
| EUS-guided hepaticogastrostomy |
| EUS-guided choledochoduodenostomy |
| EUS-guided pancreaticogastrostomy |
| EUS-guided pancreaticoduodenostomy |
| *Anterograde access and downstream drainage* |
| EUS-guided anterograde transpapillary stent placement |
| EUS-guided anterograde transanastomotic stent placement |

## EQUIPMENT REQUIRED
### Echoendoscopes

Standard CLA echoendoscopes are commercially available with 2 channel sizes: small (standard) and large (therapeutic). The therapeutic CLA echoendoscope with a channel of 3.7 or 3.8 mm enables the passage of accessories of up to 11F. The forward-view CLA scope, which has overlapping endoscopic and EUS fields, has a 3.7-mm channel. Accessories exit along the same axis as the echoendoscope, enabling direct visualization of the accessory as it exists the channel, similar to a standard gastroscope. A potential drawback of the scope is the lack of an elevator to facilitate stent insertion and to clamp down on a guidewire during over-the-wire exchanges.

### Fine-Needle Aspiration Needles for Ductal Access

A conventional FNA needle can be used to access the bile or pancreatic duct. The choice of needle size depends on the clinical context, the goal of the procedure, and the ductal anatomy. Most operators use a 19-gauge (G) needle, through which a 0.035-in, 400 to 450 cm long wire can be inserted. The drawback of the 19-G needle is its relative stiffness, which results in a very tangential angle of puncture. The elevator, when activated, has virtually no effect on the puncture angle. It is also difficult to penetrate indurated tissue with the 19-G needle. Modified blunt-tipped access needles may avoid inadvertent shearing of the wire on the bevel of the needle. The 22-G needle has greater flexibility, but it only accepts an 0.018-in guidewire, which lacks the stability and trackability required for over-the-wire intervention. The 0.018-in wire is also hard to steer and see on fluoroscopy. The 22-G needle may be preferred when targeting a nondilated duct (eg, intrahepatic or pancreatic) or when puncture with the 19-G fails. The 0.018-in wire may need to be exchanged for a 0.035-in wire through a catheter. A 25-G needle does not accept a wire, but it might be considered when the goal is a diagnostic cholangiogram or pancreatogram, especially in a patient with a coagulation disorder or low platelet count. Injection of saline may distend the duct making access with a larger needle easier. An alternative to using the FNA needle to achieve ductal access is the diathermic needle knife with removable inner needle (Zimmon needle knife, Cook Medical, Bloomington, IN, USA). Pure cutting current is applied during puncture to penetrate tissue. The advantage of using the needle knife is the ability to immediately exchange the inner needle for a guidewire. A drawback of the needle knife is the limited visibility of only the needle at the catheter tip, both on ultrasound and fluoroscopy. Another drawback is the risk of diathermy trauma to tissue. Although a continuous stainless steel needle will maintain the predicted trajectory path as it is advanced, the more flexible needle knife catheter may veer off axis into a neighboring structure, which may be a major vessel.

### Guidewires

The guidewires used in EACP are the same as those used in ERCP. The authors routinely start with the 0.035-in hydrophilic Glidewire (Terumo, Somerset, NJ) inserted through a 19-G needle. As in ERCP, the hydrophilic Glidewire has excellent steerability to negotiate tortuous ducts and high-grade strictures. The low coefficient of friction, however, is a drawback for over-the-wire exchange of accessories. During the rendezvous procedure, extreme care must be taken that the Glidewire does not slip back during the withdrawal of the echoendoscope and insertion of the duodenoscope. One can exchange the Glidewire through a standard ERCP catheter for a stiffer instrumentation wire, but this requires advancement of the catheter across the bowel lumen and obstruction. A 22-G needle will only accept a 0.018-in guidewire, but this is very limited by the lack of stability and trackability required for over-the-wire intervention. In the United States, the hydrophilic Glidewire is only available in a 0.020-in size, which creates too much friction within the 22-G needle. Manufacturers have modified guidewires in various ways (reduced diameter, longer flexible hydrophilic tips, stiffer instrumentation shafts) to obviate wire exchanges.

### Stents

The choice of stent type, size, and length depends on the ductal anatomy. Again, as in ERCP, straight and pigtail plastic stents or self-expandable metal stents (SEMS) can be used. Pigtail stents minimize the risk of stent migration (especially into the duct), but the pigtail end makes stent insertion more difficult owing to a weakened coaxial transfer of force. The authors, therefore, prefer to use straight stents for transenteric drainage, which also allows stent retrieval or exchanging the stent over the wire without loss of ductal access. Covered SEMS have been used for transenteric drainage but may migrate, particularly with shortening.[5] The covering may block drainage of a secondary duct (eg, cystic duct or intrahepatic branch). Uncovered SEMS are generally unsuited for transenteric drainage because of leakage between the struts. Uncovered SEMS can be placed in exchange for a temporary plastic stent after the fistula tract has matured. The authors always use SEMS when a malignant stricture can be traversed and drained downstream. This practice is justified because plastic stent clogging is likely to require a repeat EACP procedure.

More recently, specialized stents have been developed for specific purposes in transenteric drainage (see section "Lumen-apposing transluminal stent"). These stents create a lumen-apposing transenteric anastomosis to allow secure leak-free drainage and through-the-stent endoscopic interventions.

### PATIENT CONSIDERATIONS FOR ENDOSCOPIC ULTRASOUND–GUIDED ANTEROGRADE CHOLANGIOPANCREATOGRAPHY

The decision to pursue EACP should be made on a case-by-case basis at the time of failed ERCP by the endoscopist, taking into account the underlying clinical indication and condition of each patient. All patients in whom EACP procedures are considered must be suitable for EUS-guided FNA (EUS-FNA) and therapeutic ERCP (eg, no bleeding diatheses, large-volume ascites, or other condition precluding EUS-FNA or therapeutic ERCP). Ideally, all procedures should be performed under monitored anesthesia care with propofol or general anesthesia to allow adequate time for completion of the interventions. Antibiotics (ciprofloxacin or a third-generation cephalosporin) are routinely administered before EACP to minimize the risk of peritonitis from leakage of ductal or enteric contents at the transmural puncture site. Oral antibiotics are continued for a minimum of 3 days after the procedure. High-resolution fluoroscopy requirements are no different than for ERCP.

## TECHNICAL PROCEDURAL STEPS

It is helpful to fluoroscopically assess the position of the echoendoscope before puncturing the targeted duct. The exit path of the needle should be oriented toward the downstream portion of the duct. To access the left hepatic bile duct, the scope is positioned in the proximal stomach along the lesser curve. To access the proximal and distal extrahepatic bile ducts, the scope is positioned in the midstomach and duodenal bulb, respectively. In the duodenal bulb, it may be necessary to shift from a long to a short position; in the long position the needle tends to orient toward the upstream bifurcation, whereas in the short position the needle orients toward the downstream ampulla. A trade-off of the short position is that it can be unstable, with a tendency for the echoendoscope to fall back into the stomach. Transhepatic access has the advantage of protection afforded by the liver parenchyma against complications of a bile leak (as is well known from percutaneous transhepatic access). Extrahepatic access has the advantage of easier, more direct access, usually from the duodenal bulb where the bile duct runs along the duodenal wall as it emerges from the pancreatic head (this is also the location used by surgeons to create a choledochoduodenostomy). The portal vein is usually deep to the bile duct and, therefore, not in the needle path.

The pancreatic duct, which is inaccessible to the interventional radiologist, can be punctured at virtually any point along its length from the stomach to the duodenal bulb. It is easiest to access the junction of the neck to body region from the stomach. The initial puncture point should not be too close to the stricture in order to have some distance to steer the guidewire through the stricture. Analogous to transhepatic drainage, the pancreatic parenchyma surrounding the pancreatic duct is thought to protect against complications of a possible leak from the pancreatic duct.

There are distinct strategies for EACP interventions, depending on the bowel and biliary anatomy. These strategies can either be anterograde downstream across the obstruction or anterograde upstream drainage across the bowel wall (see **Box 2**). In patients with an endoscopically accessible papilla, EUS-guided transpapillary wire placement for rendezvous ERCP can be performed. In patients in whom the papilla cannot be accessed (eg, gastric outlet obstruction or surgical bypass), direct EUS-guided therapy is feasible.

## OUTCOMES
### Transpapillary Rendezvous Procedure (Anterograde Access and Retrograde Drainage)

The rendezvous procedure is derived from the percutaneous technique[6] whereby a guidewire is passed anterograde across the stricture and papilla (or surgical anastomosis) for subsequent rendezvous retrograde drainage by ERCP (**Fig. 1**). The rendezvous procedure is limited by 2 requirements: (1) an endoscopically accessible papilla (or bilioenteric anastomosis) and (2) successful passage of the guidewire across the stricture into the downstream small bowel. Traditional percutaneous access under fluoroscopic guidance is substituted for transgastric or transduodenal access under

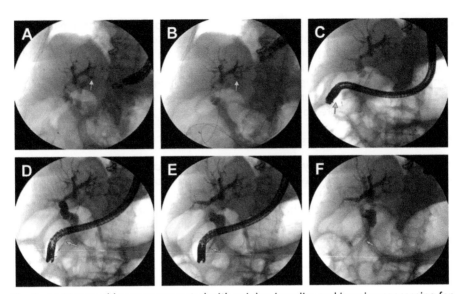

**Fig. 1.** An 81-year-old woman presented with painless jaundice and imaging concerning for a pancreatic mass. An EUS was performed, which demonstrated a mass in the pancreatic head. FNA was diagnostic for adenocarcinoma. An ERCP was attempted; however, despite multiple attempts including a precut sphincterotomy, deep cannulation could not be achieved. The patient subsequently underwent an EUS-guided rendezvous procedure. (*A*) Left intrahepatic puncture with a 19-G needle (*arrow*) under EUS guidance. (*B*) 0.035-in guidewire passed anterograde through the needle (*arrow*), across the obstruction and into the duodenum. (*C*) Capture of the guidewire (*arrow*) by a duodenoscope. (*D*) Stent catheter (*arrow*) placed into the bile duct. (*E*) 10 mm × 6-cm self-expandable metal biliary stent partially deployed (*arrow*). (*F*) Fully deployed stent (*arrow*).

EUS guidance. This procedure minimizes the role of interventional radiology and should be considered an advanced cannulation technique for ERCP. More than 300 cases of successful EUS-guided rendezvous procedures performed for pancreatobiliary obstructions have been reported in the literature (**Table 1**).[5,7–18] Success rates vary between 35% and 98% in the largest cases series. EUS-guided puncture of the duct and ductography are accomplished in most cases. Failure is mainly caused by the inability to steer a guidewire across the stricture. Rescue upstream transenteric drainage can be performed to drain the obstructed duct. When combining attempted EUS-guided rendezvous and upstream drainage in cases of failure, the overall drainage success rate is 87%. The reported complication rates are 12% to 22% and include bile leaks, self-resolving pneumoperitoneum, subcapsular hematoma, and postprocedural pancreatitis.

### Anterograde Access and Downstream Transductal Drainage

This strategy is derived from percutaneous internal stent drainage performed by interventional radiologists.[19,20] The prerequisite for downstream drainage is the successful traversal of the obstruction with a guidewire. The authors have reported a series of 5 patients who underwent anterograde biliary SEMS placement because of nontraversable high-grade duodenal strictures (n = 4) and an endoscopically unreachable hepaticojejunostomy (n = 1).[21] The SEMS was successfully deployed with a decrease in bilirubin levels in all cases. No postprocedural complications were noted after a median follow-up of 9.2 months. Puspok and colleagues[22] have previously described a

**Table 1**
**Studies evaluating EUS-guided rendezvous**

| | No. of Cases | Technical Success (%) | Clinical Success (%) | Procedural Complications |
|---|---|---|---|---|
| Mallery et al,[5] 2004 | 2 | 100 | 100 | Transient fever (1) |
| Kahaleh et al,[7] 2004 | 5 | 60 | 80 | None |
| Kahaleh et al,[8] 2005 | 6 | 67 | 83 | None |
| Kahaleh et al,[9] 2006 | 23 | 78 | 91 | Bleeding (1)<br>Bile leak (1)<br>Pneumoperitoneum (2) |
| Tarantino et al,[10] 2008 | 8 | 50 | 50 | None |
| Brauer et al,[11] 2009 | 20 | 35 | 90 | None |
| Maranki et al,[12] 2009 | 49 | 65 | 84 | Bleeding (1)<br>Bile leak (1)<br>Pneumoperitoneum (4) |
| Iwashita et al,[13] 2012 | 40 | 73 | 73 | Pancreatitis (1), abdominal pain (2), pneumoperitoneum (1), and sepsis (1) |
| Shah et al,[14] 2012 | 50 | 86 | 75 | Pancreatitis (4), perforation (1), subcapsular hematoma (1) Bile leak (1) |
| Dhir et al,[15] 2012 | 58 | 98.3 | 98.3 | Adverse events (2) |
| Vila et al,[16] 2012 | 60 | 68.3 | 68.3 | Biloma (3), bleeding (2), perforation (2), cholangitis (2), pancreatitis (4) |
| Khashab et al,[17] 2013 | 13 | 100 | 100 | Pancreatitis (1), cholecystitis (1) |
| Park do et al,[18] 2013 | 20 | 80 | 80 | Pancreatitis (1), peritonitis (1) |

successful EUS-guided transhepatic SEMS in a single patient with a malignant biliary obstruction following gastrectomy and Roux-en-Y anastomosis. Bories and colleagues[23] successfully placed a SEMS transhepatically and under EUS guidance in 2 patients. However, these procedures were performed in a 2-stage fashion with initial creation of a hepaticogastrostomy tract followed by anterograde placement of a SEMS in a second separate procedure.

The authors' success with anterograde drainage for malignant obstruction has led them to apply a similar approach for benign disease. An alternative to ERCP is particularly attractive in post–gastric bypass patients harboring biliary stones. Hurdles to successful ERCP include the need for deep enteroscopy to reach the ampulla, difficult bile duct cannulation using a forward viewing scope, and limitations imposed by a longer length and smaller channel size of the enteroscope. The authors reported technical success of EUS-guided anterograde balloon sphincteroplasty and anterograde stone extraction in 4 out of 6 patients.[24] Park do and colleagues[25] have described a case report of EUS-guided transhepatic anterograde balloon dilation for a benign bilioenteric anastomotic stricture. The available data on EUS-guided downstream transductal interventions are summarized in **Table 2**.[14,18,21,24–29]

**Table 2**
Anterograde access and downstream transductal drainage

| | No. of Cases | Puncture and Dilatation Device | Stent Placed | Technical Success (%) | Clinical Success (%) | Complications |
|---|---|---|---|---|---|---|
| Nguyen-Tang et al,[21] 2010 | 5 | 19-G needle | SEMS | 100 | 100 | None |
| Park do et al,[25] 2012 | 1 | 19-G needle | Anterograde stricturoplasty | 100 | 100 | None |
| Weilert et al,[24] 2011 | 6 | 19-G needle | Anterograde sphincteroplasty | 67 | 67 | Subcapsular hematoma (1) |
| Artifon et al,[26] 2011 | 1 | 19-G needle | SEMS | 100 | 100 | None |
| Shah et al,[14] 2012 | 16 | 19-G needle | SEMS, anterograde sphincteroplasty | 81 | 81 | Hepatic hematoma |
| Iwashita et al,[27] 2013 | 7 | 19-G needle | Anterograde sphincteroplasty SEMS | 86 | 86 | Adverse events (2) |
| Park do et al,[18] 2013 | 14 | 19-G needle | — | 57 | 57 | None |
| Weilert,[28] 2014 | 7 | 19-G needle | SEMS/anterograde sphincteroplasty | 86 | 86 | Bile leak (1) |
| Saxena et al,[29] 2014 | 2 | 19-G needle | SEMS | 100 | 100 | None |

### Anterograde Access and Upstream Transenteric Drainage (Hepaticogastrostomy and Choledochoduodenostomy)

Upstream transenteric drainage is performed when the stricture cannot be traversed with a wire or when the ampulla or surgical anastomosis cannot be reached with an endoscope. Creating a fistula upstream from the obstructing stricture may afford longer stent patency rates because of the elimination of tumor ingrowth and overgrowth. For hepaticogastrostomy, a long plastic stent has the advantage that it will not block drainage of duct radicals; but there may be leakage alongside the stent, especially if tract dilation exceeded the diameter of the stent. A covered metal stent will provide an effective seal against leakage of bile between the liver and stomach, but the covering may block drainage of duct radicals. Metal stents will foreshorten and may migrate. Placement of a long plastic pigtail stent through the expandable stent may help reduce the risk of stent migration. An alternative approach is to first place a straight plastic stent to allow a mature tract to form and exchange this several weeks later over the wire for an uncovered SEMS.

The available data on *EUS-guided hepaticogastrostomy* is summarized in **Table 3**.[9,12,14,16,17,23,28,30–48] More than 300 cases have been reported in the literature with a high rate of technical success exceeding 90%. Both plastic and metal stents have been used for transenteric drainage. The overall complication rate is 22% and includes cholangitis, biloma, ileus, and stent occlusion. Because of nonadherence of the liver to the stomach wall and constant movement between the two organs, fatal migration or dislodgement of a transhepatic stent can occur.[49] Isayama and colleagues[50] observed proximal stent migration in 2 of 5 patients after hepatogastric placement of an 8-cm fully covered SEMS versus no migration in 10 patients treated with a 12-cm SEMS (1 cm uncovered at the hepatic end), suggesting that the intragastric portion needs to be at least 4 cm or longer. Giovannini and colleagues[51] reported the use of a 8- or 10-cm half-covered stent (at the gastric end, with a flared flange) in 22 patients with resolution of jaundice in 21 patients but with an 18% cholangitis rate in the first month caused by stent obstruction. The stent has a radiological marker visible on fluoroscopy at the transition zone of stent covering to guide placement of the uncovered portion within the liver, but stent shortening and migration may alter the position of the uncovered position.

The available data on *EUS-guided choledochoduodenostomy* (CD) are summarized in **Table 4**.[9–12,14,16,17,22,30,34,35,37–43,45,46,48,52–64] More than 300 cases have been reported, and the overall success rate of the procedure is high (89%). The main drawback of a choledochoenterostomy is the absence of adherence between the bile duct and the bowel wall. As seen from the literature, there is a very high risk of bile leak and pneumoperitoneum. Compounding this, intraductal pressures are higher in the extrahepatic bile duct than in the intrahepatic duct, which is compensated for by decompression after initial puncture. Early experience with plastic stents[60] was complicated by bile leakage and abandoned in preference for fully covered SEMS.[64,65] Artifon and colleagues[48] randomized 49 patients to percutaneous transhepatic drainage or CD with placement of SEMS in all, with clinical success in 91% and an adverse event rate of 16.3%, showing no significant difference between the two clinical approaches.

## ENDOSCOPIC ULTRASOUND–GUIDED PANCREATIC DUCT DRAINAGE

The main indications for EUS-guided drainage of the pancreatic duct are symptomatic obstruction caused by chronic pancreatitis, postsurgical stricture of the pancreaticojejunal anastomosis, or a ductal disruption. The puncture site varies depending on the

**Table 3**
Studies evaluating EUS-guided hepatogastric drainage

| | No. of Cases | Puncture and Dilation Devices | Stent Placed | Technical Success (%) | Clinical Success (%) | Procedural Complications |
|---|---|---|---|---|---|---|
| Burmester et al,[30] 2003 | 1 | Fistulotome | Plastic | 100 | 100 | None |
| Giovannini et al,[31] 2003 | 1 | 19-G needle Needle knife | Plastic | 100 | 100 | None |
| Kahaleh et al,[9] 2006 | 1 | 19-G/22-G needle | Plastic | 100 | 100 | None |
| Artifon et al,[32] 2007 | 1 | 19-G needle | SEMS | 100 | 100 | None |
| Will et al,[33] 2007 | 4 | 19-G needle 6F bougie and 4- or 6-mm balloon | SEMS | 100 | 75 | Cholangitis (1) |
| Bories et al,[23] 2007 | 11 | 19 G/22 G needle 6.0F or 8.5F cystotome | Plastic (7) SEMS (3) | 91 | 100 | Ileus (1) Stent occlusion (1) Biloma (1) Cholangitis (1) |
| Horaguchi et al,[34] 2009 | 6 | Non-applicable | Plastic | 100 | 100 | Cholangitis (1) |
| Maranki et al,[12] 2009 | 3 | 19-G/22-G needle | Plastic | 100 | 100 | Unknown |
| Park do et al,[35] 2009 | 9 | 19-G needle | SEMS | 100 | 100 | — |
| Park do et al,[36] 2010 | 5 | Needle knife | — | — | — | — |
| Belletrutti et al,[37] 2011 | 3 | 19-G needle | Plastic SEMS | 67 | 67 | None |
| Shah et al,[14] 2012 | 8 | 19-G needle | Plastic SEMS | 100 | 100 | Bacteremia (1) |

| Study | N | Needle | Stent | % | % | Complications |
|---|---|---|---|---|---|---|
| Ramirez-Luna et al,[38] 2011 | 2 | 19-G needle | Plastic | 100 | 100 | Stent migration (1) |
| Park do et al,[39] 2011 | 31 | 19-G needle | Plastic SEMS | 100 | 100 | 6 Complications (no detail) |
| Attasaranya et al,[40] 2012 | 16 | 19-G needle | Plastic SEMS | 81 | 81 | No data |
| Kim et al,[41] 2012 | 4 | 19-G needle | SEMS | 75 | 75 | Abdominal pain (1), stent migration (1) |
| Vila et al,[16] 2012 | 34 | Non-applicable | Non-applicable | 65 | 65 | Biloma (3), bleeding (3), perforation (2), liver hematoma (1), abscess (1) |
| Tonozuka et al,[42] 2013 | 3 | 19-G needle | SEMS | 100 | 100 | None |
| Khashab et al,[17] 2013 | 5 | 19-G needle | Plastic SEMS | 100 | 100' | No data |
| Kawakubo et al,[43] 2014 | 20 | 19-G needle | Plastic SEMS | 95 | 100 | Bile leak (2), stent migration (2), bleeding (1), cholangitis (1), biloma (1) |
| Weilert,[28] 2014 | 9 | 19-G needle | Plastic (1) SEMS (8) | 100 | 95 | Bile leak |
| Paik et al,[44] 2014 | 74 | 19-G needle | SEMS | 96 | 91 | Pneumoperitoneum (2), stent migration (6), bleeding (1), abdominal pain (1), plus (2) NA |
| Hamada et al,[45] 2014 | 3 | 19-G needle | SEMS | 100 | 100 | Bleeding (1) |
| Song et al,[46] 2014 | 10 | 19-G needle | SEMS | 100 | 100 | Pneumoperitoneum (2), bleeding (1) |
| Ogura et al,[47] 2014 | 20 | 19-G needle | SEMS | 100 | 100 | Stent migration (2), peritonitis (1) |
| Artifon et al,[48] 2015 | 25 | 19-G needle | — | 96 | 91 | Biloma (2), bleeding (3), bacteremia (1) |

**Table 4**
Studies evaluating EUS-guided choledochoduodenal drainage

| | No. of Cases | Puncture and Dilation Devices | Stent Placed | Technical Success (%) | Clinical Success (%) | Procedural Complications |
|---|---|---|---|---|---|---|
| Giovannini et al,[52] 2001 | 1 | Needle knife Dilating catheter | Plastic | 100 | 100 | None |
| Burmester et al,[30] 2003 | 2 | Fistulotome | Plastic | 50 | 100 | Bile peritonitis (1) |
| Puspok et al,[22] 2005 | 5 | Needle knife | Plastic | 80 | 100 | None |
| Kahaleh et al,[9] 2006 | 1 | 19-G needle | SEMS | 100 | 100 | Pneumoperitoneum (1) |
| Fujita et al,[53] 2007 | 1 | 19-G needle Dilating catheter | Plastic | 100 | 100 | None |
| Ang et al,[54] 2007 | 2 | Needle knife Dilating catheter | Plastic | 100 | 100 | Pneumoperitoneum (1) |
| Yamao et al,[55] 2008 | 5 | Needle knife Dilating catheter | Plastic | 100 | 100 | Pneumoperitoneum (1) |
| Tarantino et al,[10] 2008 | 4 | 19-G/22-G needle Balloon dilation | Plastic | 100 | 100 | None |
| Itoi et al,[56] 2008 | 4 | 19-G needle or needle knife Dilating catheter or balloon dilation | Plastic | 100 | 100 | Bile peritonitis (1) |
| Brauer et al,[11] 2009 | 3 | 19-G/22-G needle | Plastic | 100 | 100 | Pneumoperitoneum (1) |
| Horaguchi et al,[34] 2009 | 8 | 19-G needle | Plastic | 100 | 100 | Peritonitis (1) |
| Hanada et al,[57] 2009 | 4 | 19-G needle | Plastic | 100 | 100 | None |
| Park do et al,[35] 2009 | 4 | 19-G needle | SEMS | 100 | 100 | None |
| Iwamuro et al,[58] 2010 | 5 | Needle knife | Plastic | 100 | 100 | Abdominal pain and fever (1) |

| Study | n | Needle | Stent | % | % | Complications |
|---|---|---|---|---|---|---|
| Siddiqui et al,[59] 2011 | 8 | 19-G needle | SEMS | 100 | 100 | Duodenal perforation (1), abdominal pain (1) |
| Belletrutti et al,[37] 2011 | 4 | 19-G needle | Plastic SEMS | 100 | 100 | None |
| Shah et al,[14] 2012 | 2 | Needle knife | SEMS | 50 | 100 | Pneumoperitoneum (1) |
| Hara et al,[60] 2011 | 18 | Needle knife | Plastic | 94 | 94 | Peritonitis (2), hemobilia (1) |
| Komaki et al,[61] 2011 | 15 | 19-G needle Needle knife | Plastic | 93 | 93 | Cholangitis (4), peritonitis (2), stent migration (1) |
| Ramirez-Luna et al,[38] 2011 | 9 | 19-G needle | Plastic | 89 | 89 | Biloma (1) |
| Park do et al,[39] 2011 | 24 | 19-G needle | Plastic SEMS | 92 | 92 | No data |
| Fabbri et al,[62] 2011 | 15 | 19-G needle | SEMS | 80 | 80 | Pneumoperitoneum (1) |
| Attasaranya et al,[40] 2012 | 9 | 19-G needle | Plastic SEMS | 56 | 56 | 4 Complications (no detail) |
| Kim et al,[41] 2012 | 9 | 19-G needle | SEMS | 100 | 100 | Pneumoperitoneum (2), migration (2), peritonitis (1) |
| Song et al,[63] 2012 | 15 | 19-G needle | SEMS | 87 | 87 | Pneumoperitoneum (2), cholangitis (1) |
| Vila et al,[16] 2012 | 26 | No data | No data | 86 | 86 | Biloma (3), bleeding (1), pancreatitis (1), cholangitis (1) |
| Tonozuka et al,[42] 2013 | 4 | 19-G | SEMS | 100 | 100 | None |
| Khashab et al,[17] 2013 | 15 | 19-G/22-G needle | Plastic SEMS | 100 | 100 | — |
| Kawakubo et al,[43] 2014 | 44 | 19-G needle or needle knife | Plastic SEMS | 95 | 95 | Bile leak (3), bleeding (1), stent misplaced (1) |
| Hara et al,[64] 2013 | 18 | Needle knife | SEMS | 94 | 94 | Peritonitis (2) |
| Hamada et al,[45] 2014 | 4 | 19-G needle | Plastic SEMS | 100 | 100 | None |
| Song et al,[46] 2014 | 17 | 19-G needle | SEMS | 100 | 100 | Pneumoperitoneum (1) |
| Artifon et al,[48] 2015 | 24 | 19-G needle | SEMS | 91 | 77 | Bile leak (1), bleeding (1), perforation (1) |

site of the stenosis. In most cases the main pancreatic duct is targeted from the stomach (transgastric route). The easiest transmural access to the pancreatic duct is at the junction of the genu and body. Puncturing a nondilated or minimally dilated pancreatic duct can be difficult with a 19-G needle and may require a 22-G needle. The penetration of fibrosed pancreatic parenchyma is also facilitated by a 22-G needle. However, the 22-G needle takes only an 0.018-in wire, which is difficult to see and to guide. There is also a tendency for the guidewire to enter side branches. Drainage can be accomplished using a rendezvous approach if the stricture can be negotiated with a wire and the papilla or pancreaticojejunostomy can be reached with the endoscope. Failing this, transenteric drainage is performed. The procedure steps are similar to those of hepaticogastrostomy outlined earlier. The authors' preference is to use a straight 7F stent for transgastric drainage. The authors replace the single stent with two 7F stents if there is recurrence of symptoms.

The reported data are summarized in **Table 5**.[14,16,66–72] A total of 130 patients underwent EUS-guided pancreatic drainage. The pancreatic duct was accessed and drained in most patients via the transgastric route. The technical success rate was 91% with a complication rate of 15%. Complications included postprocedural pain, bleeding, perforations, and pancreatitis. Tessier and colleagues[69] reported stent dysfunction requiring repeat endoscopies during a median follow-up of 14.5 months in 55%.

The technical challenges relate to the fibrotic changes of chronic pancreatitis, which make needle penetration of the pancreas and tract dilation difficult. As mentioned, a 22-G needle can be used to achieve penetration and duct access but leads to a second hurdle of tract dilation for stent drainage. The smallest bougies and balloons advanced over a wire usually fail to penetrate the pancreas and will buckle. One solution is to use cautery with a double-lumen needle knife or diathermic ring device. The risks, including pancreatitis, leakage, and perforation, remain to be defined in larger studies.

## STANDARDIZED ALGORITHM FOR ENDOSCOPIC ULTRASOUND–GUIDED BILE DUCT DRAINAGE

EUS-guided biliary drainage (EUS-BD) requires fusion and integration of EUS and ERCP skills while using tools that are not specifically designed for its use, which has lead to variable approaches and techniques. Recent criticism has been raised because of its relatively high adverse event rate reported by Vila and colleagues[16] in the Spanish National Survey on EUS-guided cholangiopancreatography and transmural intervention. For biliary intervention, technical success was low at 68.9% with an adverse event rate of 22.6%. Technical failure is linked with wire manipulation as well as tract dilatation, which was also associated with adverse events. Of particular concern was a 4% mortality associated with these adverse events. Endoscopist experience was dismissed as contributing to this; however, 23 endoscopists performed 125 procedures (average of 5 cases per proceduralist only). Adverse events were also reported at 20% by Park do and colleagues,[18] whereby needle-knife use was the single risk factor for postprocedural adverse events after EUS-BD (odds ratio 12.4; $P = .01$).

These concerns have lead to the description of algorithms to standardize approaches and make reporting of adverse events more uniform with most preferring an extrahepatic access route.[17,18] The rationale for promoting this seems to be the ease of common bile duct (CBD) puncture from the duodenum with shorter and more direct wire manipulation. Initial reports of a higher adverse event rate may be caused by tract dilatation (7F or 4 mm) resulting in leak caused by nonadherence of the duodenal wall and the CBD.[39] Park do and colleagues[18] and Khashab and colleagues[17] reported subsequent lower adverse event rates of 11% and 12%,

**Table 5**
**Studies evaluating EUS-guided pancreatic drainage**

| | No. of Cases | Puncture and Dilation Device | Drainage Route | Technical Success (%) | Procedural Complications |
|---|---|---|---|---|---|
| François et al,[66] 2002 | 4 | 19-G needle Cystotome | Transgastric | 100 | None |
| Kahaleh et al,[67] 2003 | 2 | 19-G needle Balloon dilatation | Transgastric | 100 | None |
| Kahaleh et al,[68] 2007 | 13 | 19-G/22-G needle Balloon dilation | Transgastric | 83 | Bleeding (1) Perforation (1) |
| Tessier et al,[69] 2007 | 36 | 19-G/22-G needle or cystotome | Transgastric (29) Transduodenal (7) | 92 | Pancreatitis (1) Hematoma (1) |
| Will et al,[70] 2007 | 12 | 19-G needle Dilating catheter and stent retriever | Transgastric | 69 | Pain (4) Bleeding (1) Perforation (1) |
| Shah et al,[14] 2012 | 5 | 19-G needle Dilating catheter | Transgastric | 100 | Perforation (1) |
| Kurihara et al,[71] 2013 | 17 | 19-G needle | Transgastric | 82 | No data |
| Vila et al,[16] 2012 | 5 | No data | No data | 40 | Pseudocyst (1) |
| Fujii et al,[72] 2013 | 43 | 19-G needle Balloon/bougie dilatation | Transgastric | 74 | Stent dysfunction (8), abscess (1), pancreatitis (1), guidewire loss (1), abdominal pain (13) |

respectively. The rates of technical success (91% and 94%) and adverse events reported in the studies are similar to those of PTBD performed at high-volume referral centers.[73]

## LUMEN-APPOSING TRANSLUMINAL STENT

Tubular stents, conceived for lumen recanalization, have several limitations when applied to transluminal drainage. Firstly, they do not impart lumen-to-lumen anchorage. This lack of anchorage may result in leakage of bile and enteric contents if there is absence of a stricture to hold it in place. Thirdly, the length of tubular stents exceeds the anatomic requirement of a short transluminal anastomosis. The exposed stent ends may cause tissue trauma, resulting in bleeding or perforation. Finally, the longer the stent length, the more prone the stent is to clogging.

The development of a lumen-apposing, dual-anchor stent (AXIOS, Xlumena Inc, Mountain View, CA, USA) designed for transluminal bile duct drainage was first reported by Binmoeller and Shah in 2011.[74] The stent consists of double-walled flanges that are perpendicular to the lumen and hold the tissue walls in apposition (**Fig. 2**A). Fully expanded, the flange diameter is approximately twice that of the stent lumen. The stent flanges are designed to distribute pressure evenly on the lumenal wall. The stent is made of braided nitinol wire and fully covered to prevent tissue ingrowth and tract leakage as well as enable removability.

An evolutionary modification of the AXIOS delivery system is the integration of cautery into the nosecone at the catheter tip (Hot AXIOS, **Fig. 2**B).[75] Two radially distributed diathermic wires converge around the guidewire lumen to optimize the current density to provide a clean, sharp cut with minimal coagulation effect. Cautery enables transmural advancement of the stent delivery catheter into the target lumen without preliminary tract dilation. This advancement minimizes or eliminates over-the-wire exchanges of instruments during which wire access can be lost and leakage can occur. The Hot AXIOS catheter can be inserted over the wire after puncture of the target site with a 19-G FNA needle and through-the-needle wire placement or used freestyle to directly access the target lumen (Video 1). Freestyle access has the advantage of enabling a one-step access and stent deployment procedure, eliminating over-the-wire exchange entirely.

**A**                              **B**

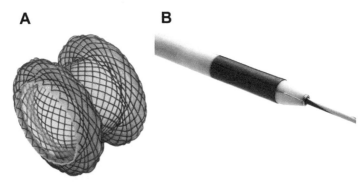

**Fig. 2.** (*A*) The AXIOS stent consists of double-walled flanges that are perpendicular to the lumen and hold the tissue walls in apposition. (*B*) Tip of the 10.8F Hot AXIOS catheter. Two radially distributed diathermic wires converge around the guidewire lumen. The catheter houses the AXIOS stent for immediate deployment after entry into the target lumen. (*Courtesy of* Xlumena Inc, Mountain View, CA; with permission.)

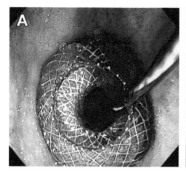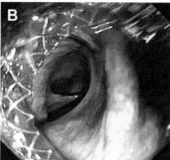

**Fig. 3.** AXIOS stent for choledochoduodenostomy. (*A*) Endoscopic view of bile draining through stent after deployment in the duodenal bulb. (*B*) Used as a conduit to access the bile duct for cholangioscopy.

Depending on the target for drainage, the AXIOS stent has been custom designed for this purpose with diameters of 6 mm and 8 mm and saddle length of 8 mm for CBD drainage or lumen diameters of 10, 15, and 20 mm for transenteric drainage of adjacent organ/collections.[76] Additionally, the stent serves as an access port for direct cholangioscopy and endoscopy-guided therapy (**Fig. 3**).

## EXTENDED DRAINAGE INDICATIONS

Having specialized access and drainage tools has allowed for a widening of potential applications to drain biliary and pancreatic structures within the reach of the therapeutic echoendoscopist, including the gallbladder, bilomas, and postsurgical abscess cavities.[77–79]

In gallbladder drainage, the use of a lumen-apposing stent reduces the risk of bile and gas leakage when adherence is lacking or indeterminate. Itoi and colleagues[80] described the use of the AXIOS lumen-apposing stent in 5 patients presenting with acute cholecystitis with clinical success in all. de la Serna-Higuera and colleagues[77] reported technical success in 11 of 13 patients who underwent gallbladder drainage using the AXIOS stent. Of these 11 patients, direct endoscopic intervention was performed in 6 patients using a standard or ultraslim endoscope, introduced into the gallbladder via the stent lumen to aspirate pus, stone, or sludge removal and for lavage. de la Serna-Higuera and colleagues[77] left the AXIOS stent in situ as a definitive treatment strategy in 10 of 11 patients because of underlying comorbidities, without further recurrence of symptoms during a median follow-up of 101 days.

Using the Hot AXIOS platform with single-step puncture and stent delivery, Teoh and colleagues[75] reported a case of EUS-guided gallbladder drainage in a patient with ongoing sepsis despite prior percutaneous drainage. The gallbladder was directly punctured freestyle, using cautery to assist the puncture, without prior needle or guidewire insertion. The investigators noted excellent maneuverability and visibility of the delivery system under EUS guidance.

## SUMMARY

EUS can assist pancreaticobiliary access using an anterograde route when conventional retrograde access fails. For biliary drainage, internal EUS-guided has numerous theoretic advantages over external percutaneous. The literature supports the feasibility of EUS-guided drainage, targeting either the intrahepatic or extrahepatic bile duct, with high technical success rates. Complication rates have been high; however, the safety profile of EAC is improving with increasing experience. Pancreatic drainage is less widely disseminated because of technical challenges related to the fibrotic changes of chronic pancreatitis and high complication rates. Stents designed for EUS-guided applications have allowed functional transluminal drainage of an obstructed pancreaticobiliary system to achieve clinical benefit to a wide spectrum of patients with both malignant and benign diseases. The complexity of EACP requires the highest levels of training in both EUS and ERCP. Training programs in pancreaticobiliary endoscopy must integrate the 2 procedures if EACP is to become widely accepted.

## SUPPLEMENTARY DATA

Supplementary data related to this article can be found online at http://dx.doi.org/10.1016/j.giec.2015.06.003.

## REFERENCES

1. Carr-Locke D. Overview of the role of ERCP in the management of diseases of the biliary tract and the pancreas. Gastrointest Endosc 2002;56:S157–60.
2. Winick A, Waybill P, Venbrux A. Complications of percutaneous transhepatic biliary interventions. Tech Vasc Interv Radiol 2001;4:200–6.
3. Smith A, Dowsett J, Russell R, et al. Randomised trial of endoscopic stenting versus surgical bypass in malignant low bile duct obstruction. Lancet 1994;344:1655–60.
4. Wiersema M, Sandusky D, Carr R. Endosonography-guided cholangiopancreatography. Gastrointest Endosc 1996;43:102–6.
5. Mallery S, Matlock J, Freeman M. EUS-guided rendezvous drainage of obstructed biliary and pancreatic ducts: report of 6 cases. Gastrointest Endosc 2004;59:100–7.
6. Dowsett J, Vaira D, Hatfield A, et al. Endoscopic biliary therapy using the combined percutaneous and endoscopic technique. Gastroenterology 1989;96:1180–6.
7. Kahaleh M, Yoshida C, Kane L, et al. Interventional EUS cholangiography: a report of five cases. Gastrointest Endosc 2004;60:138–42.
8. Kahaleh M, Wang P, Shami V, et al. EUS-guided transhepatic cholangiography: report of 6 cases. Gastrointest Endosc 2005;61:307–13.
9. Kahaleh M, Hernandez A, Tokar J, et al. Interventional EUS-guided cholangiography: evaluation of a technique in evolution. Gastrointest Endosc 2006;64:52–9.
10. Tarantino I, Barresi L, Repici A, et al. EUS-guided biliary drainage: a case series. Endoscopy 2008;40:336–9.
11. Brauer B, Chen Y, Fukami N, et al. Single-operator EUS-guided cholangiopancreatography for difficult pancreaticobiliary access (with video). Gastrointest Endosc 2009;70:471–9.
12. Maranki J, Hernandez A, Arslan B, et al. Interventional endoscopic ultrasound-guided cholangiography: long-term experience of an emerging alternative to percutaneous transhepatic cholangiography. Endoscopy 2009;41:532–8.
13. Iwashita T, Lee JG, Shinoura S, et al. Endoscopic ultrasound-guided rendezvous for biliary access after failed cannulation. Endoscopy 2012;44(1):60–5.
14. Shah J, Marson F, Weilert F, et al. Single-operator, single-session EUS-guided anterograde cholangiopancreatography in failed ERCP or inaccessible papilla. Gastrointest Endosc 2012;75(1):56–64.
15. Dhir V, Bhandari S, Bapat M, et al. Comparison of EUS-guided rendezvous and precut papillotomy techniques for biliary access (with videos). Gastrointest Endosc 2012;75(2):354–9.

16. Vila J, Perez-Miranda M, Vazquez-Sequeiros E, et al. Initial experience with EUS-guided cholangiopancreatography for biliary and pancreatic duct drainage: a Spanish national survey. Gastrointest Endosc 2012;76:1133–41.

17. Khashab M, Valeshabad A, Modayil R, et al. EUS-guided biliary drainage by using a standardized approach for malignant biliary obstruction: rendezvous versus direct transluminal techniques. Gastrointest Endosc 2013;78:734–41.

18. Park do H, Jeong S, Lee B, et al. Prospective evaluation of a treatment algorithm with enhanced guidewire manipulation protocol for EUS-guided biliary drainage after failed ERCP. Gastrointest Endosc 2013;78:91–101.

19. Stoker J, Lameris J, van Blankenstein M. Percutaneous metallic self-expandable endoprostheses in malignant hilar biliary obstruction. Gastrointest Endosc 1993; 39:43–9.

20. Becker C, Glattli A, Maibach R, et al. Percutaneous palliation of malignant obstructive jaundice with the wallstent endoprosthesis: follow-up and reintervention in patients with hilar and non-hilar obstruction. J Vasc Interv Radiol 1993;4: 597–604.

21. Nguyen-Tang T, Binmoeller K, Sanchez-Yague A, et al. Endoscopic ultrasound (EUS)-guided anterograde self-expandable metal stent (SEMS) placement across malignant biliary obstruction. Endoscopy 2010;42:232–6.

22. Puspok A, Lomoschitz F, Dejaco C, et al. Endoscopic ultrasound guided therapy of benign and malignant biliary obstruction: a case series. Am J Gastroenterol 2005;100:1743–7.

23. Bories E, Pesenti C, Caillol F, et al. Trans-gastric endoscopic ultrasonography-guided biliary drainage: results of a pilot study. Endoscopy 2007;39:287–91.

24. Weilert F, Binmoeller K, Marson F, et al. Endoscopic ultrasound-guided anterograde treatment of biliary stones following gastric bypass. Endoscopy 2011;43:1105–8.

25. Park do H, Jang J, Lee S, et al. EUS-guided transhepatic antegrade balloon dilation for benign bilioenteric anastomotic strictures in a patient with hepaticojejunostomy. Gastrointest Endosc 2012;75(3):692–3.

26. Artifon EL, Safatle-Ribeiro AV, Ferreira FC, et al. EUS-guided antegrade transhepatic placement of a self-expandable metal stent in hepatico-jejunal anastomosis. JOP 2011;12(6):610–3.

27. Iwashita T, Yasuda I, Doi S, et al. Endoscopic ultrasound-guided antegrade treatments for biliary disorders in patients with surgically altered anatomy. Dig Dis Sci 2013;58(8):2417–22.

28. Weilert F. Prospective evaluation of simplified algorithm for EUS-guided intra-hepatic biliary access and anterograde interventions for failed ERCP. Surg Endosc 2014;28(11):3193–9.

29. Saxena P, Kumbhari V, Zein ME, et al. EUS-guided biliary drainage with antegrade transpapillary placement of a metal biliary stent. Gastrointest Endosc 2014. http://dx.doi.org/10.1016/j.gie.2014.06.038.

30. Burmester E, Niehaus J, Leineweber T, et al. EUS-cholangio-drainage of the bile duct: report of 4 cases. Gastrointest Endosc 2003;57:246–51.

31. Giovannini M, Dotti M, Bories E, et al. Hepaticogastrostomy by echo-endoscopy as a palliative treatment in a patient with metastatic biliary obstruction. Endoscopy 2003;35:1076–8.

32. Artifon E, Chaves D, Ishioka S, et al. Echoguided hepatico-gastrostomy: a case report. Clinics (Sao Paulo) 2007;62:799–802.

33. Will U, Thieme A, Fueldner F, et al. Treatment of biliary obstruction in selected patients by endoscopic ultrasonography (EUS)-guided transluminal biliary drainage. Endoscopy 2007;39:292–5.

34. Horaguchi J, Fujita N, Noda Y, et al. Endosonography-guided biliary drainage in cases with difficult transpapillary endoscopic biliary drainage. Dig Endosc 2009; 21(4):239–44.
35. Park do H, Koo JE, Oh J, et al. EUS-guided biliary drainage with one-step placement of a fully covered metal stent for malignant biliary obstruction: a prospective feasibility study. Am J Gastroenterol 2009;104(9):2168–74.
36. Park do H, Song T, Eum J, et al. EUS-guided hepaticogastrostomy with fully covered metal stent as the biliary diversion technique fro an occluded biliary metal stent after failed ERCP. Gastrointest Endosc 2010;71(2):413–9.
37. Belletrutti PJ, DiMaio CJ, Gerdes H, et al. Endoscopic ultrasound guided biliary drainage in patients with unapproachable ampullae due to malignant duodenal obstruction. J Gastrointest Cancer 2011;42(3):137–42.
38. Ramirez-Luna MA, Tellez-Avila FI, Giovannini M, et al. Endoscopic ultrasound-guided biliodigestive drainage is a good alternative in patients with unresectable cancer. Endoscopy 2011;43(9):826–30.
39. Park do H, Jang JW, Lee SS, et al. EUS-guided biliary drainage with transluminal stenting after failed ERCP: predictors of adverse events and long-term results. Gastrointest Endosc 2011;74(6):1276–84.
40. Attasaranya S, Netinasunton N, Jongboonyanuparp T, et al. The spectrum of endoscopic ultrasound intervention in biliary diseases: a single center's experience in 31 cases. Gastroenterol Res Pract 2012;2012:680753.
41. Kim TH, Kim SH, Oh HJ, et al. Endoscopic ultrasound-guided biliary drainage with placement of a fully covered metal stent for malignant biliary obstruction. World J Gastroenterol 2012;18(20):2526–32.
42. Tonozuka R, Itoi T, Sofuni A, et al. Endoscopic double stenting for the treatment of malignant biliary and duodenal obstruction due to pancreatic cancer. Dig Endosc 2013;25(Suppl 2):100–8.
43. Kawakubo K, Isayama H, Kato H, et al. Multicenter retrospective study of endoscopic ultrasound-guided biliary drainage for malignant biliary obstruction in Japan. J Hepatobiliary Pancreat Sci 2014;21(5):328–34.
44. Paik WH, Park do H, Choi JH, et al. Simplified fistula dilation technique and modified stent deployment maneuver for EUS-guided hepaticogastrostomy. World J Gastroenterol 2014;20(17):5051–9.
45. Hamada T, Isayama H, Nakai Y, et al. Transmural biliary drainage can be an alternative to transpapillary drainage in patients with an indwelling duodenal stent. Dig Dis Sci 2014;59(8):1931–8.
46. Song TJ, Lee SS, Park do H, et al. Preliminary report on a new hybrid metal stent for EUS-guided biliary drainage (with videos). Gastrointest Endosc 2014;80(4):707–11.
47. Ogura T, Kurisu Y, Masuda D, et al. Novel method of endoscopic ultrasound-guided hepaticogastrostomy to prevent stent dysfunction. J Gastroenterol Hepatol 2014;29(10):1815–21.
48. Artifon E, Marson F, Gaidhane M, et al. Hepaticogastrostomy or choledochoduodenostomy for distal malignant biliary obstruction after failed ERCP: is there any difference? Gastrointest Endosc 2015;81(4):950–9.
49. Martins F, Rossini L, Ferrari A. Migration of a covered metallic stent following endoscopic ultrasound-guided hepaticogastroscotomy: fatal complication. Endoscopy 2010;42:E126–7.
50. Isayama H, Nakai Y, Kawakubo K, et al. Feasibility and efficacy of a 12-cm long covered metallic stent for EUS-guided hepaticogastrostomy (EUS-HGS) for unresectable malignant biliary obstruction. Gastrointest Endosc 2013;77(5S):AB423.

51. Giovannini M, Pesenti C, Bories E, et al. EUS guided hepatico-gastrostomy using a new design partially covered stent (GIOBOR stent). Gastrointest Endosc 2012; 75(4S):AB441.

52. Giovannini M, Moutardier V, Pesenti C, et al. Endoscopic ultrasound-guided bilio-duodenal anastomosis: a new technique for biliary drainage. Endoscopy 2001; 33:898–900.

53. Fujita N, Noda Y, Kobayashi G, et al. Histological changes at an endosonography-guided biliary drainage site: a case report. World J Gastroenterol 2007;13:5512–5.

54. Ang T, Teo E, Fock K. EUS-guided transduodenal biliary drainage in unresectable pancreatic cancer with obstructive jaundice. JOP 2007;8:438–43.

55. Yamao K, Bhatia V, Mizuno N, et al. EUS-guided choledochoduodenostomy for palliative biliary drainage in patients with malignant biliary obstruction: results of long-term follow-up. Endoscopy 2008;40:340–2.

56. Itoi T, Itokawa F, Sofuni A, et al. Endoscopic ultrasound-guided choledochoduodenostomy in patients with failed endoscopic retrograde cholangiopancreatography. World J Gastroenterol 2008;14:6078–82.

57. Hanada K, Iiboshi T, Ishii Y. Endoscopic ultrasound-guided choledochoduodenostomy for palliative biliary drainage in cases with inoperable pancreas head carcinoma. Dig Endosc 2009;21(Suppl 1):S75–8.

58. Iwamuro M, Kawamoto H, Harada R, et al. Combined duodenal stent placement and endoscopic ultrasonography-guided biliary drainage for malignant duodenal obstruction with biliary stricture. Dig Endosc 2010;22(3):236–40.

59. Siddiqui AA, Sreenarasimhaiah J, Lara LF, et al. Endoscopic ultrasound-guided transduodenal placement of a fully covered metal stent for palliative biliary drainage in patients with malignant biliary obstruction. Surg Endosc 2011;25(2):549–55.

60. Hara K, Yamao K, Niwa Y. Prospective clinical study of EUS-guided choledochoduodenostomy for malignant lower biliary tract obstruction. Am J Gastroenterol 2011;106(7):1239–45.

61. Komaki T, Kitano M, Sakamoto H, et al. Endoscopic ultrasonography-guided biliary drainage: evaluation of a choledochoduodenostomy technique. Pancreatology 2011;11(Suppl 2):47–51.

62. Fabbri C, Luigiano C, Fuccio L, et al. EUS-guided biliary drainage with placement of a new partially covered biliary stent for palliation of malignant biliary obstruction: a case series. Endoscopy 2011;43(5):438–41.

63. Song TJ, Hyun YS, Lee SS, et al. Endoscopic ultrasound-guided choledochoduodenostomies with fully covered self-expandable metallic stents. World J Gastroenterol 2012;18(32):4435–40.

64. Hara K, Yamao K, Hijioka S, et al. Prospective clinical study of endoscopic ultrasound-guided choledochoduodenostomy with direct metallic stent placement using forward-viewing echoendoscope. Endoscopy 2013;45:392–6.

65. Itoi T, Yamao K. EUS 2008 working group document: evaluation of EUS-guided choledochoduodenostomy (with video). Gastrointest Endosc 2009;69:S8–12.

66. François E, Kahaleh M, Giovannini M, et al. EUS-guided pancreaticogastrostomy. Gastrointest Endosc 2002;56:128–33.

67. Kahaleh M, Yoshida C, Yeaton P. EUS anterograde pancreatography with gastropancreatic duct stent placement: review of two cases. Gastrointest Endosc 2003; 58:919–23.

68. Kahaleh M, Hernandez A, Tokar J, et al. EUS-guided pancreaticogastrostomy: analysis of its efficacy to drain inaccessible pancreatic ducts. Gastrointest Endosc 2007;65:224–30.

69. Tessier G, Bories E, Arvanitakis M, et al. EUS-guided pancreato-gastrostomy and pancreatobulbostomy for the treatment of pain in patients with pancreatic ductal dilatation inaccessible for transpapillary endoscopic therapy. Gastrointest Endosc 2007;65:233–41.

70. Will U, Fueldner F, Thieme A, et al. Transgastric pancreatography and EUS-guided drainage of the pancreatic duct. J Hepatobiliary Pancreat Surg 2007; 14:377–82.

71. Kurihara T, Itoi T, Sofuni A, et al. Endoscopic ultrasonography-guided pancreatic duct drainage after failed endoscopic retrograde cholangiopancreatography in patients with malignant and benign pancreatic duct obstructions. Dig Endosc 2013;25(Suppl 2):109–16.

72. Fujii LL, Topazian MD, Abu Dayyeh BK, et al. EUS-guided pancreatic duct intervention: outcomes of a single tertiary-care referral center experience. Gastrointest Endosc 2013;78(6):854–64.e1.

73. Tapping C, Byass O, Tapping CR, et al. Percutaneous transhepatic biliary drainage (PTBD) with or without stenting-complications, re-stent rate and a new risk stratification score. Eur Radiol 2011;21:1948–55.

74. Binmoeller K, Shah J. A novel lumen-apposing stent for transluminal fluid collections. Endoscopy 2011;43:337–42.

75. Teoh A, Binmoeller K, Lau J. Single-step EUS-guided puncture and delivery of a lumen-apposing stent for gallbladder drainage using a novel cautery-tipped stent delivery system. Gastrointest Endosc 2014;80(6):1171.

76. Itoi T, Binmoeller K. EUS-guided choledochoduodenostomy by using a biflanged lumen-apposing metal stent. Gastrointest Endosc 2014;79(5):715.

77. de la Serna-Higuera C, Perez-Miranda M, Gil-Simon P, et al. EUS-guided transenteric gallbladder drainage with a new fistula-forming, lumen-apposing metal stent. Gastrointest Endosc 2013;77(2):303–8.

78. Consiglieri CF, Escobar I, Gornals JB. EUS-guided transesophageal drainage of a mediastinal abscess using a diabolo-shaped lumen-apposing metal stent. Gastrointest Endosc 2015;81(1):221–2.

79. Alcaide N, Vargas-Garcia AL, de la Serna-Higuera C, et al. EUS-guided drainage of liver abscess by using a lumen-apposing metal stent (with video). Gastrointest Endosc 2013;78(6):941–2 [discussion: 942].

80. Itoi T, Binmoeller K, Shah J, et al. Clinical evaluation of a novel lumen-apposing metal stent for endosonography-guided pancreatic pseudocyst and gallbladder drainage. Gastrointest Endosc 2012;75:870–6.

# United States Postal Service

## Statement of Ownership, Management, and Circulation
### (All Periodicals Publications Except Requestor Publications)

| 1. Publication Title | 2. Publication Number | 3. Filing Date |
|---|---|---|
| Gastrointestinal Endoscopy Clinics of North America | 0 1 2 - 6 0 0 3 | 9/18/15 |

| 4. Issue Frequency | 5. Number of Issues Published Annually | 6. Annual Subscription Price |
|---|---|---|
| Jan, Apr, Jul, Oct | 4 | $335.00 |

7. Complete Mailing Address of Known Office of Publication *(Not printer)* *(Street, city, county, state, and ZIP+4®)*

Elsevier Inc.
360 Park Avenue South
New York, NY 10010-1710

Contact Person
Stephen R. Bushing

Telephone *(Include area code)*
215-239-3688

8. Complete Mailing Address of Headquarters or General Business Office of Publisher *(Not printer)*

Elsevier Inc., 360 Park Avenue South, New York, NY 10010-1710

9. Full Names and Complete Mailing Addresses of Publisher, Editor, and Managing Editor *(Do not leave blank)*

Publisher *(Name and complete mailing address)*

Linda Belfus, Elsevier Inc., 1600 John F. Kennedy Blvd., Suite 1800, Philadelphia, PA 19103

Editor *(Name and complete mailing address)*

Kerry Holland, Elsevier Inc., 1600 John F. Kennedy Blvd., Suite 1800, Philadelphia, PA 19103-2899

Managing Editor *(Name and complete mailing address)*

Adrianne Brigido, Elsevier Inc., 1600 John F. Kennedy Blvd., Suite 1800, Philadelphia, PA 19103-2899

10. Owner *(Do not leave blank. If the publication is owned by a corporation, give the name and address of the corporation immediately followed by the names and addresses of all stockholders owning or holding 1 percent or more of the total amount of stock. If not owned by a corporation, give the names and addresses of the individual owners. If owned by a partnership or other unincorporated firm, give its name and address as well as those of each individual owner. If the publication is published by a nonprofit organization, give its name and address.)*

| Full Name | Complete Mailing Address |
|---|---|
| Wholly owned subsidiary of | 1600 John F. Kennedy Blvd. Ste. 1800 |
| Reed/Elsevier, US holdings | Philadelphia, PA 19103-2899 |

11. Known Bondholders, Mortgagees, and Other Security Holders Owning or Holding 1 Percent or More of Total Amount of Bonds, Mortgages, or Other Securities. If none, check box ☐ None

| Full Name | Complete Mailing Address |
|---|---|
| N/A | |

12. Tax Status *(For completion by nonprofit organizations authorized to mail at nonprofit rates) (Check one)*
The purpose, function, and nonprofit status of this organization and the exempt status for federal income tax purposes:
☐ Has Not Changed During Preceding 12 Months
☐ Has Changed During Preceding 12 Months *(Publisher must submit explanation of change with this statement)*

| 13. Publication Title | 14. Issue Date for Circulation Data Below |
|---|---|
| Gastrointestinal Endoscopy Clinics of North America | July 2015 |

| 15. Extent and Nature of Circulation | | | Average No. Copies Each Issue During Preceding 12 Months | No. Copies of Single Issue Published Nearest to Filing Date |
|---|---|---|---|---|
| a. Total Number of Copies *(Net press run)* | | | 432 | 424 |
| b. Legitimate Paid and/Or Requested Distribution *(By Mail and Outside the Mail )* | (1) | Mailed Outside-County Paid/Requested Mail Subscriptions stated on PS Form 3541. *(Include paid distribution above nominal rate, advertiser's proof copies and exchange copies)* | 179 | 137 |
| | (2) | Mailed In-County Paid/Requested Mail Subscriptions stated on PS Form 3541. *(Include paid distribution above nominal rate, advertiser's proof copies and exchange copies)* | | |
| | (3) | Paid Distribution Outside the Mails Including Sales Through Dealers And Carriers, Street Vendors, Counter Sales, and Other Paid Distribution Outside USPS® | 55 | 62 |
| | (4) | Paid Distribution by Other Classes of Mail Through the USPS (e.g. First-Class Mail®) | | |
| c. Total Paid and/or Requested Circulation *(Sum of 15b (1), (2), (3), and (4))* | | ▶ | 234 | 199 |
| d. Free or Nominal Rate Distribution *(By Mail and Outside the Mail)* | (1) | Free or Nominal Rate Outside-County Copies included on PS Form 3541 | 58 | 44 |
| | (2) | Free or Nominal Rate In-County Copies included on PS Form 3541 | | |
| | (3) | Free or Nominal Rate Copies mailed at Other classes Through the USPS (e.g. First-Class Mail®) | | |
| | (4) | Free or Nominal Rate Distribution Outside the Mail *(Carriers or Other means)* | | |
| e. Total Nonrequested Distribution *(Sum of 15d (1), (2), (3) and (4))* | | ▶ | 58 | 44 |
| f. Total Distribution *(Sum of 15c and 15e)* | | ▶ | 292 | 243 |
| g. Copies not Distributed *(See instructions to publishers #4 (page #3))* | | ▶ | 140 | 181 |
| h. Total *(Sum of 15f and g)* | | ▶ | 432 | 424 |
| i. Percent Paid and/or Requested Circulation *(15c divided by 15f times 100)* | | | 80.14% | 81.89% |

*If you are claiming electronic copies go to line 16 on page 3. If you are not claiming Electronic copies, skip to line 17 on page 3*

| 16. Electronic Copy Circulation | Average No. Copies Each Issue During Preceding 12 Months | No. Copies of Single Issue Published Nearest to Filing Date |
|---|---|---|
| a. Paid Electronic Copies | ▶ | |
| b. Total paid Print Copies (Line 15c) + Paid Electronic copies (Line 16a) | ▶ | |
| c. Total Print Distribution (Line 15f) + Paid Electronic Copies (Line 16a) | ▶ | |
| d. Percent Paid (Both Print & Electronic copies) (16b divided by 16c X100) | ▶ | |

☐ I certify that 50% of all my distributed copies (electronic and print) are paid above a nominal price

17. Publication of Statement of Ownership
☐ If the publication is a general publication, publication of this statement is required. Will be printed in the __October 2015__ issue of this publication.

| 18. Signature and Title of Editor, Publisher, Business Manager, or Owner | Date |
|---|---|
| *Stephen R. Bushing* Stephen R. Bushing – Inventory Distribution Coordinator | September 18, 2015 |

I certify that all information furnished on this form is true and complete. I understand that anyone who furnishes false or misleading information on this form or who omits material or information requested on the form may be subject to criminal sanctions (including fines and imprisonment) and/or civil sanctions (including civil penalties).

PS Form 3526, July 2014 (Page 3 of 3) PSN 7530-01-000-9931 PRIVACY NOTICE: See our Privacy policy in www.usps.com

PS Form 3526, July 2014 (Page 1 of 3 (Instructions Page 3)) PSN 7530-01-000-9931 PRIVACY NOTICE: See our Privacy policy in www.usps.com

# Moving?

## Make sure your subscription moves with you!

To notify us of your new address, find your **Clinics Account Number** (located on your mailing label above your name), and contact customer service at:

Email: journalscustomerservice-usa@elsevier.com

800-654-2452 (subscribers in the U.S. & Canada)
314-447-8871 (subscribers outside of the U.S. & Canada)

Fax number: 314-447-8029

Elsevier Health Sciences Division
Subscription Customer Service
3251 Riverport Lane
Maryland Heights, MO 63043

*To ensure uninterrupted delivery of your subscription, please notify us at least 4 weeks in advance of move.

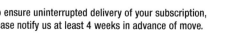